Microcirculation

Maria Dorobantu • Lina Badimon
Editors

Microcirculation

From Bench to Bedside

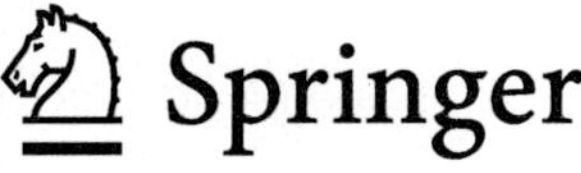

Editors
Maria Dorobantu
Department of Cardiology
Carol Davila University of Medicine
Bucharest
Romania

Lina Badimon
Cardiovascular Program-ICCC,
IR- Hospital de la Santa Creu i Sant Pau
Autonomous University of Barcelona
Barcelona
Spain

ISBN 978-3-030-28198-4 ISBN 978-3-030-28199-1 (eBook)
https://doi.org/10.1007/978-3-030-28199-1

This Springer imprint is published by the registered company Springer Nature Switzerland AG
The registered company address is: Gewerbestrasse 11, 6330 Cham, Switzerland

Contents

Introduction

In the last years we assisted to a dramatic reconsideration of microcirculation as a component of coronary physiology at least as important as the large epicardial vasculature. Extensive research was conducted in the field which allowed us to get a glimpse on the complex and intricated mechanisms of the microcirculation physiology. Importantly, structural and functional alterations of microcirculation have been described in almost all cardiovascular pathologies. Ischaemic heart disease is the most prevalent of these, but abnormal microcirculation has been also described in cardiomyopathies or in valvular heart disease.

The research is ongoing and novel information will be continuously added to our baggage of knowledge allowing us to fill the gaps of this puzzling area of medicine. However, currently we experience an unmet need to translate the results of research in the field of microcirculation into clinical practice. Alterations of microcirculatory function may be obvious in some of the clinical scenarios, but sometimes it is challenging for the physician to accurately diagnose and treat microcirculatory dysfunction.

This book aims to bring the preclinical data into the clinical arena, where it is most useful for both patients and physicians.

The book is organized in three main sections covering both theoretical and practical applications of what we are currently know about microcirculation.

The chapters in the first part explain the basic concepts of microcirculation in health and disease, including lessons from the large animal models. Specific roles of platelet function and perivascular tissue are discussed in two different chapters. The most important techniques for studying microcirculation such as dynamic testing and study through direct microscopic techniques are also covered in the first part of the book. A separate chapter is dedicated to myocardial infarction with normal coronary arteries, an entity which is frequently encountered in daily clinical practice.

The second part of the book follows a relatively innovative approach. It aims to delineate the role of microcirculatory dysfunction in specific conditions such as: ST elevation myocardial infarction, chronic angina, vasospastic angina, left ventricular hypertrophy, acute heart failure or silent cerebral damage. Each of the chapter begin with a real-life clinical case which is then followed by complex theoretical discussions related to each case. This approach is intended to get the physician closer to the intimate mechanisms of microcirculatory dysfunction.

The third part of the book is reserved for the therapeutic considerations and it covers treatment of no-reflow phenomenon, the role of lipid lowering therapies, as well as the cell strategies to stimulate angiogenesis/vasculogenesis for improvement of microcirculation.

The contributing authors are well renowned specialists with a solid background in both the preclinical and clinical areas.

We consider this book to be a valuable tool for all specialists who work in the various fields related to normal and dysfunctional microcirculation.

Part I
Coronary Microcirculation: Theoretical Aspects

Chapter 1
Basic Concepts of the Microcirculation

Cor de Wit

Introduction

The heart receives its perfusion through the coronary circulation, which consists of large conductance vessels (epicardial coronary arteries), that can be visualized during coronary angiography, and small arteries and arterioles. These latter vessels, that exhibit a diameter below 500 μm and are thus too small to be seen in angiography, comprise the arterial part of the coronary microcirculation. They form together with the capillaries that originate from the arterioles and the draining venules as well as the small veins the microcirculatory network. These vessels serve different tasks and their structure follows the respective function.

Functional Compartments Along the Coronary Vascular Tree

Large Arteries Provide Conduction Pathways

Large epicardial coronary arteries exhibit a capacitance function and offer only minimal resistance to blood flow (in the range of 10% of the total resistance within the coronary circulation). These arteries possess a pronounced flow-induced dilation that helps to maintain minimal resistance at this level of the coronary tree also during high flow conditions. In case, the endothelium-dependent dilation upon flow is compromised relative resistance may increase substantially resulting in increased

C. de Wit (✉)
Institut für Physiologie, Universität zu Lübeck, Lübeck, Germany

Deutsches Zentrum für Herz-Kreislauf-Forschung (DZHK) e.V. (German Center for Cardiovascular Research), partner site Hamburg/Kiel/Lübeck, Lübeck, Germany
e-mail: dewit@uni-luebeck.de

M. Dorobantu, L. Badimon (eds.), *Microcirculation*,
https://doi.org/10.1007/978-3-030-28199-1_1

pressure drop along the epicardial arteries that may even be further accentuated if a vessel exhibits additionally stenotic areas. During systole these arteries are distended by the enhanced transmural pressure. The blood that is stored in the artery during its distension is released again during diastole when pressure decreases due to enhanced blood flow into the microcirculation. Taken together, apart from providing a flow pathway, two main features of these arteries support the physiologic function of the coronary circulation, firstly, the dilation and thus resistance decrease during high flow and secondly, the storage and the release of blood with changing pressures during the rhythmic contractions of the heart.

High Resistance and Active Dilation in the Microcirculation

Small arteries and arterioles exhibit substantial resistance and control thus physiologically coronary blood flow [1, 2]. They do so despite the large number of arterioles because of their small diameter since conductivity (the reciprocal of resistance) increases with the fourth power of the radius (Poiseuille's law). Thus, vascular diameter is the most powerful variable controlling resistance. Functionally, the high resistance residing in these vessels translates into the largest pressure drop along this part of the coronary vascular tree. Basically, a vessel with a smaller diameter provides less space for the separation of fluid layers during laminar flow and thus velocity differences between separate layers are becoming larger. The larger differences in velocity enhance the frictional resistance of the flowing blood which must be overcome by the driving pressure. The result is enhanced energy dissipation and thus a larger pressure drop along a certain length of the vessel. This can be offset by dilation and a subsequent increase in the number of separate fluid layers during laminar flow [3]. In fact, arteriolar dilation is the physiologic response to cope with enhanced tissue needs for oxygen that provides increased blood flow through the coronary vascular bed without the need to raise driving pressure. A prerequisite for a dilation is a substantial amount of preconstriction because a vessel can only decrease the level of constriction force which then results in distension by the transmural pressure. Nevertheless, this process is often named dilation implying an active dilatory process and as a matter of fact this makes sense because several mechanisms actively induce the lessening of constriction force as will be outlined below. Taken together, the function of these small arteries and the arterioles is to provide a high resistance that is subject to substantial regulation. These processes include a preconstriction, the so-called vascular tone, and mechanisms that relax the constriction. As these are active processes they are named active dilations. It is worth noting that small arteries residing outside of the heart, are named extra-cardial or intermediate arteries and exhibit diameters larger than 100 μm. Thus, they possess relatively less resistance than the arterioles residing in the cardiac tissue. In the narrow sense of the word these intermediate arteries do not belong to the microcirculation, however, the definition of coronary microcirculation varies between authors [4–6]. On a larger time scale, these vessels are subject of chronic adaptations which is referred to as vascular remodelling. The vascular system of the heart is expanded in size and number of microvessels during growth or exercise training while sustained reduction of physical activity leads to involution [7].

Branching Pattern Increases the Number of Vessels and Capillaries Provide Large Areas for Diffusional Exchange

The heart exhibits a dense network of capillaries [8]. The cardiomyocytes are surrounded by reticular capillaries. Thus, the diffusional distance for oxygen is very small which enables the high oxygen extraction that is characteristic for the coronary circulation already in individuals at rest. Coronary arteries branch into small and intermediate arteries in a tree-like fashion and these vessels have been functionally named ‘distributing vessels’ as opposed to ‘delivering vessels’. Their branching pattern is decisively distinct in that distributing vessels give rise to daughter vessels that are considerably smaller in diameter and their own diameter decreases only to small degree (nonuniform branching). In contrast, delivering vessels branch more uniformly, i.e. two daughter vessels of a comparable diameter arise [9, 10]. The functional distinction does not directly translate into absolute diameter values, which means that there are vessels of similar diameter that serve, however, a different purpose. These considerations underscore the difficult distinction between ‘distribution’ and ‘delivery’ only by diameter measurements. In any case, the delivering arterioles dive into the tissue, the true microcirculation begins and arterioles exhibit diameters smaller than 100 μm. They divide by dichotomous, uniform branching into further arterioles and this results finally in a terminale arteriole [11]. However, the formation of the capillary network does not follow this same branching pattern. A recent study by Kaneko and coworkers [12] demonstrated by 3-dimensional reconstruction of the intramyocardial vessels after consecutive serial sectioning of the human heart that capillaries emerge by two distinct mechanisms: Firstly, by dichotomous branching from a terminal arteriole and, secondly, a precapillary sinus emerged from a terminal arteriole that gave rise to a larger number of capillaries. All these capillaries form many anastomoses within the bundle before draining into a venule. Cardiomyocytes were found running in parallel to the capillaries and thereby, in fact, surrounded in a longitudinal direction by capillaries. The arrangement of the terminal arteriole, the capillaries arising from it, and the draining venules appeared to form a microcirculatory unit serving to nourish a certain small number of cardiomyocytes. Interestingly, the authors observed myocardial micronecroses and their size matched the size of the microcirculatory unit [12]. This suggests that a terminal arteriole feeds a specific tissue region and such a microcirculatory unit allows the adjustment of perfusion in a confined region providing locally restricted changes of oxygen delivery depending on the needs of the tissue.

Origin of High Resting Tone

Vessels require a level of preconstriction in order to exhibit a capacity to dilate and decrease resistance to allow enhanced blood flow if required. The preconstriction gives rise to the so-called basal vascular tone that is specifically large in small arteries and arterioles. This is not achieved by sympathetic activity and alpha-adrenergic receptor activation since blockade of such receptors exerts hardly any change in coronary blood flow in humans at rest [13]. The basal vascular tone originates from a constriction of the vessel in response to a transmural pressure increase (pressure-induced constriction) which is also known as Bayliss effect or myogenic vasoconstriction. It is named 'myogenic' because it is intrinsic to the smooth muscle itself, i.e. independent of exogenous influence (e.g. nerve activity or hormones) or the endothelium although the myogenic constriction may well be modulated by these factors. Since the myogenic constriction also acts in the reverse direction, i.e. lower transmural pressure induces conversely a reduced constriction force which results in a distension (dilation) of the vessel the myogenic reactivity adopts the resistance along a vascular segment according to inflow pressure. Thus, organ perfusion and also capillary pressure remains virtually constant despite variations in the pressure head (within certain limits).

The myogenic tone and the myogenic response originate from a mechanical stimulus emanating from the circumferential stretch on the vessel wall imposed by the transmural pressure leading to an altered wall tension that, in turn, generates intracellular signals that modulate the contractile state of the vascular smooth muscle cells (Fig. 1.1). Modelling suggests that indeed arteriolar wall tension (rather than radius or distension) is the parameter driving the myogenic response and the sensor is required to be arranged in series (rather than in parallel) with the contractile elements. Thus, the response (constriction) abrogates its own stimulus (wall tension) in a negative feedback loop mechanism providing a limit for the response. Interestingly, such a setup provides 'a relatively close regulation of blood flow even though flow is not the regulated variable' [14–18].

However, the mechanosensor responsible for assessing the alteration of wall tension is rather elusive. From experimental data, different hypotheses have been developed that include mechanosensitive, stretch-activated ion channels that open upon distension of the plasma membrane causing depolarisation such as transient receptor potential (TRP) channels, specifically TRPC6 and TRPM4 [19–21], receptor mediated processes that involve mechanosensitiveGq/11-coupled receptors such as the angiotensin1 receptor [22–24], extracellular matrix elements such as integrins acting as mechanosensors [25, 26], the translocation of enzymes and concomitant change of enzyme acitivity (e.g. sphingosine kinase) [27], but also cytoskeletal proteins that may act as mechanosensors. A new family of mechanosensitive ion channels (Piezo channels) has been very recently discovered [28] and their structure

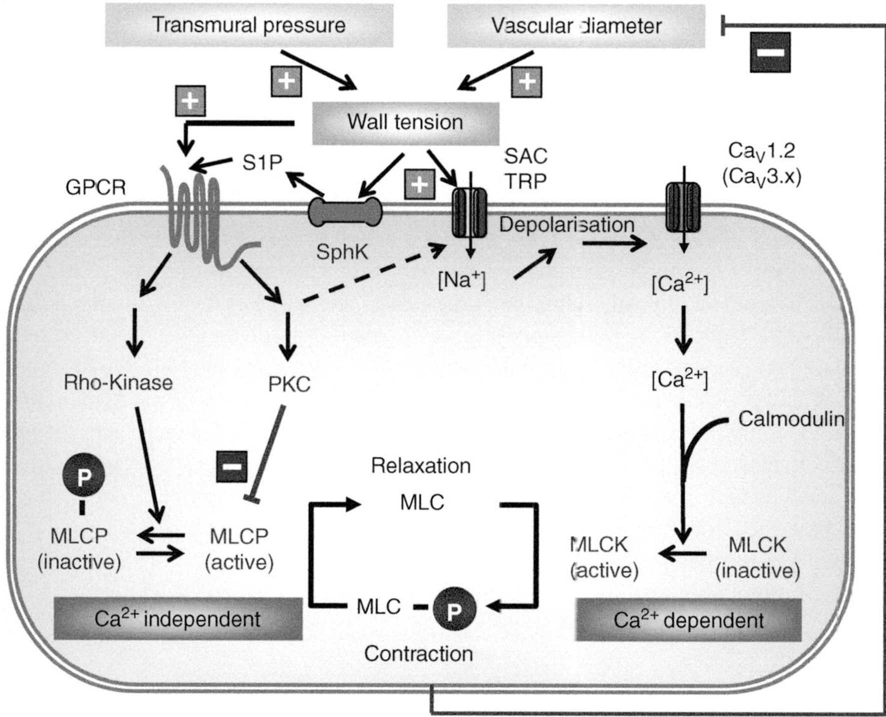

Fig. 1.1 Mechanisms of myogenic responses in vascular smooth muscle. Wall tension is the product of transmural pressure and vascular diameter according to the law of Laplace and tension itself is the most likely stimulus for myogenic responses. The mechanotransducers in smooth muscle cells are not clearly identified but mechanosensitive ion channels (SAC or TRP), GPCR or activation of enzymes (sphingosine kinase) have been implicated in the response. Ion channel activation induces a depolarisation which leads to increases in cytosolic Ca^{2+} through activation of voltage-dependent Ca^{2+} channels and subsequently via Ca^{2+}-dependent mechanisms to an enhanced phosphorylation of MLC by MLCK that translates into contraction. The product of sphingosine kinase (sphingosine-1-phosphate) may act through its GPCR receptors. Other GPCR (e.g. angiotensin receptors) have also been demonstrated to contribute without the need of the respective agonist. The intracellular signalling mechanism involves Ca^{2+} independent mechanisms targeting the activity of MLCP, that is either directly phosphorylated and inactivated (Rho-kinase) or is inhibited via other molecules (PKC). Inhibition of MLCP also enhances MLC phosphorylation. However, molecules activated through GPCR may also activate TRP channels and thus invoking Ca^{2+}-dependent contraction. In both cases (Ca^{2+}-dependent and Ca^{2+}-independent), the ensuing contraction decreases vascular diameter and thereby impacts in a negative feedback manner on the initial stimulus. Abreviations used: Voltage-dependent Ca^{2+} channels (CaV), G-protein coupled receptor (GPCR), myosin light chain kinase (MLCK), myosin light chain phosphatase (MLCP), myosin light chain (MLC), protein kinase C (PKC), transient receptor potential channels (TRP), stretch-activated channels (SAC), sphingosine kinase (SphK), sphingosine-1-phosphate (S1P). The symbol P indicates protein phosphorylation, enzyme names are printed in blue, arrows indicate activation or increase, red lines indicate inhibition

been examined [29]. They play a role in various mechanotransduction processes [30] and we will see in the future if they are also important in vascular smooth muscle as has already been shown for endothelial cells [31].

The evolving change of contractile force in vascular smooth muscle invokes Ca^{2+}-dependent and Ca^{2+}-independent signalling pathways. The change in membrane potential modulates the activity of voltage-dependent L-type Ca^{2+}-channels (primarily $Ca_V1.2$) [32, 33] and potentially also involves the activity of other voltage-dependent Ca^{2+} channels (T-type, $Ca_V3.x$). Thus, a depolarisation in response to pressure increase (and vice versa for pressure decrease) activates Ca^{2+} channels with subsequent Ca^{2+} influx activating the myosin light-chain kinase after formation of the Ca^{2+}-calmodulin-complex that leads to the phosphorylation of myosin light-chain (MLC), the cornerstone of the myogenic response, and subsequent force development [34]. On the other hand, MLC phosphorylation may also be increased if the activity of the MLC phosphatase is inhibited. This constriction is thus independent of MLC kinase activity and of its activator, the intracellular Ca^{2+} level. Hence this type of constriction is named Ca^{2+}-independent constriction and represents a Ca^{2+}sensitisation, i.e. constriction takes place at a constant Ca^{2+} level. It has recently been demonstrated that such Ca^{2+}-independent mechanisms also contribute to myogenic responses and involve the activation of protein kinase C (PKC) and RhoA/Rho kinase [35].

Metabolically Induced Dilatory Pathways

The myocardium releases signalling molecules or modulates the concentration of molecules in the local environment by oxygen consumption, metabolism and electrical activity that act either directly on the smooth muscle cells or onto endothelial cells which then affect through diverse mechanisms the contractile state of the adjacent vascular smooth muscle. The coronary microcirculation is highly responsive to such dilator stimuli and by the ensuing active dilation coronary blood flow increases up to ~fivefold with high oxygen demand [36–38].

Adenosine was first proposed as a metabolite to contribute to coronary vasomotor regulation by Berne in 1963 [39, 40]. Our knowledge about this local purinergic metabolite has evolved considerably and it became clear that adenosine is not required at all or contributes only to a minor degree in the regulation of coronary flow at rest or during exercise [41–43]. Nevertheless it is a powerful dilator acting through the activation of ATP-dependent K^+ channels and possibly also voltage-dependent K^+ channels, probably by a direct effect on smooth muscle through adenosine receptors (most likely A2A and A2B) [44]. It may exert a function in coronary arterioles during ischemia [45]. In addition, during compromised endothelial function metabolically generated signals may step in and secure appropriate blood supply [38].

Another interesting metabolite is the carbon dioxide that is produced at enhanced rates during cardiac exercise [42]. As carbon dioxide chemically reacts with water to form protons and bicarbonate, pH changes may also have a role in this setting. Although it is an attractive hypothesis that molecules emerging from enhanced metabolism drive concomitantly vascular dilation, the simple observation that neither coronary venous carbon dioxide tension nor pH is changing during exercise refutes the idea that these two metabolites play a significant role [43, 46]. Moreover, it is hard to imagine that these substances reach the decisive site of regulation, namely the precapillary arterioles.

Very recently, a new metabolic pathway was suggested that involves a specific voltage-dependent K^+ channel ($K_V1.5$). This channel exhibits, in addition to its voltage-dependency, a specific oxygen- and redox-sensitivity [47]. In mice deficient for this channel myocardial blood flow upon circulatory stress (systemic norepinephrine infusion) was significantly lower although cardiac load was similar (or even higher). Interestingly, at high cardiac work loads tissue oxygen tensions dropped in $K_V1.5$ deficient mice. This phenotype was rescued after expression of this channel specifically in vascular smooth muscle cells [48]. These observations led the authors to conclude that vascular smooth muscle $K_V1.5$ activation is required to couple myocardial blood flow to cardiac metabolism. Together with their previous work it was hypothetised that hydrogen peroxide (H_2O_2) released from mitochondria (at enhanced rates during high metabolism) is the feed-forward link between metabolism and flow in the heart [49, 50]. The effector of H_2O_2 is the $K_V1.5$ in smooth muscle cells and its activation induces a hyperpolarisation as the membrane potential approaches the K^+ equilibrium potential with enhanced K^+ conductance of the membrane. Other K_V channels may also contribute in this coupling of metabolism and flow through H_2O_2 release, as recent data implicate also the $K_V1.3$ in this interesting signalling pathway [51].

The sympathetic activity acts as an additional feed-forward system in the regulation of myocardial blood flow. During stress such as exercise the enhanced workload of the heart is generated by the enhanced sympathetic activity that results in beta-adrenoceptor-mediated increases in heart rate and contractility. This activation simultaneously produces feedforward beta-adrenoceptor-mediated coronary vasodilation thus matching coronary blood flow to expected enhanced oxygen demand [52, 53] and may account for up to 25% of the increase in flow observed in dogs during exercise [54]. Herein, norepinephrine has the largest role and epinephrine contributes only to a small amount. It involves both, beta1- and beta2-receptors (in pigs) [55]. However, pigs are somewhat different than humans (or dogs) with respect to the presence of adrenergic receptors in the coronary circulation. They lack significant alpha-adrenergic resistance vessel control which is, however, the case in humans (and dogs) even during exercise or in coronary artery diseases [56].

The Role of the Endothelium

The endothelium located at the interface between the blood stream and the vascular smooth muscle or (in capillaries) the surrounding tissue modulates the contractile state of the smooth muscle through multiple mechanisms in addition to its signalling function towards the flowing blood. It releases vasodilators that act in the vicinity of their production [57] but it also integrates the vessel wall into a functional syncitium [58, 59]. The role of the endothelium is also decisive in the coronary microcirculation and alterations of endothelial function are summarized in the clinical term 'endothelial dysfunction' [57, 60–63]. Its function can be interrogated clinically by stimulating the endothelium either mechanically (flow) or pharmacologically (e.g. acetylcholine) and provoke endothelium-dependent dilator responses [64]. In the following I will highlight the main mechanisms that induce endothelium-dependent dilations (Fig. 1.2) that are reviewed in detail in numerous excellent publications [4, 65–69].

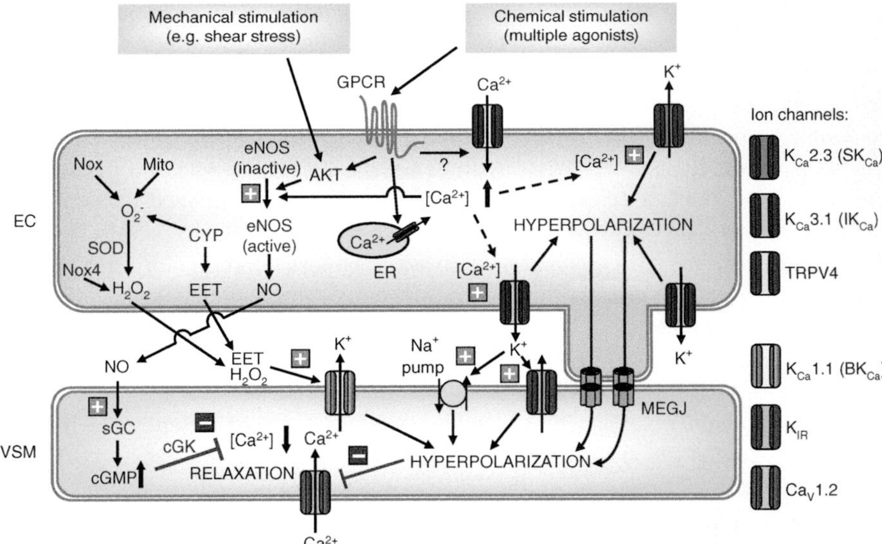

Fig. 1.2 Endothelium dependent dilations. Endothelial cells are stimulated by mechanical forces and a multitude of different agonists and both stimuli lead to cytosolic Ca^{2+} increase and/or activation of protein kinases (such as AKT). This activates eNOS and endothelial Ca^{2+}-dependent K^+ channels inducing endothelial hyperpolarisation. NO diffuses into the smooth muscle cell and activates a pathway invoking sGC, cGMP and cGK that leads to a decrease in smooth muscle Ca^{2+}. This is also achieved by smooth muscle hyperpolarisation through inhibition of voltage-dependent Ca^{2+} channels. Smooth muscle hyperpolarisation is initiated by multiple mechanisms originating from endothelial cells (EDH-type dilation) that include direct current transfer through myoendothelial gap junctions, but also chemical factors (EET, H_2O_2) may contribute. They transfer the signal through the extracellular space and subsequently activate the smooth muscle Ca^{2+}-dependent K^+ channel (BKCa). The signalling pathways interact in endothelial cells which leads to different relative importance of the distinct EDH pathways depending on many factors including age and disease. For further details see text. Abreviations used: Voltage-dependent Ca^{2+} channel (Ca_V), cGMP-dependent kinase (cGK), cytochrome-p450 oxidase (CYP), endothelial cell (EC), epoxyeicosatrienoic acids (EET), endothelial nitric oxide synthase (eNOS), endoplasmatic reticulum (ER), G-protein coupled receptor (GPCR), hydrogen peroxide (H_2O_2), Ca^{2+}-dependent K^+ channel (K_{Ca}) with small, intermediate or large (big) conductance (SK_{Ca}, IK_{Ca}, BK_{Ca}, respectively), inward rectifier K^+ channel (K_{IR}), myoendothelial gap junctions (MEGJ), mitochondria (mito), NADPH oxidase (Nox), soluble guanylate cyclase (sGC), superoxide dismutase (SOD), transient receptor potential channel type V4 (TRPV4), vascular smooth muscle (VSM). Enzyme names are printed in blue, arrows indicate activation or increase, red lines indicate inhibition

Nitric Oxide

The best-known dilator released from endothelial cells is nitric oxide (NO) [69]. The endothelial NO synthase (eNOS, NOSIII) is the major source of endothelium-derived NO. The enzyme is localized in small invaginations of the plasma membrane containing caveolin-1 protein and thus these areas are called caveolae. Herein, a signalling complex (signalosome) is found that modulates eNOS activity. Releasing eNOS from caveolin-1 by increases of intracellular Ca^{2+} that interferes after binding to calmodulin with the caveolin-1 interaction enhances its activity drastically. However, activation of eNOS can also be achieved by its phosphorylation that can be elicited by a multitude of kinases including AKT and protein kinase A [70]. This explains the numerous physiologic stimuli that result in eNOS activation including physical forces (shear stress), circulating hormones (catecholamines), platelet products (serotonin, adenosine diphosphate), autacoids (histamine, bradykinin), thrombin and also acetylcholine, although the physiologic relevance of the latter stimulus is questionable [69]. NO is produced by the transfer of electrons derived from NADPH through flavins in the reductase domain of eNOS to the cofactor heme that is bound at the oxygenase domain of eNOS. This electron transfer allows oxygen to bind and further catalyse the stepwise synthesis of NO from *L*-arginine. The electron transfer between the domains requires a conformational change that is enabled by Ca^{2+}-calmodulin that binds to the linker of these two domains [71]. The complex interactions of eNOS also with other proteins in the signalosome may become dysregulated (also termed 'endothelial dysfunction') and result in so-called eNOS uncoupling. This term refers to an electron transfer that is uncoupled from L-arginine oxidation and results in the generation of superoxide anions and hydrogen peroxide instead of NO [70].

NO diffuses freely from its site of production and reaches its target the soluble guanylate cyclase (sGC) that is located in the cytosol of the vascular smooth muscle (but also in platelets). sGC is a heterodimeric hemoprotein composed of an alpha- and a beta-subunit. NO binds to the heme group thereby enhancing the catalytic activity of sGC drastically and increasing the generation of cyclic guanosine monophosphate (cGMP) from GTP [72, 73]. This second messenger activates cGMP dependent protein kinases (cGK) which in turn, induce relaxation of smooth muscle [74, 75]. This is achieved through Ca^{2+}-dependent as well as Ca^{2+}-independent mechanisms. Important targets of the cGK are the inositol-1,4,5-trisphosphate (IP3) receptor I-associated protein (IRAG) which phosphorylation inhibits IP3-induced Ca^{2+} release from intracellular stores, the large-conductance Ca^{2+}-activated K^+ channel (KCa1.1) which activation hyperpolarizes the smooth muscle cell and the myosin light chain phosphatase (MLCP) that is activated and reduces Ca^{2+} sensitivity by decreasing the MLC phosphorylation.

The importance of NO seems to be pronounced in larger arteries and small arteries in which NO mediates the well-known flow-induced dilation. An increase of wall shear stress is an adequate stimulus for the augmentation of endothelial NO release with increasing flow due to downstream dilation [76]. The ensuing dilation tends to bring back the stimulus to initial values (negative feedback) and, functionally important, prevents the energy dissipation along the length of the vessel during high flow. By keeping wall shear stress constant, the pressure decrease along a certain length of the conduction pathway remains unchanged and virtually independent of flow. This mechanism prevents that larger upstream arteries adopt a larger fraction of the total resistance in face of a downstream dilation and concurrent flow increase. In case upstream dilation fails, these upstream vessels with their now relatively enhanced resistance would limit flow increases during exercise. In fact, during exercise inhibition of NO synthase reduced myocardial flow increases, however, the effects were small and sometimes even absent [37]. The role of NO at resting conditions is even more difficult to validate as a diminished dilator influence of NO in small arteries may be counterbalanced by a compensatory dilation of arterioles. However, there is ample evidence in dogs supporting this view, i.e. a role for NO in small arteries and a lack of a physiologic dilator function of NO in arterioles [77]. The fact that arterioles dilate in spite of blockade of NO synthesis argues that other dilator mechanisms are present in these vessels.

Endothelium-Dependent Hyperpolarisation

A further mechanism initiated by endothelial cells induces vascular smooth muscle relaxation. It is related to smooth muscle hyperpolarisation and was consequently termed endothelium-dependent hyperpolarising factor (EDHF) under the assumption that a transferable factor released from endothelial cells (not being NO or a prostaglandin) is responsible for this effect in smooth muscle. In search for this factor, a number of distinct chemical molecules have been proposed to act as transferable mediator. The suggestions included potassium ions (K^+), epoxyeicosatrienoic acids (EETs), hydrogen peroxide (H_2O_2), C-type natriuretic peptide (CNP), hydrogen sulfide (H_2S), but also adenosine. However, this is a 'sticky' business as plasma membranes have to be crossed and it is difficult to imagine that several of these compounds are easily and quickly transferable in the required amounts. Moreover, some postulated EDHFs may rather modulate another mechanism that is acting as 'the EDH principle' (e.g. modify endothelial hyperpolarisation or gap junctional coupling, see below) and are therefore wrongly implied to be an EDHF. The view that it is indeed a factor that diffuses through the extracellular space has recently been challenged and a direct communication pathway was suggested that is provided by intercellular channels (myoendothelial gap junctions). Through such channels that connect the cytoplasms of adjacent cells charge is transferred electrotonically from endothelial cells into smooth muscle driven by an initial endothelial hyperpolarization. The amount of charge transferred initiates a certain level of membrane potential change and consequently the hyperpolarisation depends on the conductivity (the inverse of resistance) of the intercellular channels. With this new concept the term EDHF was replaced by the phrase endothelium-dependent hyperpolarisation (EDH) and EDH-type dilation which includes also the idea of an actual factor being transferred [66]. Whatever the exact nature is, smooth muscle hyperpolarisation reduces the opening probability of voltage-dependent Ca^{2+} channels and thereby induces relaxation. In the following some of these dilator principles will be explained mechanistically.

Most of the distinct hypotheses agree on the initial event to elicit EDH-type dilations and this is the hyperpolarisation of endothelial cells. Upon endothelial stimulation and activation of different G-protein coupled receptors intracellular Ca^{2+} increases, which may even be a very localized event and this leads to subsequent activation of Ca^{2+}-dependent K^+-channels (KCa) [78, 79]. This family of channels comprise three subgroups, that are functionally differentiated by their conductance into small, intermediate, and large conductance channels (SKCa, IKCa, BKCa). Alternative names are KCa1.1 (BKCa), mainly expressed in vascular smooth muscle, and KCa2.3 (SKCa) as well as KCa3.1 (IKCa) [80]. These two latter channels are expressed only in endothelial cells and are implicated in the initially required endothelial hyperpolarisation during EDH-type dilations as genetic deletion of the channels or their blockade consistently affects EDH-type dilations [81–85] (for review see [4]). Although both channels support a similar functional response they may serve different functions that is also implied by their subcellular location [66, 86]. The endothelial hyperpolarisation sets the stage for the first EDHF to be discussed, namely potassium ions (K^+). The opening of the endothelial KCa results in an efflux of K^+ due to the chemical driving force which is opposed by the electrical force due to the ensuing hyperpolarisation of the membrane. A critical question herein is the amount of K^+ that leaves the endothelial cell because the change of the potential does not require a huge amount of K^+ to flow across the membrane. In any case, the idea of K^+ acting as an EDHF is based on the fact, that extracellular K^+ increases inside the vessel wall that then leads to the activation of K^+ channels in the membrane of the smooth muscle cell, in this case the inward rectifier K^+ channel (KIR) that is activated by increased extracellular K^+ concentrations. Furthermore, extracellular K^+ increases activate the sodium pump that in itself is electrogenic by pumping three sodium ions out of cell while only pumping two potassium ions to the inside. However, it is questionable that such pumping affects the membrane potential except for an alteration of the ion concentrations since the membrane potential is governed by conductance for ions and not active transfer of ions across the membrane. This hypothesis was initially developed during experiments in the rat hepatic artery [87] but thereafter also demonstrated to govern responses in other vessels and modulated depending on the external conditions [88–91]. However, it was not demonstrated in coronary arteries to the best of my knowledge although endothelial KCa have been identified in coronaries by these investigators [92].

Specifically in coronary arteries, a wealth of experimental data suggest that EETs and H_2O_2 represent an EDHF or are at least important modifiers of the EDH-type dilation [4, 93]. Upon mechanical stimuli and physiologic agonists endothelial cells synthesize via activation of cytochrome-P450 epoxygenases EET regioisomers from arachidonic acid and various lipids in the cell membrane [94]. These EETs are all degraded by the soluble epoxide hydrolase (sEH) which hydrates them to the corresponding diols (dihydroxyepoxyeicosatrienoic acids) that mostly lack biological activity [95]. Interestingly, sEH can be pharmacologically targeted and thereby biological actions of EETs prolonged [96–98]. EETs bind to a selective receptor that leads in a GTP-dependent ADP-ribosylation dependent process to subsequent activation of a smooth muscle K^+ channel, in this case the large-conductance Ca^{2+}-dependent K^+ channel KCa1.1 (BKCa), and thereby hyperpolarisation [99]. On the other hand, EETs may also act in an autocrine fashion on endothelial cells themselves by activation of a specific TRP channel (TRPV4) fostering Ca^{2+} influx and thereby boosting endothelial hyperpolarisation through further activation of the aforementioned KCa2.3 (SKCa) and KCa3.1 (IKCa) [99]. However, CYP epoxygenases also produce reactive oxygen species (ROS), namely superoxide anions (O_2^-), during EET synthesis [100]. Other relevant sources of superoxide production in endothelial cells by reduction of molecular O_2 are NADPH oxidases (Nox), the mitochondrial electron transport chain [101], and uncoupled NOS (see above). These superoxide anions may either react with NO to form $ONOO^-$, the reaction which is referred to when highlighting the property of ROS to reduce NO bioavailability. Alternatively, superoxide anion may be reduced by superoxide dismutase (SOD) to form hydrogen peroxide (H_2O_2). This uncharged molecule in itself has been established to act as EDHF, being also produced directly from the Nox isoform Nox4 [102, 103], and induce dilation through the activation of smooth muscle KCa1.1 (BKCa) [104]. However, recently K_V channels have also been shown to be activated by H_2O_2 (see section above). The role of EETs in this setting may therefore be reconciled in as much as they act to foster H_2O_2 production through TRPV4 and Ca^{2+} signalling and, in addition, by modulating myoendothelial gap junctional communication (see below).

A further important mechanism that has been demonstrated to underlie EDH-type dilations is the electrotonic transfer of charge through myoendothelial gap junctions (MEGJ) [4, 66, 79, 105] although it has yet to be proven that this mechanism contributes also in arteriolar dilations in vivo [106–108]. Cells of the vessel wall are interconnected by gap junctions, which are built by connexin proteins [106, 109]. They form a pathway between adjacent cells connecting their cytoplasms that allows ions, but also signalling molecules such as cyclic nucleotides, to pass. The conductivity for ions leads to the passage of ions according to the respective driving force which is (at comparable ionic intracellular concentrations) the potential difference between the connected cells. Gap junctions not only connect endothelial to smooth muscle cells, but they also interconnect endothelial and smooth muscle cells themselves. In fact, endothelial cells are very well coupled with low intercellular resistance and thus potential changes spread readily along the endothelial cell layer over large distances and the functionally most important connexin isoform to do so is connexin40 [107, 110, 111]. This provides a longitudinal signalling pathway orchestrating cellular behaviour along the length of the vessel by conducting locally initiated dilations to remote sites [58, 112–114]. However, vascular cells are also radially coupled [115] providing a pathway to transmit an endothelial hyperpolarisation into the smooth muscle cell layer without the need of a chemical mediator. It has, however, to be considered that a substantial amount of current needs to be generated in endothelial cells and transferred in order to hyperpolarize a larger amount of smooth muscle cells [116, 117]. Direct electrotonic transfer of membrane potential changes are also underlying EDH-type dilations in coronary arterioles to a certain amount and the relative importance may also vary with physiologic environment, age, and certainly diseases that affect endothelial function [5, 118–123].

After this brief summary of the endothelial factors to influence the contractile state of the smooth muscle it needs to be highlighted that these various mechanisms not only differ between vessels from distinct vascular beds, but even with a specific vascular bed such as the coronaries the mechanism may change with age and even more so with disease [1, 121]. In addition, these systems not only act additively, but rather redundantly, i.e. if a certain mediator is not synthetized any longer or its target is not responding (in the experimental setting using enzyme inhibitors or receptor blockers, respectively) any other pathway may take over by being activated or by being stimulated to a higher degree [124]. In fact, active interference of some of the known pathways has been additionally demonstrated as for the inhibitory interaction of H_2O_2 on CYP activity [125].

References

1. Beyer AM, Gutterman DD. Regulation of the human coronary microcirculation. J Mol Cell Cardiol. 2012;52:814–21.
2. Chilian WM, Eastham CL, Marcus ML. Microvascular distribution of coronary vascular resistance in beating left ventricle. Am J Phys. 1986;251:H779–88.
3. Zamir M. Shear forces and blood vessel radii in the cardiovascular system. J Gen Physiol. 1977;69:449–61.
4. Ellinsworth DC, Sandow SL, Shukla N, Liu Y, Jeremy JY, et al. Endothelium-derived hyperpolarization and coronary vasodilation: diverse and integrated roles of epoxyeicosatrienoic acids, hydrogen peroxide, and gap junctions. Microcirculation. 2016;23:15–32.
5. Gutterman DD, Chabowski DS, Kadlec AO, Durand MJ, Freed JK, et al. The human microcirculation: regulation of flow and beyond. Circ Res. 2016;118:157–72.
6. Pries AR, Reglin B. Coronary microcirculatory pathophysiology: can we afford it to remain a black box? Eur Heart J. 2017;38:478–88.
7. Pries AR, Badimon L, Bugiardini R, Camici PG, Dorobantu M, et al. Coronary vascular regulation, remodelling, and collateralization: mechanisms and clinical implications on behalf of the working group on coronary pathophysiology and microcirculation. Eur Heart J. 2015;36:3134–46.
8. Rakusan K, Flanagan MF, Geva T, Southern J, Van Praagh R. Morphometry of human coronary capillaries during normal growth and the effect of age in left ventricular pressure-overload hypertrophy. Circulation. 1992;86:38–46.
9. Zamir M. Distributing and delivering vessels of the human heart. J Gen Physiol. 1988;91:725–35.
10. Zamir M, Chee H. Branching characteristics of human coronary arteries. Can J Physiol Pharmacol. 1986;64:661–8.
11. Brown RE. The pattern of the microcirculatory bed in the ventricular myocardium of domestic mammals. Am J Anat. 1965;116:355–74.
12. Kaneko N, Matsuda R, Toda M, Shimamoto K. Three-dimensional reconstruction of the human capillary network and the intramyocardial micronecrosis. Am J Physiol Heart Circ Physiol. 2011;300:H754–61.

13. Heusch G, Baumgart D, Camici P, Chilian W, Gregorini L, et al. Alpha-adrenergic coronary vasoconstriction and myocardial ischemia in humans. Circulation. 2000;101:689–94.
14. Borgstrom P, Gestrelius S. Integrated myogenic and metabolic control of vascular tone in skeletal muscle during autoregulation of blood flow. Microvasc Res. 1987;33:353–76.
15. Carlson BE, Arciero JC, Secomb TW. Theoretical model of blood flow autoregulation: roles of myogenic, shear-dependent, and metabolic responses. Am J Physiol Heart Circ Physiol. 2008;295:H1572–9.
16. Cornelissen AJM, Dankelman J, VanBavel E, Spaan JAE. Balance between myogenic, flow-dependent, and metabolic flow control in coronary arterial tree: a model study. Am J Physiol Heart Circ Physiol. 2002;282:H2224–37.
17. Davis MJ. Perspective: physiological role(s) of the vascular myogenic response. Microcirculation. 2012;19:99–114.
18. Johnson PC. Autoregulation of blood flow. Circ Res. 1986;59:483–95.
19. Baylie RL, Brayden JE. TRPV channels and vascular function. Acta Physiol (Oxf). 2011;203:99–116.
20. Earley S, Brayden JE. Transient receptor potential channels in the vasculature. Physiol Rev. 2015;95:645–90.
21. Sharif-Naeini R, Dedman A, Folgering JHA, Duprat F, Patel A, et al. TRP channels and mechanosensory transduction: insights into the arterial myogenic response. Pflugers Arch. 2008;456:529–40.
22. Kauffenstein G, Laher I, Matrougui K, Guerineau NC, Henrion D. Emerging role of G protein-coupled receptors in microvascular myogenic tone. Cardiovasc Res. 2012;95:223–32.
23. Kauffenstein G, Tamareille S, Prunier F, Roy C, Ayer A, et al. Central role of P2Y6 UDP receptor in arteriolar myogenic tone. Arterioscler Thromb Vasc Biol. 2016;36:1598–606.
24. Mederos Y, Schnitzler M, Storch U, Gudermann T. Mechanosensitive Gq/11 protein-coupled receptors mediate myogenic vasoconstriction. Microcirculation. 2016;23:621–5.
25. D'Angelo G, Mogford JE, Davis GE, Davis MJ, Meininger GA. Integrin-mediated reduction in vascular smooth muscle [Ca2+](i) induced by RGD-containing peptide. Am J Phys. 1997;272:H2065–70.
26. Davis MJ, Wu X, Nurkiewicz TR, Kawasaki J, Davis GE, et al. Integrins and mechanotransduction of the vascular myogenic response. Am J Physiol Heart Circ Physiol. 2001;280:H1427–33.
27. Lidington D, Schubert R, Bolz SS. Capitalizing on diversity: an integrative approach towards the multiplicity of cellular mechanisms underlying myogenic responsiveness. Cardiovasc Res. 2013;97:404–12.
28. Coste B, Mathur J, Schmidt M, Earley TJ, Ranade S, et al. Piezo1 and Piezo2 are essential components of distinct mechanically activated cation channels. Science. 2010;330:55–60.
29. Saotome K, Murthy SE, Kefauver JM, Whitwam T, Patapoutian A, et al. Structure of the mechanically activated ion channel Piezo1. Nature. 2018;554:481–6.
30. Wang Y, Xiao B. The mechanosensitive Piezo1 channel: structural features and molecular bases underlying its ion permeation and mechanotransduction. J Physiol. 2018;596:969–78.
31. Wang S, Chennupati R, Kaur H, Iring A, Wettschureck N, et al. Endothelial cation channel PIEZO1 controls blood pressure by mediating flow-induced ATP release. J Clin Invest. 2016;126:4527–36.
32. Fernandez-Tenorio M, Gonzalez-Rodriguez P, Porras C, Castellano A, Moosmang S, et al. Short communication: genetic ablation of L-type Ca2+ channels abolishes depolarization-induced Ca2+ release in arterial smooth muscle. Circ Res. 2010;106:1285–9.
33. Moosmang S, Schulla V, Welling A, Feil R, Feil S, et al. Dominant role of smooth muscle L-type calcium channel Cav1.2 for blood pressure regulation. EMBO J. 2003;22:6027–34.
34. Davis MJ, Hill MA. Signaling mechanisms underlying the vascular myogenic response. Physiol Rev. 1999;79:387–423.
35. Schubert R, Lidington D, Bolz SS. The emerging role of Ca2+ sensitivity regulation in promoting myogenic vasoconstriction. Cardiovasc Res. 2008;77:8–18.

36. de Marchi SF, Gloekler S, Rimoldi SF, Rolli P, Steck H, et al. Microvascular response to metabolic and pressure challenge in the human coronary circulation. Am J Physiol Heart Circ Physiol. 2011;301:H434–41.
37. Duncker DJ, Bache RJ. Regulation of coronary blood flow during exercise. Physiol Rev. 2008;88:1009–86.
38. Duncker DJ, Bache RJ, Merkus D. Regulation of coronary resistance vessel tone in response to exercise. J Mol Cell Cardiol. 2012;52:802–13.
39. Berne RM. Cardiac nucleotides in hypoxia: possible role in regulation of coronary blood flow. Am J Phys. 1963;204:317–22.
40. Berne RM. The role of adenosine in the regulation of coroanry blood flow. Circ Res. 1980;47:807–13.
41. Bache RJ, Dai XZ, Schwartz JS, Homans DC. Role of adenosine in coronary vasodilation during exercise. Circ Res. 1988;62:846–53.
42. Deussen A, Ohanyan V, Jannasch A, Yin L, Chilian W. Mechanisms of metabolic coronary flow regulation. J Mol Cell Cardiol. 2012;52:794–801.
43. Duncker DJ, Stubenitsky R, Verdouw PD. Role of adenosine in the regulation of coronary blood flow in swine at rest and during treadmill exercise. Am J Phys. 1998;275:H1663–72.
44. Layland J, Carrick D, Lee M, Oldroyd K, Berry C. Adenosine: physiology, pharmacology, and clinical applications. JACC Cardiovasc Interv. 2014;7:581–91.
45. Berwick ZC, Payne GA, Lynch B, Dick GM, Sturek M, et al. Contribution of adenosine A(2A) and A(2B) receptors to ischemic coronary dilation: role of K(V) and K(ATP) channels. Microcirculation. 2010;17:600–7.
46. Tune JD, Richmond KN, Gorman MW, Feigl EO. Role of nitric oxide and adenosine in control of coronary blood flow in exercising dogs. Circulation. 2000;101:2942–8.
47. Weir EK, Lopez-Barneo J, Buckler KJ, Archer SL. Acute oxygen-sensing mechanisms. N Engl J Med. 2005;353:2042–55.
48. Ohanyan V, Yin L, Bardakjian R, Kolz C, Enrick M, et al. Requisite role of Kv1.5 channels in coronary metabolic dilation. Circ Res. 2015;117:612–21.
49. Rogers PA, Dick GM, Knudson JD, Focardi M, Bratz IN, et al. H2O2-induced redox-sensitive coronary vasodilation is mediated by 4-aminopyridine-sensitive K+ channels. Am J Physiol Heart Circ Physiol. 2006;291:H2473–82.
50. Saitoh SI, Kiyooka T, Rocic P, Rogers PA, Zhang C, et al. Redox-dependent coronary metabolic dilation. Am J Physiol Heart Circ Physiol. 2007;293:H3720–5.
51. Ohanyan V, Yin L, Bardakjian R, Kolz C, Enrick M, et al. Kv1.3 channels facilitate the connection between metabolism and blood flow in the heart. Microcirculation. 2017;24:e12334.
52. Duncker DJ, Stubenitsky R, Verdouw PD. Autonomic control of vasomotion in the porcine coronary circulation during treadmill exercise - evidence for feed-forward beta-adrenergic control. Circ Res. 1998;82:1312–22.
53. Gorman MW, Tune JD, Richmond KN, Feigl EO. Feedforward sympathetic coronary vasodilation in exercising dogs. J Appl Physiol. 2000;89:1892–902.
54. Gorman MW, Tune JD, Richmond KN, Feigl EO. Quantitative analysis of feedforward sympathetic coronary vasodilation in exercising dogs. J Appl Physiol. 2000;89:1903–11.
55. Gao F, de Beer VJ, Hoekstra M, Xiao C, Duncker DJ, et al. Both beta1- and beta2-adrenoceptors contribute to feedforward coronary resistance vessel dilation during exercise. Am J Physiol Heart Circ Physiol. 2010;298:H921–9.
56. Heusch G. The paradox of alpha-adrenergic coronary vasoconstriction revisited. J Mol Cell Cardiol. 2011;51:16–23.
57. Vanhoutte PM, Shimokawa H, Feletou M, Tang EHC. Endothelial dysfunction and vascular disease - a 30th anniversary update. Acta Physiol (Oxf). 2017;219:22–96.
58. de Wit C. Connexins pave the way for vascular communication. News Physiol Sci. 2004;19:148–53.
59. Schmidt K, Windler R, de Wit C. Communication through gap junctions in the endothelium. Adv Pharmacol. 2016;77:209–40.

60. Badimon L, Bugiardini R, Cenko E, Cubedo J, Dorobantu M, et al. Position paper of the European Society of Cardiology-working group of coronary pathophysiology and microcirculation: obesity and heart disease. Eur Heart J. 2017;38:1951–8.
61. Camici PG, d'Amati G, Rimoldi O. Coronary microvascular dysfunction: mechanisms and functional assessment. Nat Rev Cardiol. 2015;12:48–62.
62. Crea F, Camici PG, Bairey Merz CN. Coronary microvascular dysfunction: an update. Eur Heart J. 2014;35:1101–11.
63. Gimbrone MAJ, Garcia-Cardena G. Endothelial cell dysfunction and the pathobiology of atherosclerosis. Circ Res. 2016;118:620–36.
64. Pries AR, Habazettl H, Ambrosio G, Hansen PR, Kaski JC, et al. A review of methods for assessment of coronary microvascular disease in both clinical and experimental settings. Cardiovasc Res. 2008;80:165–74.
65. de Wit C, Wolfle SE. EDHF and gap junctions: important regulators of vascular tone within the microcirculation. Curr Pharm Biotechnol. 2007;8:11–25.
66. Garland CJ, Dora KA. EDH: endothelium-dependent hyperpolarization and microvascular signalling. Acta Physiol (Oxf). 2017;219:152–61.
67. Leung SWS, Vanhoutte PM. Endothelium-dependent hyperpolarization: age, gender and blood pressure, do they matter? Acta Physiol (Oxf). 2017;219:108–23.
68. Murrant CL, Lamb IR, Novielli NM. Capillary endothelial cells as coordinators of skeletal muscle blood flow during active hyperemia. Microcirculation. 2017;24:e12348.
69. Vanhoutte PM, Zhao Y, Xu A, Leung SWS. Thirty years of saying NO: sources, fate, actions, and misfortunes of the endothelium-derived vasodilator mediator. Circ Res. 2016;119:375–96.
70. Siragusa M, Fleming I. The eNOS signalosome and its link to endothelial dysfunction. Pflugers Arch. 2016;468:1125–37.
71. Campbell MG, Smith BC, Potter CS, Carragher B, Marletta MA. Molecular architecture of mammalian nitric oxide synthases. Proc Natl Acad Sci U S A. 2014;111:E3614–23.
72. Friebe A, Koesling D. The function of NO-sensitive guanylyl cyclase: what we can learn from genetic mouse models. Nitric Oxide. 2009;21:149–56.
73. Thunemann M, Wen L, Hillenbrand M, Vachaviolos IA, Feil S, et al. Transgenic mice for cGMP imaging. Circ Res. 2013;113:365–71.
74. Hofmann F, Feil R, Kleppisch T, Schlossmann J. Function of cGMP-dependent protein kinases as revealed by gene deletion. Physiol Rev. 2006;86:1–23.
75. Koeppen M, Feil R, Siegl D, Feil S, Hofmann F, et al. cGMP-dependent protein kinase mediates NO- but not acetylcholine-induced dilations in resistance vessels in vivo. Hypertension. 2004;44:952–5.
76. Pohl U, de Wit C. A unique role of NO in the control of blood flow. News Physiol Sci. 1999;14:74–80.
77. Jones CJ, Kuo L, Davis MJ, DeFily DV, Chilian WM. Role of nitric oxide in the coronary microvascular responses to adenosine and increased metabolic demand. Circulation. 1995;91:1807–13.
78. Busse R, Edwards G, Feletou M, Fleming I, Vanhoutte PM, et al. EDHF: bringing the concepts together. Trends Pharmacol Sci. 2002;23:374–80.
79. de Wit C, Griffith TM. Connexins and gap junctions in the EDHF phenomenon and conducted vasomotor responses. Pflugers Arch. 2010;459:897–914.
80. Wulff H, Kohler R. Endothelial small-conductance and intermediate-conductance KCa channels: an update on their pharmacology and usefulness as cardiovascular targets. J Cardiovasc Pharmacol. 2013;61:102–12.
81. Batenburg WW, Garrelds IM, van Kats JP, Saxena PR, Danser AHJ. Mediators of bradykinin-induced vasorelaxation in human coronary microarteries. Hypertension. 2004;43:488–92.
82. Brahler S, Kaistha A, Schmidt VJ, Wolfle SE, Busch C, et al. Genetic deficit of SK3 and IK1 channels disrupts the endothelium-derived hyperpolarizing factor vasodilator pathway and causes hypertension. Circulation. 2009;119:2323–32.

83. Crane GJ, Gallagher N, Dora KA, Garland CJ. Small- and intermediate-conductance calcium-activated K+ channels provide different facets of endothelium-dependent hyperpolarization in rat mesenteric artery. J Physiol. 2003;553:183–9.
84. Miura H, Liu Y, Gutterman DD. Human coronary arteriolar dilation to bradykinin depends on membrane hyperpolarization - contribution of nitric oxide and Ca2+–activated K+ channels. Circulation. 1999;99:3132–8.
85. Si H, Heyken WT, Wolfle SE, Tysiac M, Schubert R, et al. Impaired endothelium-derived hyperpolarizing factor-mediated dilations and increased blood pressure in mice deficient of the intermediate-conductance Ca2+-activated K+ channel. Circ Res. 2006;99:537–44.
86. Milkau M, Kohler R, de Wit C. Crucial importance of the endothelial K+ channel SK3 and connexin40 in arteriolar dilations during skeletal muscle contraction. FASEB J. 2010;24:3572–9.
87. Edwards G, Dora KA, Gardener MJ, Garland CJ, Weston AH. K+ is an endothelium-derived hyperpolarizing factor in rat arteries. Nature. 1998;396:269–72.
88. Dora KA, Gallagher NT, McNeish A, Garland CJ. Modulation of endothelial cell KCa3.1 channels during endothelium-derived hyperpolarizing factor signaling in mesenteric resistance arteries. Circ Res. 2008;102:1247–55.
89. Edwards G, Feletou M, Weston AH. Endothelium-derived hyperpolarising factors and associated pathways: a synopsis. Pflugers Arch. 2010;459:863–79.
90. Richards GR, Weston AH, Burnham MP, Feletou M, Vanhoutte PM, et al. Suppression of K+-induced hyperpolarization by phenylephrine in rat mesenteric artery: relevance to studies of endothelium-derived hyperpolarizing factor. Br J Pharmacol. 2001;134:1–5.
91. Weston AH, Richards GR, Burnham MP, Feletou M, Vanhoutte PM, et al. K+-induced hyperpolarization in rat mesenteric artery: identification, localization and role of Na+/K+-ATPases. Br J Pharmacol. 2002;136:918–26.
92. Burnham MP, Bychkov R, Feletou M, Richards GR, Vanhoutte PM, et al. Characterization of an apamin-sensitive small-conductance Ca(2+)-activated K(+) channel in porcine coronary artery endothelium: relevance to EDHF. Br J Pharmacol. 2002;135:1133–43.
93. Fisslthaler B, Popp R, Kiss L, Potente M, Harder DR, et al. Cytochrome P4502C is an EDHF synthase in coronary arteries. Nature. 1999;401:493–7.
94. Fleming I. The pharmacology of the cytochrome P450 epoxygenase/soluble epoxide hydrolase axis in the vasculature and cardiovascular disease. Pharmacol Rev. 2014;66:1106–40.
95. Fleming I. The factor in EDHF: cytochrome P450 derived lipid mediators and vascular signaling. Vasc Pharmacol. 2016;86:31–40.
96. Imig JD. Epoxides and soluble epoxide hydrolase in cardiovascular physiology. Physiol Rev. 2012;92:101–30.
97. Oparil S, Schmieder RE. New approaches in the treatment of hypertension. Circ Res. 2015;116:1074–95.
98. Sun D, Cuevas AJ, Gotlinger K, Hwang SH, Hammock BD, et al. Soluble epoxide hydrolase-dependent regulation of myogenic response and blood pressure. Am J Physiol Heart Circ Physiol. 2014;306:H1146–53.
99. Campbell WB, Fleming I. Epoxyeicosatrienoic acids and endothelium-dependent responses. Pflugers Arch. 2010;459:881–95.
100. Fleming I, Michaelis UR, Bredenkotter D, Fisslthaler B, Dehghani F, et al. Endothelium-derived hyperpolarizing factor synthase (Cytochrome P4502C9) is a functionally significant source of reactive oxygen species in coronary arteries. Circ Res. 2001;88:44–51.
101. Zinkevich NS, Fancher IS, Gutterman DD, Phillips SA. Roles of NADPH oxidase and mitochondria in flow-induced vasodilation of human adipose arterioles: ROS-induced ROS release in coronary artery disease. Microcirculation. 2017;24:e12380.
102. Ray R, Murdoch CE, Wang M, Santos CX, Zhang M, et al. Endothelial Nox4 NADPH oxidase enhances vasodilatation and reduces blood pressure in vivo. Arterioscler Thromb Vasc Biol. 2011;31:1368–76.
103. Schroder K, Zhang M, Benkhoff S, Mieth A, Pliquett R, et al. Nox4 is a protective reactive oxygen species generating vascular NADPH oxidase. Circ Res. 2012;110:1217–25.

104. Liu Y, Bubolz AH, Mendoza S, Zhang DX, Gutterman DD. H2O2 is the transferrable factor mediating flow-induced dilation in human coronary arterioles. Circ Res. 2011;108:566–73.
105. Griffith TM. Endothelium-dependent smooth muscle hyperpolarization: do gap junctions provide a unifying hypothesis? Br J Pharmacol. 2004;141:881–903.
106. de Wit C, Boettcher M, Schmidt VJ. Signaling across myoendothelial gap junctions - fact or fiction? Cell Commun Adhes. 2008;15:231–45.
107. Jobs A, Schmidt K, Schmidt VJ, Lubkemeier I, van Veen TAB, et al. Defective Cx40 maintains Cx37 expression but intact Cx40 is crucial for conducted dilations irrespective of hypertension. Hypertension. 2012;60:1422–9.
108. Siegl D, Koeppen M, Wolfle SE, Pohl U, de Wit C. Myoendothelial coupling is not prominent in arterioles within the mouse cremaster microcirculation in vivo. Circ Res. 2005;97:781–8.
109. Schmidt VJ, Wolfle SE, Boettcher M, de Wit C. Gap junctions synchronize vascular tone within the microcirculation. Pharmacol Rep. 2008;60:68–74.
110. de Wit C, Roos F, Bolz SS, Kirchhoff S, Kruger O, et al. Impaired conduction of vasodilation along arterioles in connexin40 deficient mice. Circ Res. 2000;86:649–55.
111. Wolfle SE, Schmidt VJ, Hoepfl B, Gebert A, Alcolea S, et al. Connexin45 cannot replace the function of connexin40 in conducting endothelium-dependent dilations along arterioles. Circ Res. 2007;101:1292–9.
112. Bagher P, Segal SS. Regulation of blood flow in the microcirculation: role of conducted vasodilation. Acta Physiol (Oxf). 2011;202:271–84.
113. Segal SS. Regulation of blood flow in the microcirculation. Microcirculation. 2005;12:33–45.
114. Welsh DG, Tran CHT, Hald BO, Sancho M. The conducted vasomotor response: function, biophysical basis, and pharmacological control. Annu Rev Pharmacol Toxicol. 2018;58:391–410.
115. Straub AC, Zeigler AC, Isakson BE. The myoendothelial junction: connections that deliver the message. Physiology (Bethesda). 2014;29:242–9.
116. Hald BO, Jacobsen JCB, Sandow SL, Holstein-Rathlou NH, Welsh DG. Less is more: minimal expression of myoendothelial gap junctions optimizes cell-cell communication in virtual arterioles. J Physiol. 2014;592:3243–55.
117. Hald BO, Welsh DG, Holstein-Rathlou NH, Jacobsen JCB. Origins of variation in conducted vasomotor responses. Pflugers Arch. 2015;467:2055–67.
118. Beyer AM, Durand MJ, Hockenberry J, Gamblin TC, Phillips SA, et al. An acute rise in intraluminal pressure shifts the mediator of flow-mediated dilation from nitric oxide to hydrogen peroxide in human arterioles. Am J Physiol Heart Circ Physiol. 2014;307:H1587–93.
119. Beyer AM, Zinkevich N, Miller B, Liu Y, Wittenburg AL, et al. Transition in the mechanism of flow-mediated dilation with aging and development of coronary artery disease. Basic Res Cardiol. 2017;112:5.
120. Boettcher M, de Wit C. Distinct endothelium-derived hyperpolarizing factors emerge in vitro and in vivo and are mediated in part via connexin 40-dependent myoendothelial coupling. Hypertension. 2011;57:802–8.
121. Durand MJ, Gutterman DD. Diversity in mechanisms of endothelium-dependent vasodilation in health and disease. Microcirculation. 2013;20:239–47.
122. Freed JK, Beyer AM, LoGiudice JA, Hockenberry JC, Gutterman DD. Ceramide changes the mediator of flow-induced vasodilation from nitric oxide to hydrogen peroxide in the human microcirculation. Circ Res. 2014;115:525–32.
123. LeBlanc AJ, Hoying JB. Adaptation of the coronary microcirculation in aging. Microcirculation. 2016;23:157–67.
124. Duncker DJ, Merkus D. Exercise hyperaemia in the heart: the search for the dilator mechanism. J Physiol. 2007;583:847–54.
125. Larsen BT, Gutterman DD, Sato A, Toyama K, Campbell WB, et al. Hydrogen peroxide inhibits cytochrome p450 epoxygenases: interaction between two endothelium-derived hyperpolarizing factors. Circ Res. 2008;102:59–67.

Chapter 2
Coronary Microvascular Dysfunction in Cardiovascular Disease: Lessons from Large Animal Models

Oana Sorop, Jens van de Wouw, Daphne Merkus, and Dirk J. Duncker

Introduction

Perfusion of the left ventricle is tightly matched to the demands of the working myocardium to maintain a consistently high level of myocardial oxygen extraction. Consequently, an increase in myocardial oxygen demand must be met by a commensurate increase in coronary blood flow [1–3]. The coronary microvasculature plays a key role in regulating coronary blood flow, involving both acute and chronic adaptations of the coronary microvasculature via regulation of vascular smooth muscle tone and structural changes in microvascular diameter and densities, respectively.

Understanding the factors regulating these microvascular adaptation processes, and particularly how these factors are affected by various diseases and how they contribute to myocardial perfusion abnormalities, has been the study subject of many research groups. As a result of these research efforts in the last 50 years, our understanding of the regulation of coronary microvascular function in health and disease has advanced substantially. A significant contribution to our current knowledge has come from experimental studies involving large animal models—particularly swine—which demonstrate a remarkably similar cardiovascular anatomy and physiology as humans. In this chapter we will discuss the factors regulating coronary microvascular tone under healthy physiological circumstances, and the role of

O. Sorop · J. van de Wouw · D. J. Duncker (✉)
Division of Experimental Cardiology, Department of Cardiology, Thoraxcenter, Erasmus MC, University Medical Center Rotterdam, Rotterdam, The Netherlands
e-mail: o.sorop@erasmusmc.nl; j.vandewouw@erasmusmc.nl; d.duncker@erasmusmc.nl

D. Merkus
Division of Experimental Cardiology, Department of Cardiology, Thoraxcenter, Erasmus MC, University Medical Center Rotterdam, Rotterdam, The Netherlands

Walter-Brendel-Centre of Experimental Medicine, University Hospital, LMU Munich, Munich, Germany
e-mail: d.merkus@erasmusmc.nl

M. Dorobantu, L. Badimon (eds.), *Microcirculation*,
https://doi.org/10.1007/978-3-030-28199-1_2

microvascular dysfunction in obstructive and non-obstructive coronary artery disease, as studied in large animal models and confirmed in human studies.

Physiological Control of Coronary Microvascular Tone

Since left ventricular myocardial oxygen extraction is already well above 70% at rest, any increase in oxygen demand must principally be met by an increase in myocardial oxygen delivery and hence in coronary blood flow. Such an increase is achieved by a reduction in basal vascular tone, leading to an increase in vascular diameter and, consequently, resulting in a decrease in vascular resistance. Resistance of the coronary vasculature is the most important determinant of myocardial perfusion and is the sum of both active (vascular tone) and passive (vascular structure) factors. At rest, approximately 75% of total coronary resistance resides in the coronary small arteries and arterioles, i.e. arterial vessels <200 μm in diameter [4]. Coronary vascular resistance is controlled by a variety of mechanisms including passive mechanical factors (extravascular compression by the contracting myocardium, distension by intravascular pressure), and active changes in smooth muscle tone through the myogenic response (in response to changes in perfusion pressure), and under the influence of metabolic, endothelial, and neurohumoral factors, acting in concert to ensure an optimal level of vascular tone. These regulatory factors exert variable influences on different segments of the microvasculature [5, 6]. For example, during metabolic hyperemia, the smallest arterioles (<100 μm diameter), appear to be most sensitive to the effects of myocyte-derived metabolites, while myogenic mechanisms and flow-mediated dilation dictate the tone of more upstream small arteries (100–400 μm). These factors act synergistically to optimize the distribution of vascular tone along the vascular tree and hence myocardial perfusion. Figure 2.1 summarizes the most important factors influencing coronary microvascular tone. Blood-borne and endothelium-derived factors as well as metabolic and neurohumoral influences act in concert to regulate coronary microvascular tone.

Endothelial Mechanisms

The endothelial layer of the vasculature releases a variety of vasoactive substances with potent effects on vascular tone through different signaling pathways. The strong vasodilator effects of nitric oxide (NO), prostaglandins, and endothelium-derived hyperpolarizing factors (EDHF), including epoxyeicosatrienoic acids (EETs), and hydrogen peroxide (H_2O_2) are counterbalanced by the production and release of potent vasoconstrictors such as endothelin-1 (ET-1).

Endothelium-derived NO is produced by endothelial NO synthase (eNOS) and is released abluminally to the vascular smooth muscle layer, where it binds to soluble guanylyl cyclase, increasing cyclic guanosine monophosphate (cGMP) production

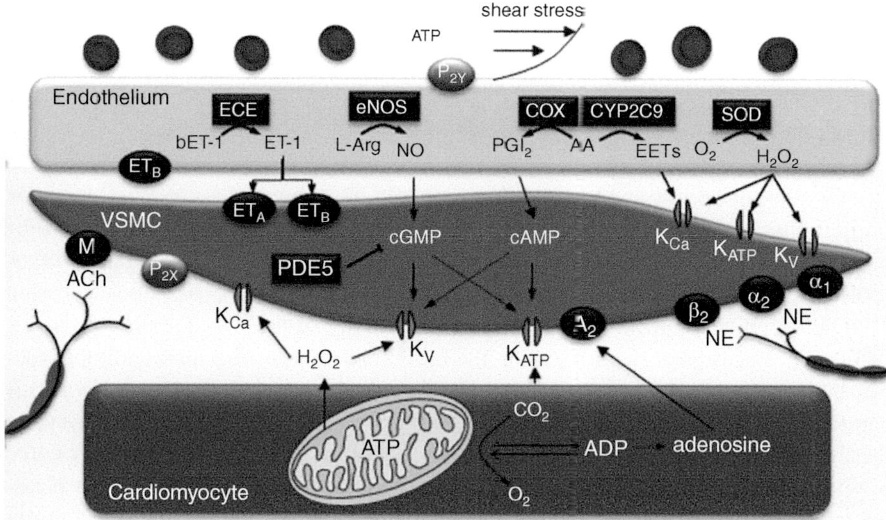

Fig. 2.1 Schematic drawing of endothelium, vascular smooth muscle cell (VSMC) and cardiomyocyte illustrating mechanisms for control of vasomotor tone and diameter. Abbreviations: *ATP* adenosine triphosphate, P_{2y} purinergic receptor type 2y, *SOD* superoxide dismutase, O_2^- superoxide anion, H_2O_2 hydrogen peroxide, *eNOS* endothelial nitric oxide synthase, *L-arg* L-arginine, *NO* nitric oxide, *COX* cyclooxygenase, PGI_2 prostacyclin, *AA* arachidonic acid, *CYP2C9* cytochrome P450 2C9, *EETs* epoxyeicosatrienoic acids, *ECE* endothelin-converting enzyme, *bET-1* big endothelin-1, *ET-1* endothelin-1, ET_A endothelin type A receptor, ET_B endothelin type B receptor, *M* muscarinic receptor, *ACh* acetylcholine, P_2 purinergic receptor type 2, *PDE5* phosphodiesterase, K_{Ca} calcium-activated K^+ channel; 5, K_V voltage-gated K^+ channel, K_{ATP} ATP-sensitive K^+ channel, A_2 adenosine receptor 2, β_2 β_2-adrenergic receptor, *NE* norepinephrine, α_1 α_1-adrenergic receptor, α_2 α_2-adrenergic receptor, CO_2 carbon dioxide, O_2 oxygen, *ADP* adenosine diphosphate

and causing relaxation through a reduction in intracellular calcium. The release of NO is not only generated via biochemical mechanisms in response to several agonists, but also in response to an increase in shear stress, resulting in vasodilation. Furthermore, nitrites are converted to NO when oxygen concentrations are low [7]. Prostacyclin (PGI_2), which is the major active metabolite of arachidonic acid in the vascular endothelium, is also a potent vasodilator of coronary arteries, however, it appears to be less important for the regulation of coronary blood flow during acute myocardial ischemia [8]. Endothelium-dependent hyperpolarization is an additional endothelium-dependent vasodilator mechanism that is activated in response to certain agonists as well as to shear stress, acting via hyperpolarization of vascular smooth muscle through opening of calcium-activated potassium channels (K_{Ca}). Different candidates have been proposed as potential EDHFs, including endothelium-derived H_2O_2 and cytochrome P-450 epoxygenase metabolites EETs [9].

The endothelin family contains three isoforms, ET-1, ET-2, and ET-3, with ET-1 as the most abundant in the coronary vascular tree [10]. ET-1 is an extremely potent vasoconstrictor that is derived from the enzymatic cleavage of a larger precursor molecule (big–endothelin) via endothelin-converting enzyme (ECE). ET-1 results in potent and long-lasting vasoconstriction by binding to its local receptor ET_A on coronary vascular smooth muscle cells (VSMCs). The binding to the ET_B receptor on VSMCs also results in constriction, whereas binding to the ET_B receptor on endothelial cells results in vasodilation via NO production [10]. Cyclooxygenase (COX)-derived constrictors such as prostaglandin $F_{2\alpha}$ and thromboxane A_2 have also been shown to vasoconstrict the coronary circulation [11]. Although these vasoconstrictors do not appear to play an important role in coronary flow regulation under normal physiologic conditions, a pathophysiologic role has been shown for thromboxane A_2 during endothelial injury, coronary artery disease, and coronary vasospasm [6, 11].

In addition to their direct vasoactive effect, many of these endothelium-derived factors have also paracrine effects on the blood cells and/or the surrounding tissue. For instance, endothelial NO is able to diffuse to the parenchymal tissue where it can inhibit mitochondrial metabolism, reducing the production of reactive oxygen species (ROS), and inhibiting inflammation, as well as inhibiting myocyte hypertrophy via activation of PKG [12]. Furthermore, luminally released NO inhibits platelet activation and expression of adhesion molecules, thereby inhibiting thrombosis and vascular inflammation [12]. In conditions of reduced NO bioavailability, such as in metabolic diseases and ischemia, the release of ET-1, thromboxane A_2, and ROS are increased, resulting in decreased angiogenesis, increased cardiomyocyte apoptosis and altered cardiomyocyte contractility [12].

Neurohumoral Influences

Evaluation of the direct effects of sympathetic and parasympathetic stimulation on coronary vascular resistance during resting conditions is complicated by the concomitant changes in myocardial metabolism leading to alterations in coronary blood flow that can easily mask the direct vascular autonomic influences on the coronary resistance vessels. During exercise, the contribution of the autonomic nervous system to coronary resistance vessel tone increases, with data from dogs and swine suggesting that sympathetic activity contributes to exercise hyperemia through beta-adrenoceptor mediated coronary vasodilation that outweighs the alpha-adrenoceptor mediated coronary vasoconstriction [1]. Increased sympathetic activity has been associated with insulin resistance, involved in the development of several diseases including diabetes mellitus, obesity, metabolic syndrome, and ischemic heart disease, possibly resulting in increased coronary vasoconstriction [13]. Furthermore, obese subjects have been shown to have increased levels of circulating noradrenaline as compared to lean subjects [13].

The physiological role of vagal nerve control of coronary tone is uncertain, however, coronary resistance arteries of humans and dogs are known to dilate to acetylcholine resulting in increases in coronary blood flow [3]. This process is dependent on a healthy endothelium, as endothelial dysfunction results in an attenuation of acetylcholine-induced dilation, or even constriction. Furthermore, there is an interaction between the sympathetic and parasympathetic regulation of coronary vascular tone as data in swine indicate that during exercise, beta-adrenergic vasodilation was supported by withdrawal of muscarinic receptor-mediated inhibition of beta-adrenergic coronary vasodilation [1].

Myocardial Metabolism

Perhaps the most important physiological mechanism regulating coronary vascular resistance is metabolic activity of the heart. The heart relies entirely on aerobic metabolism to convert energetic substrates into energy (ATP), in order to maintain normal cardiac pump function. Hence a proper balance between oxygen supply and demand is essential. Since myocardial oxygen extraction is already very high at rest, metabolic control of coronary resistance vessels must ensure adequate myocardial oxygen delivery, as blood flow must increase in proportion to the increase in myocardial oxygen consumption during high myocardial metabolic demand. Although it is generally agreed that tissue-derived metabolites play an important role in the regulation of coronary microvascular resistance in the face of increased metabolic demand, the exact nature of these factors and the mechanisms responsible for local microvascular metabolic tone control remain incompletely understood [2]. Dissolved oxygen and CO_2 have been proposed in the past as possible mediators, however more recent data failed to support these hypotheses [2]. Adenosine was also initially proposed as a metabolic-derived mediator of vasodilation, however, additional studies only supported a role for adenosine during myocardial ischemia but not during physiological conditions [1]. More recently proposed mechanisms include adenine nucleotides, released from erythrocytes under hypoxic conditions, and H_2O_2 produced by mitochondria and acting via Kv1.5, and Kv1.3 channels, as key mediators coupling the coronary flow to metabolism in the heart [14]. For an in-depth review of these mechanisms the reader is referred elsewhere [15].

Intraluminal Forces: Myogenic Regulation and Flow-Mediated Control

The myogenic response is a regulatory mechanism acting in the intact coronary circulation that contributes to coronary autoregulation, i.e. the ability to maintain blood flow within a narrow range despite changes in perfusion pressure. The myogenic response is typically studied ex vivo using pressure myography methods and has been shown to be endothelium-independent and particularly pronounced in coronary arterioles of ~100 μm in diameter [1]. Coronary resistance vessels constrict in response to an increase in transmural distending pressure and dilate in response to a decrease in pressure. Furthermore, subendocardial arterioles have been shown to have reduced myogenic responses as compared to subepicardial arterioles, which is possibly related to the drop in arterial perfusion pressure across the left ventricular myocardial wall, in conjunction with the greater compressive forces of the subendocardial vessels. The myogenic response is of particular importance in post stenotic areas. The signaling mechanisms for the myogenic response include multiple types of molecules, including stretch-activated channels and voltage-operated Ca^{2+} channels, resulting in an inward Na^{+} or Ca^{2+} current and activation of protein kinase C and/or Rho-A kinase [16]. Mechanosensing of pressure may involve integrins that link the extracellular matrix to the cytoskeleton [17].

Shear stress is another important physical vasoactive stimulus in both conduit and resistance vessels. Vasodilation in response to an increase flow (i.e. laminar shear) is termed 'flow-mediated dilation', and is well conserved across species and vascular beds. It is one of the most important factors protecting the vascular integrity and preventing endothelial damage and plaque formation that typically occurs at sites with turbulent or low flow. The magnitude of endothelium-dependent dilation and the underlying mechanism depend strongly on the species, vascular bed, vessel size, and age. Conduit vessels rely primarily on NO while the microcirculation utilizes a variety of mediators, such as NO, prostacyclin, and EDHF. In the human coronary circulation, the arteriolar flow-mediated dilation evolves throughout life from prostacyclin in the young, to NO in adulthood and to H_2O_2 later in life and/or with onset of CAD [18]. Furthermore, blunted flow-mediated dilation occurs with age, as shown in both humans and animal models [6]. Mechanosensing of shear by the endothelial cells is thought to result from multiple cellular components, such as directly by integrins and indirectly by cell-cell adhesions, nuclear conformation changes and cellular-ECM adhesion sites as well as components of the endothelial glycocalyx [19].

Vascular Structure

Coronary microvascular resistance as well as vasoconstrictor and vasodilator reserve are highly dependent on the biomechanical properties of the vasculature. The inner vascular diameter, and its modulation by all the factors described above is limited by the thickness and structure of the vascular layers, in particular the VSMC organization and the perivascular matrix. Chronic increases in active tone due to either myogenic autoregulation or biochemical factors [20], can result in structural remodeling of the vessel wall, either hypertrophic or eutrophic, hampering the vasodilator capacity of the particular vascular segment. The mechanisms of the different types of coronary vascular remodeling have been studied and reviewed elsewhere, [11, 20] (Fig. 2.2), and are beyond the scope of this chapter. However, it is important to realize that different disease entities, particularly metabolic syndrome and hypertension can have a large impact on coronary microvascular structure and hence on vascular resistance and myocardial perfusion.

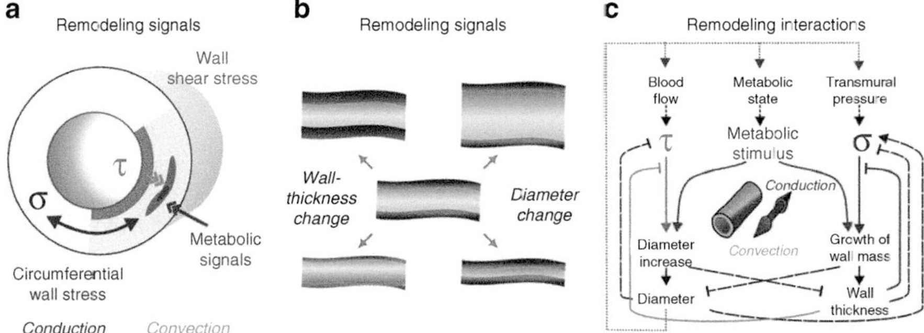

Fig. 2.2 Mechanisms of vascular remodeling: (**a**) endothelial wall shear (τ), circumferential wall stress (σ), and metabolic signals may act as vasoconstrictor or vasodilator stimuli resulting in changes in vascular diameter and wall mass (**b**). (**c**) Model connecting the hemodynamic (pressure, flow) and metabolic state with the derived stimuli (τ, σ, and metabolic stimuli) and their effects on the vascular diameter or wall mass. Lines indicate biological reactions (solid) and physical relations (dashed). With permission from [11]

Coronary Microvascular Dysfunction in Obstructive Coronary Artery Disease

For many years, ischemic heart disease has been considered to be a "large vessel" disease, caused in the majority of patients by an epicardial coronary artery obstruction. The latter is typically due to plaque deposition in one of the large coronary arteries that, when severe enough, compromises blood flow and oxygen delivery to the myocardium perfused by the obstructed artery. In recent years, the coronary microcirculation has become increasingly recognized as a key player in ischemic heart disease, as nearly half of the patients undergoing coronary angiography for typical angina complaints or have a positive stress test, do not have an obstructive coronary artery lesion [21].

Coronary Artery Stenosis

In the healthy heart, during increased metabolic demand, the microvasculature dilates allowing an up to fivefold increase in coronary blood flow [22]. In contrast, when an epicardial artery stenosis develops due to atherosclerosis, total coronary vascular resistance increases and maximal coronary blood flow decreases. This is to a significant degree due to the pressure loss produced by the proximal artery stenosis [23]. However, there is also evidence that abnormalities in the control of coronary microvascular tone and in microvascular structure, contribute to the reductions in coronary flow reserve (CFR) in patients undergoing catheterization for suspected coronary artery disease [22]. In fact, in a large group of patients—of all

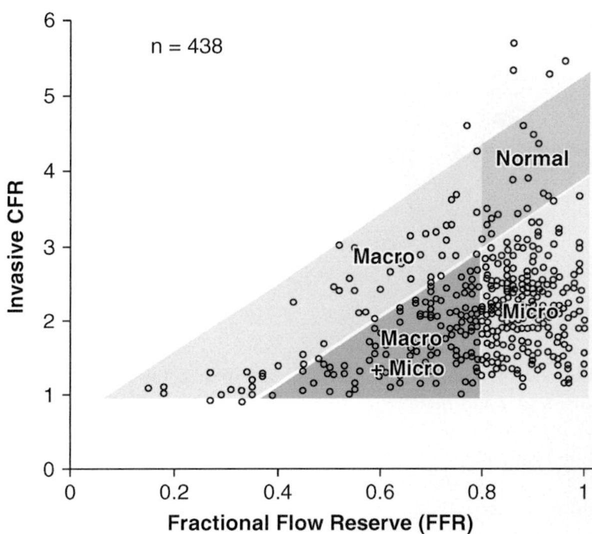

Fig. 2.3 Invasive measurements of individual coronary flow reserve (CFR) and fractional flow reserve values in 438 patients. A FFR value below 0.8 identifies patients with combined macro- and microvascular abnormalities, while a large majority of the group (blue) showed low values of CFR despite a normal FFR, indicative of microvascular problems. Adapted with permission from [22]

ages—presenting with a wide spectrum of coronary atherosclerotic disease (see Fig. 2.3), many patients with a hemodynamically significant coronary artery stenosis (FFR < 0.8) had a CFR below 2.0, suggesting the additional presence of diffuse microvascular disease distal to the coronary artery stenosis. Moreover, a large majority (Micro, light blue) had a fractional flow reserve (FFR) >0.8 and a CFR <3.0, suggestive of diffuse microvascular disease in the absence of a flow-limiting epicardial stenosis [22].

The increased resistance produced by a chronic coronary artery obstruction with >75% reduction in vascular cross-sectional area, results in a drop in perfusion pressure of the distal microvascular bed, triggering both structural and functional alterations [23]. The reduction in perfusion pressure of the distal (subendocardial) microcirculation has been shown, in swine, to contribute to inward hypertrophic and eutrophic remodeling of the resistance arteries (Fig. 2.4) [24, 25], as well as microvascular (200–500 μm diameter) and capillary rarefaction both in the subepicardium and the subendocardium [26].

Microvascular (arteriolar and capillary) densities and diameters may not only vary in time during the progression of a coronary occlusion, but may also be influenced by cardiovascular medication of the patients. Thus, inward remodeling of isolated arterioles at low intraluminal pressure was prevented by incubation with calcium antagonist amlodipine [27]. These observations may explain the findings of Verhoeff et al. [28] showing a maintained or even slight reduction in minimal microvascular resistance upon revascularization in patients with a coronary artery stenosis. Capillary rarefaction is especially important as it is one of the important factors determining myocardial functional recovery following coronary revascularization [29]. Thus, myocardial biopsies in patient with a chronic stenosis subjected to revascularization show that segments with low capillary density show poor recovery, while segments with high capillary density show good functional recovery [29].

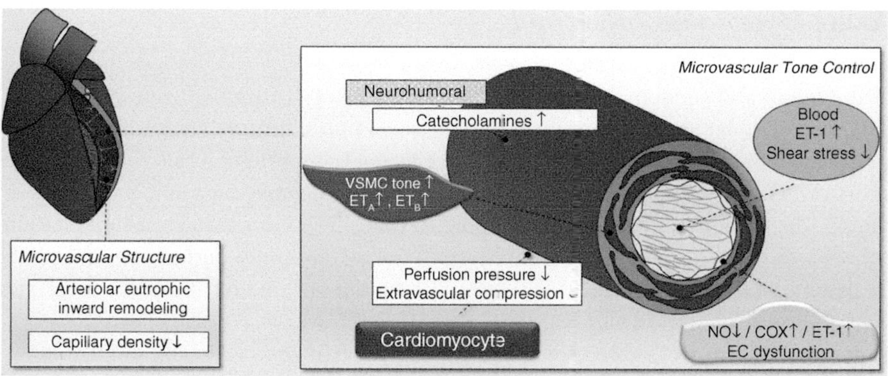

Fig. 2.4 Microvascular dysfunction distal to a chronic artery stenosis. Abbreviations: *ET-1* endothelin-1, *VSMC* vascular smooth muscle cell, ET_A endothelin receptor A, ET_B endothelin receptor B, *NO* nitric oxide, *COX* cyclooxygenase, *EC* endothelial cell

Interestingly, areas with normal microvascular density did not necessarily show a better functional recovery as compared to low capillary density, which may be due to the fact that other hemodynamic factors as well as vascular functional integrity also play a role in the recovery of tissue viability and hence functional recovery after revascularization. The microvascular abnormalities can persist long after revascularization, as 4 weeks after revascularization of hibernating myocardium in swine, abnormal blood flow in response to intracoronary dobutamine infusion were still documented despite normalized basal flow [30]. These findings suggest that perturbations in flow responses contributed to the delayed and incomplete myocardial functional recovery in the revascularized region. Vascular remodeling at the arteriolar level may also be related to alterations in microvascular (endothelial) function, as increased vasoconstrictor response to ET-1 was documented distal to a chronic occlusion of the left descending coronary artery in swine (Fig. 2.4), while this was not seen in the remote area [25]. Interestingly, in these animals, the vasodilator response to bradykinin was preserved in subendocardial arterioles, although the contribution of NO to the bradykinin response was impaired suggestive of preserved endothelial responsiveness, but with a shift in mediators from NO to prostanoids and/or EDHF. Similarly, the contribution of prostanoids to the regulation of coronary microvascular tone in humans has been shown to increase with the progression of coronary artery disease. Distal to angiographically minimally diseased coronary arteries inhibition of prostanoid production induces mild vasoconstriction [31] whereas vasoconstriction is most pronounced in patients with coronary artery disease at rest [32]. Importantly, abnormal coronary vasomotion, endothelial dysfunction and coronary vasospasm were shown to be important predictors of adverse outcome in patients with atherosclerosis and suspected ischemia [33]. In conclusion, there is increasing evidence that in patients with obstructive coronary artery disease, the distal microvascular bed undergoes functional and structural changes that likely contribute to the abnormalities in myocardial perfusion.

Acute Myocardial Infarction

A complete and sudden occlusion of a coronary artery results in acute myocardial infarction (AMI) and subsequent tissue necrosis unless timely revascularization is performed and blood flow is restored. Indeed, timely reperfusion remains the single most effective treatment for AMI to salvage ischemic myocardium, and improve ventricular function and clinical outcome to date [34]. Coronary revascularization by percutaneous coronary intervention (PCI) is a commonly performed procedure in patients with ischemic heart disease, with an annual rate of 992 procedures per one million adults in the United States alone [35]. However, coronary revascularization may not always lead to effective coronary reperfusion, as in a significant number of patients revascularization does not result in alleviation of ischemia—as indicated by electrocardiographic changes—or improvement in perfusion [36]. These observations are confirmed by experimental studies demonstrating incomplete reperfusion of infarcted areas following ischemia-reperfusion [37, 38]. This state of severe myocardial tissue hypoperfusion without angiographic evidence of a residual proximal coronary artery obstruction is termed 'no-reflow'. The pathophysiological mechanisms behind this phenomenon remain incompletely understood, however, one important underlying cause of "no-reflow" is microvascular obstruction [39]. Microvascular obstruction may be caused by various mechanisms, intrinsic or extrinsic to the coronary microcirculation, including irreversible damage to the microvasculature captured under the term 'reperfusion-related no-reflow', or direct embolization of the distal microvasculature following the percutaneous intervention, termed 'interventional no-reflow' [39]. While in the first situation, the area of no-reflow is confined to the infarcted area, "interventional no reflow" may also impact parts of the myocardium not irreversibly damaged by the prolonged ischemia prior to the procedure. Moreover, these two phenomena can also contribute to the no-reflow phenomenon in a synergistic manner, as established microvascular dysfunction due to preexisting comorbidities or ischemia can exacerbate the effects of post-interventional microvascular occlusion [39].

In reperfusion-related no-reflow, coronary microvascular endothelial damage resulting from either ischemia-reperfusion and/or the associated comorbidities such as metabolic dysregulation, hypertension, aging and dyslipidemia, is thought to play a critical role [40]. However, other mechanisms have also been proposed to contribute, including activation of inflammatory pathways, myocyte edema, platelet activation or leucocyte infiltration [39]. In addition to the microcirculatory functional and structural alterations produced by risk factors, ischemia-reperfusion injury to the endothelium plays a central role in the pathophysiology of no-reflow. Interruption of blood flow followed by its acute restoration results in endothelial dysfunction leading to alterations in the balance between the different vasoregulatory pathways as summarized in Fig. 2.5.

Indeed, in the coronary microvasculature of dogs, ischemia-reperfusion resulted in endothelial dysfunction and impaired dilation to acetylcholine and ADP [41] while in swine, 1h ischemia followed by 1h reperfusion resulted in impaired

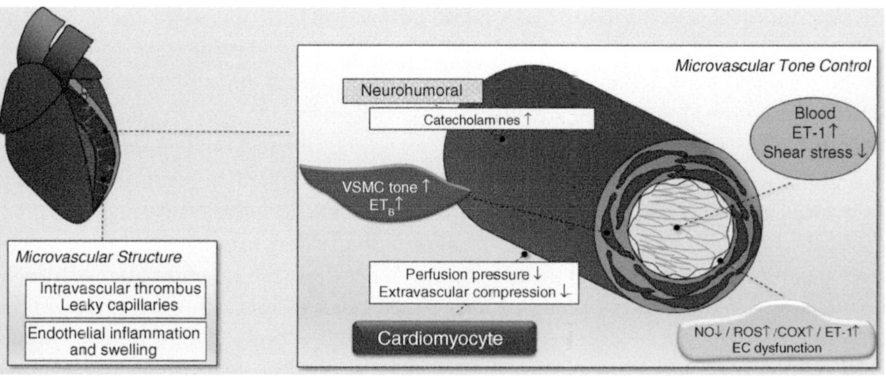

Fig. 2.5 Microvascular dysfunction in the 'no-reflow' area. Abbreviations: *ET-1* endothelin-1, *VSMC* vascular smooth muscle cell, *ET_B* endothelin receptor B, *NO* nitric oxide, *ROS* reactive oxygen species, *COX* cyclooxygenase, *EC* endothelial cell

relaxation to serotonin, and bradykinin in coronary microvessels [42], consistent with impaired endothelial nitric oxide production. Furthermore, an increase in vasoconstrictor influence of ET-1, mainly via the ET_B receptor [43], and activation of thromboxane A_2 synthase promoting arterial vasoconstriction have been documented in the coronary arteries of rodents, following ischemia-reperfusion. These findings are in line with human studies showing increased levels of serotonin and thromboxane A_2 in coronary sinus aspirate of post-PCI patients, which induced vasoconstriction of coronary microvessels [44]. Additionally, in the ischemic vasculature relying on anaerobic metabolism, sudden influx of oxygen induced by the reperfusion results in increased oxidative stress, aggravating the endothelial damage. The mechanisms responsible for the production of reactive oxygen species (ROS) include xanthine oxidase, NADPH oxidase as well as uncoupled eNOS [45].

With increasing severity of ischemia-reperfusion injury, even more extensive microvascular injury occurs, with increased vascular permeability, thinning of the capillary wall and loss of viable cell-cell junctions, leading to edema and even intramyocardial hemorrhage [46]. Although there is no evidence that no-reflow contributes to secondary cardiomyocyte damage, it may affect infarct healing responses—i.e. lead to infarct thinning and may thus aggravate post-infarct remodeling [38].

Post Myocardial Infarction-Remodeled Myocardium

In patients with a large myocardial infarction, (MI), left ventricular (LV) function continues to deteriorate over time. Myocardial perfusion abnormalities, resulting in impaired myocardial oxygen delivery to the non-infarcted regions have been suggested to contribute to the progression of LV dysfunction after MI [47]. Indeed, a significant reduction in CFR has been shown in the surviving remodeled LV myocardium in patients with overt heart failure [48]. In line with these clinical observations, in a swine model of post-MI remodeling, the increase in coronary blood flow and myocardial oxygen delivery was impaired during increased oxygen demand produced by exercise, resulting in perturbations in myocardial oxygen balance [49, 50]. The reduction in flow reserve and the impaired oxygen delivery during exercise are likely caused by structural and functional changes in the coronary microvasculature and by altered mechanical effects of the surrounding myocardium. Since the coronary vasculature is perfused principally during diastole, coronary perfusion can be impeded as a result of changes in LV diastolic function after MI, such as elevated LV diastolic pressures and reduced rates of relaxation [49]. Structural changes of the remote coronary vasculature involve both inward, hypertrophic remodeling of the existing vessels [51], as well as lengthening of the coronary vascular tree in post-MI eccentric LV remodeling, that is accompanied by an unchanged arteriolar density and even a decreased capillary density in the remote remodeled myocardium [49].

The increased extravascular compression and structural changes in the coronary microvasculature result in an increased minimal coronary microvascular resistance and a decreased myocardial perfusion, particularly in the subendocardial layers as maximal subendocardial blood flow was blunted by 40% in anesthetized swine 3 weeks after a myocardial infarction [52]. This impairment of flow reserve is particularly important during exercise, when myocardial oxygen demand and extravascular compression increase simultaneously. Although myocardial blood flow increases during exercise in the remote coronary vasculature after MI, this increase in flow did not fully match the increase in myocardial oxygen demand, as evidenced by an increase in myocardial oxygen extraction. Moreover, myocardial blood flow was redistributed away from the subendocardium in favor of the subepicardium in post-MI as compared to normal swine [49], suggesting that the impaired oxygen delivery was particularly pronounced in the subendocardium. Impaired perfusion of the subendocardium is likely to be, at least in part, responsible for the deterioration of LV function because local interstitial edema and disruption of collagen fibers resemble the ultrastructural changes that occur with recurrent ischemia [53]. Furthermore, a decrease in maximal force development was observed in cardiomyocytes isolated from the subendocardium but not the subepicardium [54].

In addition to changes in myocardial compressive forces and structural changes in the coronary vasculature, there is also evidence that functional changes occur in the coronary microvasculature post-MI, including alterations in neurohumoral, metabolic and endothelial control of coronary resistance vessel tone [55]. The most important alterations in control of coronary resistance vessel tone in post-MI remodeled myocardium are summarized in Fig. 2.6. Oxidative stress is increased after MI, even in the remote non-infarcted myocardium, and this increased oxidative stress contributes to endothelial dysfunction not only in isolated large coronary arteries [56] but also in the coronary microvasculature [57]. Indeed, the coronary vasodilator effect of ROS-scavenging with N-2-mercaptopropionylglycine [57], as well as the DHE staining of the remote myocardium [58], was increased in swine with MI as compared to normal swine, indicating an increased production of ROS in the

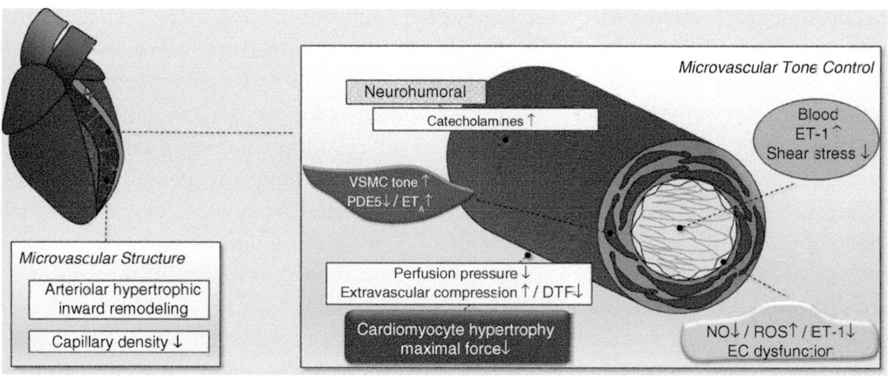

Fig. 2.6 Microvascular dysfunction in the post MI-remodeled myocardium. Abbreviations: *ET-1* endothelin-1, *VSMC* vascular smooth muscle cell, *PDE5* phosphodiesterase 5, ET_A endothelin receptor A, *DTF* diastolic time fraction, *NO* nitric oxide, *ROS* reactive oxygen species, *EC* endothelial cell

microvasculature supplying the remote myocardium. These observations are in accordance with findings that superoxide production is increased in the remote coronary arteries of rats with MI [56] as well as in monocytes/macrophages within the intima, media and adventitia in vessels with coronary artery disease [59].

The increased oxidative stress in the porcine coronary microvasculature after MI was accompanied by uncoupling of eNOS, resulting in generation of superoxide, thereby further contributing to oxidative stress [57]. Consistent with a role of eNOS in the generation of superoxide, the vasodilator effect of N-2-mercaptopropionyl-glycine in swine with MI was no longer apparent following prior eNOS inhibition. However, despite eNOS uncoupling, eNOS inhibition still resulted in significant, albeit reduced, coronary vasoconstriction at rest and during exercise [57, 60, 61], indicating eNOS-mediated NO production was still dominant over ROS production. Moreover, agonists were still capable of producing NO-dependent coronary vasodilation, although this vasodilation was impaired in the remote coronary vasculature post-MI compared to control [62]. These data are consistent with the blunted vasodilator responses to endothelium-dependent vasodilators in the coronary microvasculature of LV myocardium in clinical studies in patients with chronic heart failure [63]. A causal relationship between loss of NO-mediated vasodilation and the progression of LV dysfunction to heart failure is suggested by studies in dogs with pacing-induced dilated cardiomyopathy, in which the loss of basal NO production in the LV myocardium coincided with the progression from LV dysfunction to overt heart failure [64].

The lower levels of NO, and consequently reduced cGMP production, could potentially explain the lack of effect of PDE5-inhibition in the coronary microvasculature of CAD patients. Indeed, even in patients with mild CAD that showed little effect of PDE5-inhibition under basal conditions, PDE5-inhibition enhanced the NO-mediated vasodilation by acetylcholine of both the large epicardial coronary arteries and the coronary microvasculature [65]. Interestingly, both PDE5 mRNA expression and vasodilation produced by PDE5-inhibition were reduced in the coronary microvasculature of swine in the remote non-infarcted myocardium after MI [61], suggesting that PDE5 may be downregulated in order to prolong the bioavailability of cGMP and thereby maintain the vasodilator influence of NO. Moreover, although inhibition of eNOS did result in vasoconstriction in swine with MI, the effect of eNOS inhibition was similar in the presence and absence of PDE5 inhibition. These findings could be interpreted to suggest that in post-MI hearts the vasodilator effects of NO were no longer mediated principally via increasing cGMP, but rather could be mediated through direct inhibition of the vasoconstrictor influence of ET-1 [60, 66].

Although circulating plasma levels of ET-1 are increased after MI, the vasoconstrictor influence of endogenous as well as exogenous ET-1 on the remote coronary vasculature is reduced after MI in vivo [50]. Paradoxically, in coronary small arteries isolated from the remote myocardium of swine with MI, ET-1-induced contraction was enhanced [50], suggesting that there are factors in vivo that modulate ET-1-sensitivity of the coronary vasculature. An ET-1-mediated vasoconstrictor influence was unmasked in MI swine after inhibition of either eNOS or cyclooxygenase [60], confirming that NO, prostanoids and ET-1 interact in the regulation of coronary vasomotor tone [50]. Indeed, it has been shown that both NO and prostanoids are capable of inhibiting ET-1 production and release via a cGMP-dependent pathway [67]. Moreover, NO is capable of reducing the ET-1 receptor binding affinity in the human vasculature [68]. Consistent with the reduced eNOS activity, the suppression of ET-1 mediated coronary vasoconstriction by NO was reduced in swine with a recent MI, as compared to normal swine [60].

In contrast to the blunted influence of NO, the suppression of ET-1 by prostanoids was enhanced, while the overall vasodilator influence of prostanoids was unaltered in the remote coronary microvasculature after MI [60]. COX-1 is constitutively present in the healthy coronary vasculature [69], while COX-2 is mainly induced by shear stress and at sites of inflammation and could therefore become more important after MI. COX-1 and COX-2 end-products influence the ET-1 system on various levels, for instance thromboxane A2 stimulates the production of big-endothelin, the precursor of the vasoactive ET, while both PGE2 and PGI2 inhibit ET-1 production as well as secretion [70]. However, further experiments specifically designed to assess changes in the role of the individual COX end-products after MI are required to further investigate their role in the regulation of coronary vascular tone after MI.

Coronary Microvascular Dysfunction in Metabolic Dysregulation

Metabolic dysregulation comprises a group of conditions including metabolic syndrome (MetS), obesity, insulin resistance, diabetes mellitus, hypercholesterolemia and hypertriglyceridemia, that either alone or in combination contribute to different pathologies including coronary and peripheral artery disease, stroke and cancer [71]. The prevalence of metabolic dysregulation varies worldwide, which corresponds strongly with the prevalence of obesity, and despite a multitude of preventive programs and increased awareness of its health risks, the prevalence of obesity continues to increase [71]. In the USA, about 35% of all adults and nearly 50% of those over 60 years of age were estimated to have MetS, with a higher prevalence in women than men [72]. Importantly, the prevalence of metabolic dysregulation is also increasing in younger age groups—with about one in ten adolescents in the USA having MetS—which is associated with an increased waist circumference and high triglyceride levels, putting them at high risk of developing overt type 2 diabetes and cardiovascular problems later in life [73].

The mechanisms linking metabolic dysregulation and obesity to cardiovascular disease include microvascular dysfunction (Fig. 2.7) This is supported by clinical and experimental studies showing that metabolic diseases and obesity are associated with perturbations in the control of coronary blood flow in response to increased metabolic demand, well before overt CAD develops [23, 74–76]. Furthermore, in recent years evidence has accumulated demonstrating the involvement of microvascular dysfunction in patients with ischemia with non-obstructive coronary artery disease (INOCA) [77, 78], as well as heart failure with preserved ejection fraction [79, 80]. Indeed, MetS and obesity are associated with impaired CFR [81, 82]. These studies are supported by observations in dogs [83] and swine [84] with comorbidities, demonstrating progressive impairment of myocardial oxygen delivery during graded treadmill exercise. Also in humans, coronary flow reserve worsens with the onset of type 2 diabetes [85]. Furthermore, in young subjects, acute hyperglycemia resulted in lower adenosine-mediated increase in coronary blood flow, and altered hyperemia in response to cold press or test, suggestive of sustained endothelial dysfunction [86]. Coronary microvascular dysfunction is further evidenced by a reduction in coronary vasodilator responsiveness to various pharmacological ago-

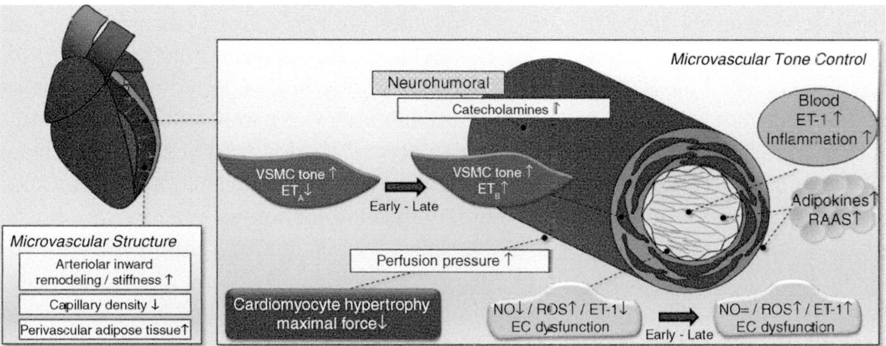

Fig. 2.7 Microvascular dysfunction in the presence of metabolic dysregulation. Abbreviations: *ET-1* endothelin-1, *VSMC* vascular smooth muscle cell, ET_A endothelin receptor A, ET_B endothelin receptor B, *RAAS* renin angiotensin aldosterone system, *NO* nitric oxide, *ROS* reactive oxygen species, *EC* endothelial cell

nists. In swine subjected to 2.5 months of hyperglycemia and hypercholesterolemia, endothelium-dependent vasodilation of isolated coronary small arteries to bradykinin was impaired, due to loss of NO. This occurred in the presence of preserved VSMC function, as evidenced by maintained vasodilation to the exogenous NO-donor SNAP (S-nitroso-N-acetylpenicillamine) [87]. Interestingly, reduced ET_A-mediated vasoconstriction to ET-1 was also observed, that was proposed to serve as a compensatory mechanism. These alterations were not noted, at this early stage, in the microvasculature of hypercholesterolemic swine in the absence of hyperglycemia, suggesting that both co-morbidities acted synergistically. The progression of coronary microvascular dysfunction was studied in the identical swine model at 15 months after induction of hyperglycemia and hypercholesterolemia [88]. At this stage of the disease, when non-obstructive atherosclerotic plaques were observed in the coronary vascular tree, the balance between the vasodilator and vasoconstrictor influences was dominated by an increased ET_B-mediated vasoconstrictor response to ET-1, while—surprisingly—the endothelium-dependent vasodilation to bradykinin was no longer reduced as compared to control. Furthermore, altered NO/EDHF balance was documented in these animals. Thus, the EDHF contribution to the dilation was reduced in the coronary circulation of swine exposed to 15 months of metabolic dysregulation [88]. Interestingly, at this stage, the microvascular alterations were also observed in non-diabetic, hypercholesterolemic swine. Taken together, these two studies [87, 88] clearly demonstrate the temporal changes in coronary microvascular dysfunction, thereby highlighting the importance of longitudinal studies when investigating perturbations in the control of coronary microvascular tone. Similar to our observations in overt diabetes and hypercholesterolemia, obesity has also been shown to increase coronary microvascular sensitivity to vasoconstrictors, including ET-1, prostaglandin H2 or thromboxane A_2, in both animal models [75] and humans [89].

In addition to well documented endothelial dysfunction, smooth muscle cell function has also been shown to be altered by metabolic dysregulation (Fig. 2.7). Thus, 16 weeks of high fat diet in obese Ossabawswine with MetS, resulted in increased coronary vascular tone that was mediated by altered electromechanical coupling between K_V and $Ca_{V1.2}$ channels in the smooth muscle cells [90]. Conversely, in swine with familiar hypercholesterolemia, impaired coronary endothelium dependent dilation to ATP, measured in vivo was paralleled by a compensatory increase in smooth muscle cell sensitivity to NO-donor sodium nitroprusside. This increased VSMC sensitivity was confirmed in isolated coronary arterioles ex vivo together with impaired dilatation to the endothelium-dependent vasodilator bradykinin, and possibly acted as a compensatory mechanism for reduced NO bioavailability [84]. This reduction in NO bioavailability was likely due to increased oxidative stress due to eNOS uncoupling and elevated NOX or xanthine oxidase activity [91, 92].

Increased sympathetic activity in metabolic dysregulation has also been documented by numerous studies both in patients and animal models, showing increased plasma catecholamines, that may result in exaggerated alpha-adrenergic coronary vasoconstriction [93]. Furthermore, there is substantial evidence for activation of the renin angiotensin aldosterone system (RAAS) associated with adipose-tissue-derived angiotensinogen, the major precursor of angiotensin, leading to increased angiotensin II-mediated vasoconstriction in the coronary circulation [94].

Additionally, adipocyte-derived free fatty acids and leptin also lead to increased adrenergic tone [94]. Indeed, the presence of adipose tissue was associated with microvascular dysfunction, as CFR was impaired in patients with metabolic dysregulation and correlated with increased amounts of epicardial fat tissue. Moreover, epicardial fat tissue deposition was a predictor of worse CFR even after accounting for the presence or absence of MetS [95]. Peripheral and perivascular adipose tissue-derived adipokines such as leptin, resistin, IL-6 and TNF-α are potent pro-inflammatory molecules promoting oxidative stress in the endothelium and altering endothelial function and NO bioavailability either directly or via increasing ET-1 production [96]. Furthermore, leptin derived from perivascular fat was also shown to promote coronary arterial vasoconstriction and smooth muscle cell proliferation via Rho kinase signaling [97]. Additionally, adipocyte-derived circulating free fatty acids (FFA) and hyperglycemia-induced advanced glycation end products (AGE) lead to increased oxidative stress limiting NO bioavailability, and increasing production of vasoconstrictor factors such as thromboxane and ET-1 [98].

Finally, not only changes in microvascular function have been documented in metabolic dysregulation, but microvascular structure is also affected. In Ossabaw swine, 16 weeks of MetS induced by a high fat/high fructose diet resulted in impaired myocardial perfusion and blunted response to adenosine, associated with reduced microvascular density [99]. In a similar model, 6 months of MetS and high-fat diet resulted in impaired hyperemic flow associated with augmented coronary myogenic tone, hypertrophic inward remodeling of the coronary resistance arteries and capillary rarefaction [100]. Similar stiffening of the small arteries was also observed in swine after 15 months of high fat diet with or without diabetes, although hypertrophy of the vascular wall was not present [88]. Together with microvascular dysfunction, structural abnormalities and reductions in vascular density may play a key role in the perfusion abnormalities and may thereby contribute to myocardial ischemia during exercise, as observed in humans [78] and animals [83, 84] with co-morbidities.

Conclusions

Coronary microvascular dysfunction, i.e. perturbations in microvascular structure and function, is an intricate part of ischemic heart disease. Here we summarized and discussed the coronary microvascular dysfunction observed in patients and large animal models of stable obstructive CAD, acute MI, post-MI ventricular remodeling, and in animals exposed to a variety of co-morbidities. Coronary microvascular dysfunction appears to be most strongly associated with endothelial dysfunction (loss of NO and increased ET-1) in conjunction with arterial (inward) remodeling and reduced capillary densities. Together these alterations in coronary microvascular tone control and architecture contribute to the observed decreases in coronary flow reserve and perturbations in myocardial oxygen supply during increased myocardial oxygen demand, thereby promoting myocardial ischemia. Consequently, coronary microvascular dysfunction remains an important target for therapeutic interventions.

References

1. Duncker DJ, Bache RJ. Regulation of coronary blood flow during exercise. Physiol Rev. 2008;88(3):1009–86.
2. Goodwill AG, Dick GM, Kiel AM, Tune JD. Regulation of coronary blood flow. Compr Physiol. 2017;7(2):321–82.
3. Laughlin MH, Davis MJ, Secher NH, van Lieshout JJ, Arce-Esquivel AA, Simmons GH, Bender SB, Padilla J, Bache RJ, Merkus D, Duncker DJ. Peripheral circulation. Compr Physiol. 2012;2(1):321–447.
4. Chilian WM, Eastham CL, Marcus ML. Microvascular distribution of coronary vascular resistance in beating left ventricle. Am J Phys. 1986;251(4 Pt 2):H779–88.
5. Jones CJ, Kuo L, Davis MJ, Chilian WM. Distribution and control of coronary microvascular resistance. Adv Exp Med Biol. 1993;346:181–8.
6. Duncker DJC, Canty JM Jr. Coronary blood flow and myocardial ischemia. In: Braunwald E, editor. Braunwald's heart disease: a textbook of cardiovascular medicine. Philadelphia: Elsevier; 2018.
7. Zweier JL, Wang P, Samouilov A, Kuppusamy P. Enzyme-independent formation of nitric oxide in biological tissues. Nat Med. 1995;1(8):804–9.
8. Duncker DJ, Bache RJ. Regulation of coronary vasomotor tone under normal conditions and during acute myocardial hypoperfusion. Pharmacol Ther. 2000;86(1):87–110.
9. Fleming I. The factor in EDHF: cytochrome P450 derived lipid mediators and vascular signaling. Vasc Pharmacol. 2016;86:31–40.
10. Dhaun N, Webb DJ. Endothelins in cardiovascular biology and therapeutics. Nat Rev Cardiol. 2019;16(8):491–502.
11. Pries AR, Badimon L, Bugiardini R, Camici PG, Dorobantu M, Duncker DJ, Escaned J, Koller A, Piek JJ, de Wit C. Coronary vascular regulation, remodelling, and collateralization: mechanisms and clinical implications on behalf of the working group on coronary pathophysiology and microcirculation. Eur Heart J. 2015;36(45):3134–46.
12. Zhang CH, Rogers PA, Merkus D, Muller-Delp JM, Tiefenbacher CP, Potter B, Knudson JD, Rocic P, Chilian WM. Regulation of coronary microvascular resistance in health and disease. In: Tuma RF, Duran WN, Ley K, editors. Handbook of physiology: microcirculation. Boston: Elsevier; 2008.
13. Thorp AA, Schlaich MP. Relevance of sympathetic nervous system activation in obesity and metabolic syndrome. J Diabetes Res. 2015;2015:341583.
14. Ohanyan V, Yin L, Bardakjian R, Kolz C, Enrick M, Hakobyan T, Luli J, Graham K, Khayata M, Logan S, Kmetz J, Chilian WM. Kv1.3 channels facilitate the connection between metabolism and blood flow in the heart. Microcirculation. 2017;24(4):e12334.
15. Jackson WF. KV channels and the regulation of vascular smooth muscle tone. Microcirculation. 2018;25(1):e12421.
16. Baek EB, Kim SJ. Mechanisms of myogenic response: Ca(2+)-dependent and -independent signaling. J Smooth Muscle Res. 2011;47(2):55–65.
17. Davis MJ, Wu X, Nurkiewicz TR, Kawasaki J, Davis GE, Hill MA, Meininger GA. Integrins and mechanotransduction of the vascular myogenic response. Am J Physiol Heart Circ Physiol. 2001;280(4):H1427–33.

18. Beyer AM, Zinkevich N, Miller B, Liu Y, Wittenburg AL Mitchell M, Galdieri R, Sorokin A, Gutterman DD. Transition in the mechanism of flow-mediated dilation with aging and development of coronary artery disease. Basic Res Cardiol. 2017;112(1):5.
19. Davies PF. Hemodynamic shear stress and the endothelium in cardiovascular pathophysiology. Nat Clin Pract Cardiovasc Med. 2009;6(1):16–26.
20. VanBavel E, Bakker EN, Pistea A, Sorop O, Spaan JA. Mechanics of microvascular remodeling. Clin Hemorheol Microcirc. 2006;34(1–2):35–41.
21. Patel MR, Peterson ED, Dai D, Brennan JM, Redberg RF, Anderson HV, Brindis RG, Douglas PS. Low diagnostic yield of elective coronary angiography. N Engl J Med. 2010;362(10):886–95.
22. Johnson NP, Kirkeeide RL, Gould KL. Is discordance of coronary flow reserve and fractional flow reserve due to methodology or clinically relevant coronary pathophysiology? JACC Cardiovasc Imaging. 2012;5(2):193–202.
23. Duncker DJ, Koller A, Merkus D, Canty JM Jr. Regulation of coronary blood flow in health and ischemic heart disease. Prog Cardiovasc Dis. 2015;57(5):409–22.
24. Canty JM Jr, Suzuki G. Myocardial perfusion and contraction in acute ischemia and chronic ischemic heart disease. J Mol Cell Cardiol. 2012;52(4):822–31.
25. Sorop O, Merkus D, de Beer VJ, Houweling B, Pistea A, McFalls EO, Boomsma F, van Beusekom HM, van der Giessen WJ, VanBavel E, Duncker DJ. Functional and structural adaptations of coronary microvessels distal to a chronic coronary artery stenosis. Circ Res. 2008;102(7):795–803.
26. Urbieta Caceres VH, Lin J, Zhu XY, Favreau FD, Gibson ME, Crane JA, Lerman A, Lerman LO. Early experimental hypertension preserves the myocardial microvasculature but aggravates cardiac injury distal to chronic coronary artery obstruction. Am J Physiol Heart Circ Physiol. 2011;300(2):H693–701.
27. Sorop O, Bakker EN, Pistea A, Spaan JA, VanBavel E. Calcium channel blockade prevents pressure-dependent inward remodeling in isolated subendocardial resistance vessels. Am J Physiol Heart Circ Physiol. 2006;291(3):H1236–45.
28. Verhoeff BJ, Siebes M, Meuwissen M, Atasever B, Voskuil M, de Winter RJ, Koch KT, Tijssen JG, Spaan JA, Piek JJ. Influence of percutaneous coronary intervention on coronary microvascular resistance index. Circulation. 2005;111(1):76–82.
29. Shimoni S, Frangogiannis NG, Aggeli CJ, Shan K, Quinones MA, Espada R, Letsou GV, Lawrie GM, Winters WL, Reardon MJ, Zoghbi WA. Microvascular structural correlates of myocardial contrast echocardiography in patients with coronary artery disease and left ventricular dysfunction: implications for the assessment of myocardial hibernation. Circulation. 2002;106(8):950–6.
30. Kelly RF, Cabrera JA, Ziemba EA, Crampton M, Anderson LB, McFalls EO, Ward HB. Continued depression of maximal oxygen consumption and mitochondrial proteomic expression despite successful coronary artery bypass grafting in a swine model of hibernation. J Thorac Cardiovasc Surg. 2011;141(1):261–8.
31. Duffy SJ, Castle SF, Harper RW, Meredith IT. Contribution of vasodilator prostanoids and nitric oxide to resting flow, metabolic vasodilation, and flow-mediated dilation in human coronary circulation. Circulation. 1999;100(19):1951–7.
32. Friedman PL, Brown EJ Jr, Gunther S, Alexander RW, Barry WH, Mudge GH Jr, Grossman W. Coronary vasoconstrictor effect of indomethacin in patients with coronary-artery disease. N Engl J Med. 1981;305(20):1171–5.
33. Pepine CJ, Anderson RD, Sharaf BL, Reis SE, Smith KM, Handberg EM, Johnson BD, Sopko G, Bairey Merz CN. Coronary microvascular reactivity to adenosine predicts adverse outcome in women evaluated for suspected ischemia results from the National Heart, Lung and Blood Institute WISE (women's ischemia syndrome evaluation) study. J Am Coll Cardiol. 2010;55(25):2825–32.
34. Zijlstra F, Patel A, Jones M, Grines CL, Ellis S, Garcia E, Grinfeld L, Gibbons RJ, Ribeiro EE, Ribichini F, Granger C, Akhras F, Weaver WD, Simes RJ. Clinical characteristics and

outcome of patients with early (<2 h), intermediate (2-4 h) and late (>4 h) presentation treated by primary coronary angioplasty or thrombolytic therapy for acute myocardial infarction. Eur Heart J. 2002;23(7):550–7.
35. Kim LK, Feldman DN, Swaminathan RV, Minutello RM, Chanin J, Yang DC, Lee MK, Charitakis K, Shah A, Kaple RK, Bergman G, Singh H, Wong SC. Rate of percutaneous coronary intervention for the management of acute coronary syndromes and stable coronary artery disease in the United States (2007 to 2011). Am J Cardiol. 2014;114(7):1003–10.
36. Niccoli G, Burzotta F, Galiuto L, Crea F. Myocardial no-reflow in humans. J Am Coll Cardiol. 2009;54(4):281–92.
37. Uitterdijk A, Yetgin T, te Lintel Hekkert M, Sneep S, Krabbendam-Peters I, van Beusekom HM, Fischer TM, Cornelussen RN, Manintveld OC, Merkus D, Duncker DJ. Vagal nerve stimulation started just prior to reperfusion limits infarct size and no-reflow. Basic Res Cardiol. 2015;110(5):508.
38. Kloner RA, King KS, Harrington MG. No-reflow phenomenon in the heart and brain. Am J Physiol Heart Circ Physiol. 2018;315(3):H550–62.
39. Jaffe R, Charron T, Puley G, Dick A, Strauss BH. Microvascular obstruction and the no-reflow phenomenon after percutaneous coronary intervention. Circulation. 2008;117(24):3152–6.
40. Heusch G. The coronary circulation as a target of cardioprotection. Circ Res. 2016;118(10):1643–58.
41. Quillen JE, Sellke FW, Brooks LA, Harrison DG. Ischemia-reperfusion impairs endothelium-dependent relaxation of coronary microvessels but does not affect large arteries. Circulation. 1990;82(2):586–94.
42. Piana RN, Shafique T, Dai HB, Sellke FW. Epicardial and endocardial coronary microvascular responses: effects of ischemia-reperfusion. J Cardiovasc Pharmacol. 1994;23(4):539–46.
43. Skovsted GF, Kruse LS, Berchtold LA, Grell AS, Warfvinge K, Edvinsson L. Myocardial ischemia-reperfusion enhances transcriptional expression of endothelin-1 and vasoconstrictor ETB receptors via the protein kinase MEK-ERK1/2 signaling pathway in rat. PLoS One. 2017;12(3):e0174119.
44. Lieder HR, Baars T, Kahlert P, Kleinbongard P. Aspirate from human stented saphenous vein grafts induces epicardial coronary vasoconstriction and impairs perfusion and left ventricular function in rat bioassay hearts with pharmacologically induced endothelial dysfunction. Physiol Rep. 2016;4(15):e12874.
45. Wu MY, Yiang GT, Liao WT, Tsai AP, Cheng YL, Cheng PW, Li CY, Li CJ. Current mechanistic concepts in ischemia and reperfusion injury. Cell Physiol Biochem. 2018;46(4):1650–67.
46. de Waard GA, Hollander MR, Teunissen PF, Jansen MF, Eerenberg ES, Beek AM, Marques KM, van de Ven PM, Garrelds IM, Danser AH, Duncker DJ, van Royen N. Changes in coronary blood flow after acute myocardial infarction: insights From a patient study and an experimental porcine model. JACC Cardiovasc Interv. 2016;9(6):602–13.
47. van Veldhuisen DJ, van den Heuvel AF, Blanksma PK, Crijns HJ. Ischemia and left ventricular dysfunction: a reciprocal relation? J Cardiovasc Pharmacol. 1998;32(Suppl 1):S46–51.
48. van den Heuvel AF, Bax JJ, Blanksma PK, Vaalburg W, Crijns HJ, van Veldhuisen DJ. Abnormalities in myocardial contractility, metabolism and perfusion reserve in non-stenotic coronary segments in heart failure patients. Cardiovasc Res. 2002;55(1):97–103.
49. Haitsma DB, Bac D, Raja N, Boomsma F, Verdouw PD, Duncker DJ. Minimal impairment of myocardial blood flow responses to exercise in the remodeled left ventricle early after myocardial infarction, despite significant hemodynamic and neurohumoral alterations. Cardiovasc Res. 2001;52:471–28.
50. Merkus D, Houweling B, van den Meiracker AH, Boomsma F, Duncker DJ. Contribution of endothelin to coronary vasomotor tone is abolished after myocardial infarction. Am J Physiol Heart Circ Physiol. 2005;288(2):H871–80.
51. Zhao H, Chen H, Li H, Li D, Wang S, Han Y. Remodeling of small intramyocardial coronary arteries distal to total occlusions after myocardial infarction in pigs. Coron Artery Dis. 2013;24(6):493–500.

52. Zhang J, Wilke N, Wang Y, Zhang Y, Wang C, Eijgelshoven MH, Cho YK, Murakami Y, Ugurbil K, Bache RJ, From AH. Functional and bioenergetic consequences of postinfarction left ventricular remodeling in a new porcine model. MRI and 31 P-MRS study. Circulation. 1996;94(5):1089–100.
53. Helmer GA, McKirnan MD, Shabetai R, Boss GR, Ross JJ, Hammond HK. Regional deficits of myocardial blood flow and function in left ventricular pacing-induced heart failure. Circulation. 1996;94(9):2260–7.
54. van der Velden J, Merkus D, de Beer V, Hamdani N, Linke WA, Boontje NM, Stienen GJ, Duncker DJ. Transmural heterogeneity of myofilament function and sarcomeric protein phosphorylation in remodeled myocardium of pigs with a recent myocardial infarction. Front Physiol. 2011;2:83.
55. Duncker DJ, de Beer VJ, Merkus D. Alterations in vasomotor control of coronary resistance vessels in remodelled myocardium of swine with a recent myocardial infarction. Med Biol Eng Comput. 2008;46(5):485–97.
56. Berges A, Van Nassauw L, Timmermans JP, Vrints C. Role of nitric oxide during coronary endothelial dysfunction after myocardial infarction. Eur J Pharmacol. 2005;516(1):60–70.
57. Taverne YJ, de Beer VJ, Hoogteijling BA, Juni RP, Moens AL, Duncker DJ, Merkus D. Nitroso-redox balance in control of coronary vasomotor tone. J Appl Physiol. 2012;112(10):1644–52.
58. Boontje NM, Merkus D, Zaremba R, Versteilen A, de Waard MC, Mearini G, de Beer VJ, Carrier L, Walker LA, Niessen HW, Dobrev D, Stienen GJ, Duncker DJ, van der Velden J. Enhanced myofilament responsiveness upon beta-adrenergic stimulation in post-infarct remodeled myocardium. J Mol Cell Cardiol. 2011;50(3):487–99.
59. Cathcart MK. Regulation of superoxide anion production by NADPH oxidase in monocytes/macrophages: contributions to atherosclerosis. Arterioscler Thromb Vasc Biol. 2004;24(1):23–8.
60. de Beer VJ, Taverne YJ, Kuster DW, Najafi A, Duncker DJ, Merkus D. Prostanoids suppress the coronary vasoconstrictor influence of endothelin after myocardial infarction. Am J Physiol Heart Circ Physiol. 2011;301(3):H1080–9.
61. Merkus D, Visser M, Houweling B, Zhou Z, Nelson J, Duncker DJ. Phosphodiesterase 5 inhibition-induced coronary vasodilation is reduced after myocardial infarction. Am J Physiol Heart Circ Physiol. 2013;304(10):H1370–81.
62. Haitsma DB, Merkus D, Vermeulen J, Verdouw PD, Duncker DJ. Nitric oxide production is maintained in exercising swine with chronic left ventricular dysfunction. Am J Physiol Heart Circ Physiol. 2002;282(6):H2198–209.
63. Treasure CB, Vita JA, Cox DA, Fish RD, Gordon JB, Mudge GH, Colucci WS, Sutton MG, Selwyn AP, Alexander RW, et al. Endothelium-dependent dilation of the coronary microvasculature is impaired in dilated cardiomyopathy. Circulation. 1990;81(3):772–9.
64. Recchia FA, McConnell PI, Bernstein RD, Vogel TR, Xu X, Hintze TH. Reduced nitric oxide production and altered myocardial metabolism during the decompensation of pacing-induced heart failure in the conscious dog. Circ Res. 1998;83(10):969–79.
65. Halcox JP, Nour KR, Zalos G, Mincemoyer RA, Waclawiw M, Rivera CE, Willie G, Ellahham S, Quyyumi AA. The effect of sildenafil on human vascular function, platelet activation, and myocardial ischemia. J Am Coll Cardiol. 2002;40(7):1232–40.
66. Merkus D, Sorop O, Houweling B, Boomsma F, van den Meiracker AH, Duncker DJ. NO and prostanoids blunt endothelin-mediated coronary vasoconstrictor influence in exercising swine. Am J Physiol Heart Circ Physiol. 2006;291(5):H2075–81.
67. Kelly LK, Wedgwood S, Steinhorn RH, Black SM. Nitric oxide decreases endothelin-1 secretion through the activation of soluble guanylate cyclase. Am J Physiol Lung Cell Mol Physiol. 2004;286(5):L984–91.
68. Wiley KE, Davenport AP. Nitric oxide-mediated modulation of the endothelin-1 signalling pathway in the human cardiovascular system. Br J Pharmacol. 2001;132(1):213–20.
69. Zidar N, Dolenc-Strazar Z, Jeruc J, Jerse M, Balazic J, Gartner U, Jermol U, Zupanc T, Stajer D. Expression of cyclooxygenase-1 and cyclooxygenase-2 in the normal human heart and in myocardial infarction. Cardiovasc Pathol. 2007;16(5):300–4.

70. Prins B, Hu R, Nazario B, Pedram A, Frank H, Weber M, Levin E. Prostaglandin E2 and prostacyclin inhibit the production and secretion of endothelin from cultured endothelial cells. J Biol Chem. 1994;269(16):11938–44.
71. Sherling DH, Perumareddi P, Hennekens CH. Metabolic syndrome. J Cardiovasc Pharmacol Ther. 2017;22(4):365–7.
72. Aguilar M, Bhuket T, Torres S, Liu B, Wong RJ. Prevalence of the metabolic syndrome in the United States, 2003-2012. JAMA. 2015;313(19):1973–4.
73. Miller JM, Kaylor MB, Johannsson M, Bay C, Churilla JR. Prevalence of metabolic syndrome and individual criterion in US adolescents: 2001-2010 National Health and Nutrition Examination Survey. Metab Syndr Relat Disord. 2014;12(10):527–32.
74. Badimon L, Bugiardini R, Cenko E, Cubedo J, Dorobantu M, Duncker DJ, Estruch R, Milicic D, Tousoulis D, Vasiljevic Z, Vilahur G, de Wit C, Koller A. Position paper of the European Society of Cardiology-working group of coronary pathophysiology and microcirculation: obesity and heart disease. Eur Heart J. 2017;38(25):1951–8.
75. Berwick ZC, Dick GM, Tune JD. Heart of the matter: coronary dysfunction in metabolic syndrome. J Mol Cell Cardiol. 2012;52(4):848–56.
76. Van De Wouw J, Sorop O, Van Drie RWA, Joles JA, Merkus D, Duncker DJ. P6555 alterations in myocardial oxygen balance in exercising swine with multiple comorbiditiese. Eur Heart J. 2018;39(suppl_1):ehy566-P6555.
77. Shah SJ, Lam CSP, Svedlund S, Saraste A, Hage C, Tan RS, Beussink-Nelson L, Fermer ML, Broberg MA, Gan LM, Lund LH. Prevalence and correlates of coronary microvascular dysfunction in heart failure with preserved ejection fraction: PROMIS-HFpEF. Eur Heart J. 2018;39(37):3439–50.
78. Bairey Merz CN, Pepine CJ, Walsh MN, Fleg JL. Ischemia and no obstructive coronary artery disease (INOCA): developing evidence-based therapies and research agenda for the next decade. Circulation. 2017;135(11):1075–92.
79. Paulus WJ, Tschope C. A novel paradigm for heart failure with preserved ejection fraction: comorbidities drive myocardial dysfunction and remodeling through coronary microvascular endothelial inflammation. J Am Coll Cardiol. 2013;62(4):263–71.
80. Ter Maaten JM, Damman K, Verhaar MC, Paulus WJ, Duncker DJ, Cheng C, van Heerebeek L, Hillege HL, Lam CS, Navis G, Voors AA. Connecting heart failure with preserved ejection fraction and renal dysfunction: the role of endothelial dysfunction and inflammation. Eur J Heart Fail. 2016;18(6):588–98.
81. Pirat B, Bozbas H, Simsek V, Yildirir A, Sade LE, Gursoy Y, Altin C, Atar I, Muderrisoglu H. Impaired coronary flow reserve in patients with metabolic syndrome. Atherosclerosis. 2008;201(1):112–6.
82. Zorach B, Shaw PW, Bourque J, Kuruvilla S, Balfour PC Jr, Yang Y, Mathew R, Pan J, Gonzalez JA, Taylor AM, Meyer CH, Epstein FH, Kramer CM, Salerno M. Quantitative cardiovascular magnetic resonance perfusion imaging identifies reduced flow reserve in microvascular coronary artery disease. J Cardiovasc Magn Reson. 2018;20(1):14.
83. Setty S, Sun W, Tune JD. Coronary blood flow regulation in the prediabetic metabolic syndrome. Basic Res Cardiol. 2003;98(6):416–23.
84. Bender SB, de Beer VJ, Tharp DL, Bowles DK, Laughlin MH, Merkus D, Duncker DJ. Severe familial hypercholesterolemia impairs the regulation of coronary blood flow and oxygen supply during exercise. Basic Res Cardiol. 2016;111(6):61.
85. Schindler TH, Cardenas J, Prior JO, Facta AD, Kreissl MC, Zhang XL, Sayre J, Dahlbom M, Licinio J, Schelbert HR. Relationship between increasing body weight, insulin resistance, inflammation, adipocytokine leptin, and coronary circulatory function. J Am Coll Cardiol. 2006;47(6):1188–95.
86. Di Carli MF, Janisse J, Grunberger G, Ager J. Role of chronic hyperglycemia in the pathogenesis of coronary microvascular dysfunction in diabetes. J Am Coll Cardiol. 2003;41(8):1387–93.
87. van den Heuvel M, Sorop O, Koopmans SJ, Dekker R, de Vries R, van Beusekom HM, Eringa EC, Duncker DJ, Danser AH, van der Giessen WJ. Coronary microvascular dys-

function in a porcine model of early atherosclerosis and diabetes. Am J Physiol Heart Circ Physiol. 2012;302(1):H85–94.

88. Sorop O, van den Heuvel M, van Ditzhuijzen NS, de Beer VJ, Heinonen I, van Duin RW, Zhou Z, Koopmans SJ, Merkus D, van der Giessen WJ, Danser AH, Duncker DJ. Coronary microvascular dysfunction after long-term diabetes and hypercholesterolemia. Am J Physiol Heart Circ Physiol. 2016;311(6):H1339–51.
89. Barton M, Baretella O, Meyer MR. Obesity and risk of vascular disease: importance of endothelium-dependent vasoconstriction. Br J Pharmacol. 2012;165(3):591–602.
90. Berwick ZC, Dick GM, O'Leary HA, Bender SB, Goodwill AG, Moberly SP, Owen MK, Miller SJ, Obukhov AG, Tune JD. Contribution of electromechanical coupling between Kv and Ca v1.2 channels to coronary dysfunction in obesity. Basic Res Cardiol. 2013;108(5):370.
91. Sorop O, Heinonen I, van Kranenburg M, van de Wouw J, de Beer VJ, Nguyen ITN, Octavia Y, van Duin RWB, Stam K, van Geuns RJ, Wielopolski PA, Krestin GP, van den Meiracker AH, Verjans R, van Bilsen M, Danser AHJ, Paulus WJ, Cheng C, Linke WA, Joles JA, Verhaar MC, van der Velden J, Merkus D, Duncker DJ. Multiple common comorbidities produce left ventricular diastolic dysfunction associated with coronary microvascular dysfunction, oxidative stress, and myocardial stiffening. Cardiovasc Res. 2018;114(7):954–64.
92. Bagi Z, Feher A, Cassuto J. Microvascular responsiveness in obesity: implications for therapeutic intervention. Br J Pharmacol. 2012;165(3):544–60.
93. Grassi G, Seravalle G, Quarti-Trevano F, Scopelliti F, Dell'Oro R, Bolla G, Mancia G. Excessive sympathetic activation in heart failure with obesity and metabolic syndrome: characteristics and mechanisms. Hypertension. 2007;49(3):535–41.
94. Kachur S, Morera R, De Schutter A, Lavie CJ. Cardiovascular risk in patients with prehypertension and the metabolic syndrome. Curr Hypertens Rep. 2018;20(2):15.
95. Tok D, Cagli K, Kadife I, Turak O, Ozcan F, Basar FN, Golbasi Z, Aydogdu S. Impaired coronary flow reserve is associated with increased echocardiographic epicardial fat thickness in metabolic syndrome patients. Coron Artery Dis. 2013;24(3):191–5.
96. Bagi Z, Feher A, Cassuto J, Akula K, Labinskyy N, Kaley G, Koller A. Increased availability of angiotensin AT 1 receptors leads to sustained arterial constriction to angiotensin II in diabetes - role for Rho-kinase activation. Br J Pharmacol. 2011;163(5):1059–68.
97. Noblet JN, Goodwill AG, Sassoon DJ, Kiel AM, Tune JD. Leptin augments coronary vasoconstriction and smooth muscle proliferation via a Rho-kinase-dependent pathway. Basic Res Cardiol. 2016;111(3):25.
98. Creager MA, Luscher TF, Cosentino F, Beckman JA. Diabetes and vascular disease: pathophysiology, clinical consequences, and medical therapy: part I. Circulation. 2003;108(12):1527–32.
99. Li ZL, Woollard JR, Ebrahimi B, Crane JA, Jordan KL, Lerman A, Wang SM, Lerman LO. Transition from obesity to metabolic syndrome is associated with altered myocardial autophagy and apoptosis. Arterioscler Thromb Vasc Biol. 2012;32(5):1132–41.
100. Trask AJ, Katz PS, Kelly AP, Galantowicz ML, Cismowski MJ, West TA, Neeb ZP, Berwick ZC, Goodwill AG, Alloosh M, Tune JD, Sturek M, Lucchesi PA. Dynamic micro- and macrovascular remodeling in coronary circulation of obese Ossabaw pigs with metabolic syndrome. J Appl Physiol. 2012;113(7):1128–40.

Chapter 3
Dynamic Control of Microvessel Diameters by Metabolic Factors

Axel R. Pries and Bettina Reglin

Vascular Adaptation and Feedback Regulation

Adaptation of vessel diameters is indispensable for generation and maintenance of functionally adequate microvascular networks and thus tissue function [1, 2]. Various stimuli guiding this adaptation were identified, including circumferential stress in the vessel wall, shear stress on the endothelial cell surface, local metabolic conditions and sympathetic input.

Diameter adaptation in response to hemodynamic signals alone causes regression of complex network structures to single arterio-venous pathways due to positive feedback regulation: vessels with high flow increase their diameter leading to even higher perfusion (Fig. 3.1) [3, 6]. Thus, compensatory negative feedback mechanism increasing perfusion in low flow vessels is needed to preserve parallel flow pathways in microvascular networks in vivo guaranteeing low diffusion distances from vessel lumen to tissue cells and to maintain adequate flow distribution. Such a negative feedback can be based on local metabolic conditions, with imbalance between substrate supply and demand eliciting signals for diameter increase. Current concepts assume that decreasing oxygen partial pressures (Po_2) induces release of metabolic signal substance(s) which stimulate increase of vessel diameters and thus perfusion, restoring adequate Po_2 (Fig. 3.1).

A. R. Pries (✉)
Department of Physiology, Charité Universitätsmedizin Berlin, Berlin, Germany

Deutsches Herzzentrum Berlin, Berlin, Germany
e-mail: axel.pries@charite.de

B. Reglin
Department of Physiology, Charité Universitätsmedizin Berlin, Berlin, Germany

M. Dorobantu, L. Badimon (eds.), *Microcirculation*,
https://doi.org/10.1007/978-3-030-28199-1_3

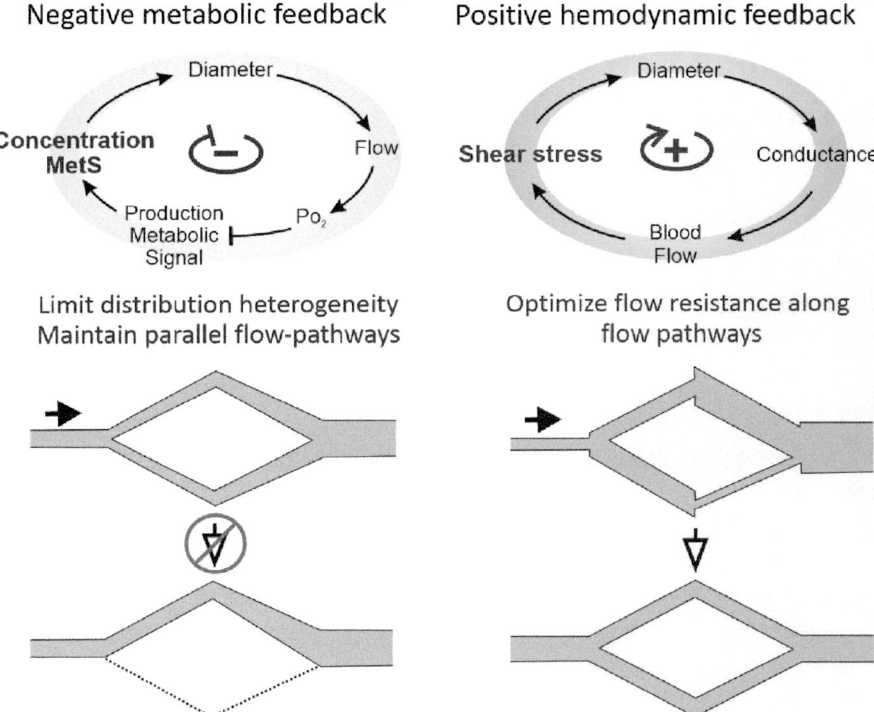

Fig. 3.1 Principle roles of metabolic and hemodynamic feedback. Arrows and blunt ends indicate stimulatory and inhibitory action. *Left*: Metabolic feedback leads to an increase of blood flow in case of insufficient oxygen supply. If local perfusion is too low to maintain adequate oxygen supply, production and concentration of a metabolic signal substance is enhanced, stimulating vessel diameter increase and increase of blood flow and oxygen supply [3, 4]. This mechanism maintains adequate flow distribution within the tissue. *Right*: The adaptation of vessel diameter to wall shear stress establishes a positive feedback: If shear stress is high, an increase in vessel diameter is elicited. This in turn leads to an increase in vascular conductance and blood flow—which leads to a further increase in shear stress. Under resting conditions, these responses tend to maintain homogeneous levels of shear stress along arteriolar and venular flow pathways [5]

Mechanisms

Studies provide evidence for different sites of oxygen dependent release of vasoactive substances, specifically the parenchymal tissue, the red blood cells (RBCs), and the vessel wall [4, 7] (Fig. 3.2). As mediators of metabolic signalling by the parenchymal tissue, substances including adenosine, CO_2, and O_2^-, phosphates, prostanoids and osmolality have been suggested [10, 11]. RBCs were shown to deliver ATP from intracellular pools in response to the local saturation of the haemoglobin with oxygen [12]. Additionally, nitric oxide (NO) as a metabolic signal substance is liberated from S-nitrosohaemoglobin in proportion to the decline of haemoglobin saturation along a vessel or reduced from nitrite mediated by deoxyhaemoglobin [13, 14].

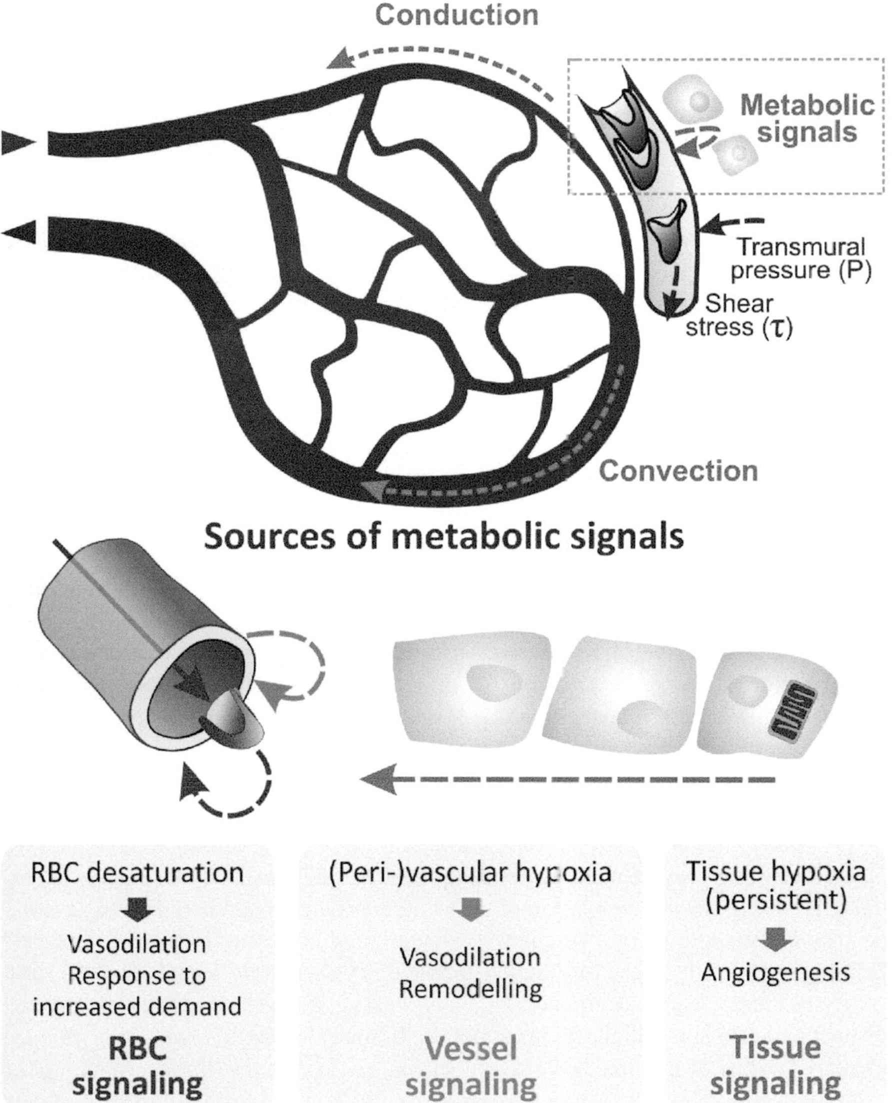

Fig. 3.2 Concepts of metabolic signalling in vessel diameter adaptation. *Upper panel*: Vascular adaptation is guided by local hemodynamic (transmural pressure and wall shear stress) and metabolic signals. The metabolic signals act not only where they are generated but are also transported with the blood in the downstream direction (convection) and elicit electric signals which travel upstream in the arteriolar vessel wall (conduction) [2, 5, 8] The remote action of these signals is essential to avoid maladaptation and the generation of arterio-veneous shunts [9]. *Lower panel*: Schematic drawing of possible origins of metabolic signals. Local oxygen levels may evoke release of metabolic signal substances (dashed arrows) from RBCs from the vessel wall (and possibly a tissue sleeve around it), and from tissue cells. These signalling pathways probably have different functional tasks [3, 4, 7]

Recent studies, using a theoretical model to simulate vessel diameter adaptation in response to hemodynamic and metabolic stimuli for microvascular networks where complete morphological and hemodynamic data sets had been measured in vivo, surprisingly suggested that a substantial component of metabolic regulation of vessel diameters can be independent of direct oxygen sensing [3, 7]. This unexpected finding is explained by the 'dilution effect': The effective concentration of a metabolic signal substance delivered by the vessel wall or the tissue to the blood will increase with decreasing blood flow. This mechanism provides a simple physical 'measurement' of local blood flow rate by an 'indicator-dilution' approach. For metabolic signal substances evoking vascular diameter increase, the dilution effect provides an additional negative feedback regulation stabilizing blood flow rate in a vessel and thus tissue oxygen supply around the vessel. The dilution effect represents a very robust and simple metabolic mechanism to maintain parallel flow pathways irrespective of oxygen demand.

Origins of Metabolic Signals

Figure 3.3 compares the signalling mechanisms for different origins of metabolic signals evoking vessel diameter increase. In 'Vessel' signalling, the dilution effect and Po_2-dependent signalling act together to provide robust negative feedback regulation, with vessel diameter increase in response to low flow and low Po_2. This provides a likely explanation for the effectiveness of 'Vessel' signalling in producing low levels of tissue hypoxia and a good agreement between experimentally measured data and simulation predictions [3, 7]. A concept for the integrated regulation by local and remote action of vessel derived metabolic signals is given in Fig. 3.4.

In 'Tissue' signalling (as in 'Vessel' signalling), both the dilution effect and Po_2-based signalling provide negative feedback regulation. However, there can be a partial decoupling since oxygenation of tissue cells is determined both by the vascular perfusion depending on vascular diameter and by the diffusion distance. Consequently, an increase of vascular diameter by metabolic signals derived from the tissue cannot lead to adequate tissue oxygenation if vessel density is too low and diffusion distances too high. In this situation, tissue cells would continue to produce increased levels of the metabolic signal substance despite the diameter increase of existing vessels [7]. However, such 'Tissue' signals are indispensable to stimulate angiogenesis upon insufficient vessel density [3, 15].

In 'RBC' signalling, metabolic substances are generated in proportion to the number of RBCs in the vessel, which, in turn, depends on vessel volume and haematocrit [12, 16, 17]. Thus, reductions in vessel diameter and reduction of haematocrit in low-flow vessels reduce the possible amount of metabolic signal substance in small vessels thus establishing a strong positive feedback loop overriding the negative feedback regulations.

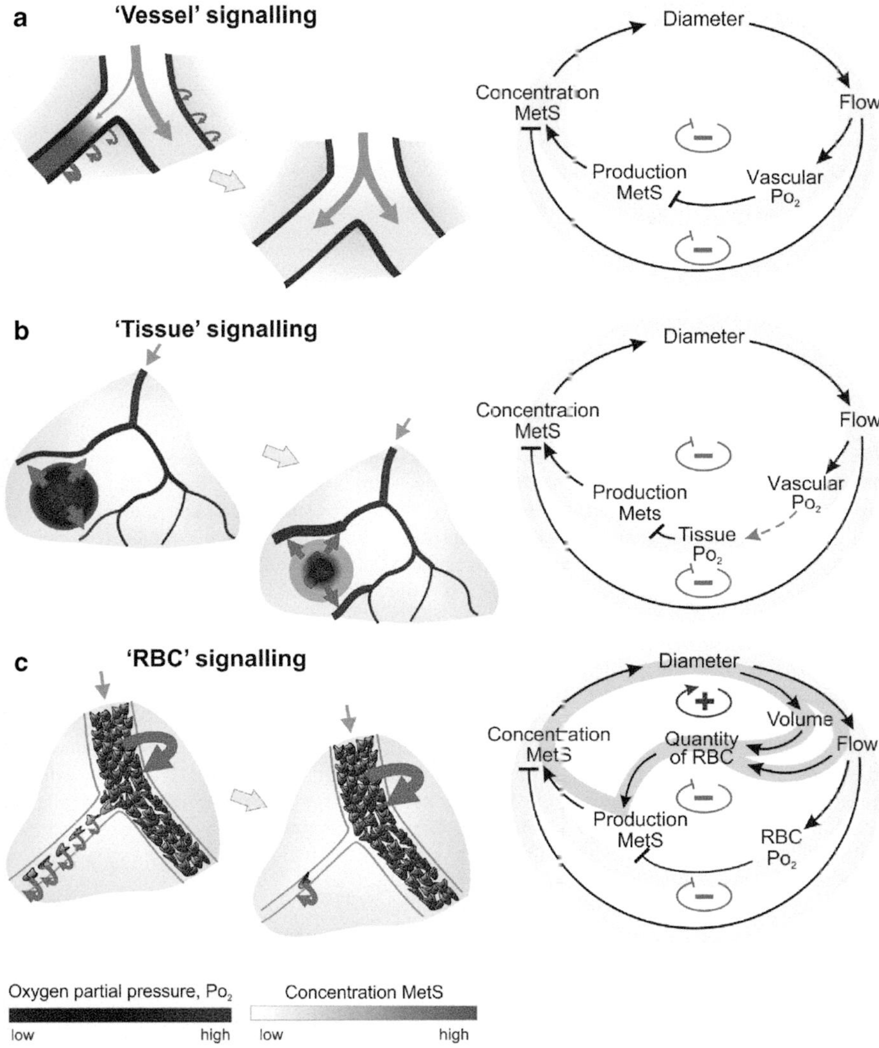

Fig. 3.3 Summary of feedback loops involved in metabolic signalling. *Left*: Schematic diagrams of vessels and perivascular parenchyma showing effects of metabolic signalling from various sources in underperfusion (green arrows indicate metabolic signal substance release). *Right*: Feedback loops ('–', blue: negative, '+', red: positive). Arrows and blunt ends indicate stimulatory and inhibitory action. (**a**) In 'Vessel' signalling, both dilution effect and Po_2-based mechanisms contribute to negative feedback control (*light blue shading*). (**b**) In 'Tissue' signalling, negative feedback regulation is compromised (dashed lines) for larger diffusion distances since the corresponding decrease in tissue Po_2 cannot be effectively counteracted by an increase of vessel diameters (diffusion limited oxygen transport). (**c**) In 'RBC' signalling, decreases in intravascular volume or blood flow lower the number of RBC and thus the metabolic stimulus level for a given oxygenation. This positive feedback (*red shading*) counteracts the negative feedback loops established by 'dilution effect' and oxygen dependent signalling

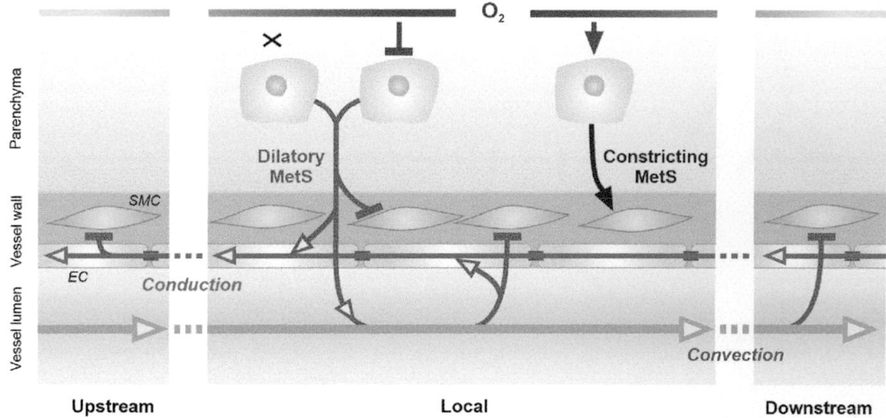

Fig. 3.4 Schematic pathways of metabolic vascular signalling in a microvessel. Shown is a cross section with the perivascular parenchyma with three exemplary cells (*top*), the vessel wall consisting of a smooth muscle (*SMC*) and an endothelial (*EC*) layer (*middle*), and the vascular lumen with flow from left to right (*bottom*). Arrows indicate stimulation while blunt ends indicate inhibition for those pathways capable to mediate stable regulation of microvascular diameters (*oxygen: red; constricting signals: purple; dilatory signals: orange; conduction via endothelial connexions: blue; convection of MetS with the blood: green*). The *middle column* gives a local site of the vessel while the *left* and *right columns* represent regions of the vessel upstream or downstream from the local site. At the local site, perivascular cells can react to oxygen levels in three ways: The leftmost cell (*black cross*) does produce a dilatory or growth inducing metabolic signalling substance (*MetS*) irrespective of oxygen availability or Po_2. The middle cell also produces a dilatory or growth inducing MetS but here production of the MetS is suppressed by high oxygen availability (oxygen sensitive dilatator). The right cell is stimulated by high oxygen availability to produce a constricting or growth inhibiting MetS. While constricting signals can provide stable regulation only locally, dilatory signals allow vascular reactions downstream (via convection with the blood stream) and upstream (via conduction along the vessel wall), which are both necessary to allow stable vascular adaptation in vascular networks [3, 7, 9]

Steady State Versus Increased Demand

The positive and negative feedback characteristics of different regulatory pathways determine their possible impact on vessel diameter adaptation under resting conditions and in situations of strong transient increase in demand, as in exercise. Under resting conditions, the central task of metabolic signaling is to provide adequate distribution of perfusion within the tissue. To balance the positive feedback from wall shear stress signaling which could cause maldistribution, a strong negative feedback from metabolic signaling is needed [9]. Metabolic signaling by the vessel wall or by a perivascular tissue sleeve is best suited for this task, since it is the only mode providing pure and robust negative feedback regulation [3, 4, 7].

In contrast to resting conditions, the main task of diameter adaptation during transient increases of demand, e.g. due to exercise, is to allow a substantial perfusion increase. While problematic for steady state diameter control, the positive feedback of RBC signalling might be helpful under such conditions (Fig. 3.5) [3]. Vessel or tissue metabolic signaling stimulated by an increased demand mediates an initial

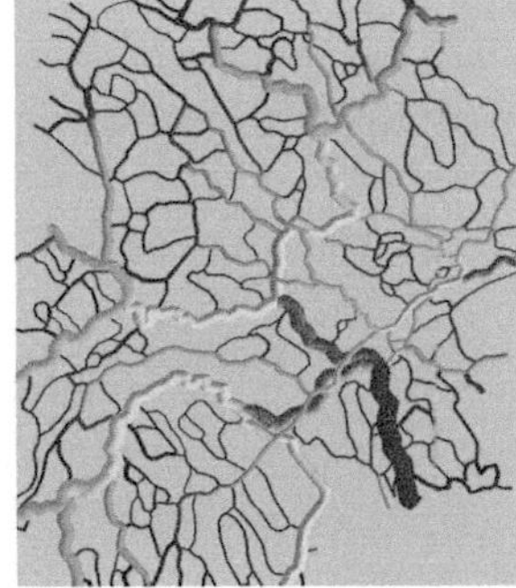

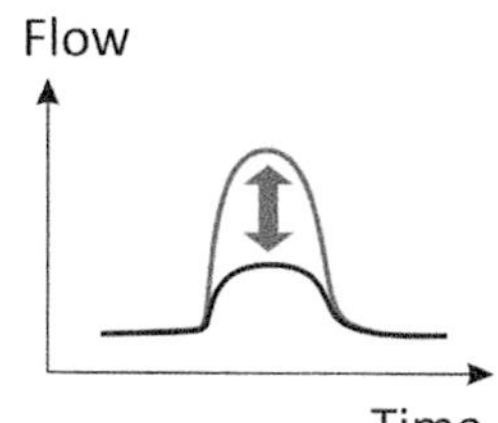

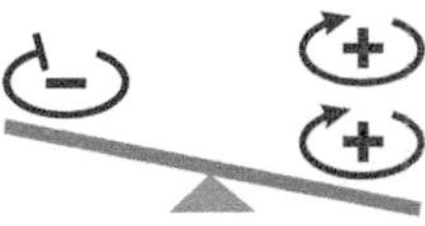

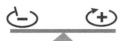

Fig. 3.5 Roles of different signalling mechanisms in the control of vascular diameter at rest and during increased demand. *Steady state*: Due to the heterogeneity of microvascular networks, malperfusion can only be avoided if the positive shear stress feedback is balanced by a strong negative metabolic feedback [5]. *Increased demand*: Transient phases of increased oxygen demand, e.g. during exercise, call for a strong increase of blood flow which requires a strong positive feedback to amplify initial increases of flow. Here, the positive metabolic feedback via RBC signalling may play a relevant role

increase of vessel diameter. The reduced flow resistance together with an increased blood pressure leads to a raise in perfusion and wall shear stress. This, in turn, leads to a further increase in vessel diameter and blood flow [18] amplifying the initial response and recruiting upstream resistance vessels into the response. Metabolic signaling by RBCs may provide a further boost: the increase of perfusion causes an increasing amount of RBC and thus metabolic signaling structures to travel through the tissue releasing an increased amount of metabolic vasodilating signals.

Pathophysiolgical Implications

Tissue function, notably in cardiac myocytes, is crucially dependent on adequate perfusion and oxygen supply under rest and under all levels of increased workload. In turn, an inadequate blood flow or flow distribution, leading to unmet tissue demand and thus global or local hypoxia constitutes ischemic heart disease [19]. Here, a relevant difference exists between the situation with epicardial stenoses as compared to microvascular disturbances [8, 20]. Permanent epicardial stenoses usually result from atherosclerotic lesions in the arterial wall and cause underperfusion in larger regions downstream.

On the other hand, there is increasing evidence that cardiac ischemic conditions can also be caused by vascular malfunction occuring in vessel with diameters below about 300 μm, the microcirculation. This is obvious from situations where a recanalization of arterial stenoses does not result in a satisfactory increase in myocardial perfusion ('myocardial no reflow') [21] suggesting that an epicardial stenosis can be accompanied with increased flow resistance in the microvascular compartment [22, 23]. Such microvascular malfunction or 'coronary microvascular dysfunction' [22–24] is obvious from the observation of angina symptoms in patients with apparently normal or near normal coronary angiograms [25, 26]. While there have been different denominations for this condition ('angina with normal coronary arteries', 'microvascular angina', 'cardiac syndrome X') [22, 27–29] it is obvious that it is both not rare and not benign [30–33]. This is underlined by the fact that acute events of 'myocardial infarction with non-obstructive coronary arteries' are increasingly described (MINOCA) [28, 34–36].

Despite the obvious clinical importance of these conditions, the insight into relevant underlying pathophysiological mechanisms as well as therapeutic approaches based on such concepts is still not developed enough (see [22, 37, 38]). It is, however, clear that vascular maladaptation both acutely (e.g. in sepsis [39–41]) and chronically (e.g. in tumours [9, 42–44]) compromises tissue supply and thus function. It is thus of great importance to assess microvascular structure and function in such conditions—in patients or in relevant animal models—to describe pathological deviations and to decipher the contributions of individual adaptive mechanisms.

References

1. Pries AR, Secomb TW, Gaehtgens P. Structural adaptation and stability of microvascular networks: theory and simulations. Am J Phys. 1998;275:H349–60.
2. Pries AR, Reglin B, Secomb TW. Remodeling of blood vessels: responses of diameter and wall thickness to hemodynamic and metabolic stimuli. Hypertension. 2005;46:726–31.
3. Reglin B, Pries AR. Metabolic control of microvascular networks: oxygen sensing and beyond. J Vasc Res. 2014;51:376–92.
4. Reglin B, Secomb TW, Pries AR. Structural adaptation of microvessel diameters in response to metabolic stimuli: where are the oxygen sensors? Am J Physiol Heart Circ Physiol. 2009;297:H2206–19.
5. Pries AR, Reglin B, Secomb TW. Structural adaptation of microvascular networks: functional roles of adaptive responses. Am J Phys. 2001;281:H1015–25.
6. Rodbard S. Vascular caliber. Cardiology. 1975;60:4–49.
7. Reglin B, Secomb TW, Pries AR. Structural control of microvessel diameters: origins of metabolic signals. Front Physiol. 2017;8:813.
8. Pries AR, Badimon L, Bugiardini R, Camici PG, Dorobantu M, Duncker DJ, Escaned J, Koller A, Piek JJ, de Wit C. Coronary vascular regulation, remodelling, and collateralization: mecha-

nisms and clinical implications on behalf of the working group on coronary pathophysiology and microcirculation. Eur Heart J. 2015;36:3134–46.
9. Pries AR, Hopfner M, Le Noble F, Dewhirst MW, Secomb TW. The shunt problem: control of functional shunting in normal and tumour vasculature. Nat Rev Cancer. 2010;10:587–93.
10. Berne RM. Cardiac nucleotides in hypoxia: possible role in regulation of coronary blood flow. Am J Phys. 1963;204:317–22.
11. Golub AS, Pittman RN. Recovery of radial PO(2) profiles from phosphorescence quenching measurements in microvessels. Comp Biochem Physiol A Mol Integr Physiol. 2002;132:169–76.
12. Ellsworth ML, Ellis CG, Goldman D, Stephenson AH, Dietrich HH, Sprague RS. Erythrocytes: oxygen sensors and modulators of vascular tone. Physiology (Bethesda). 2009;24:107–16.
13. Cosby K, Partovi KS, Crawford JH, Patel RP, Reiter CD, Martyr S, Yang BK, Waclawiw MA, Zalos G, Xu X, Huang KT, Shields H, Kim-Shapiro DB, Schechter AN, Cannon RO III, Gladwin MT. Nitrite reduction to nitric oxide by deoxyhemoglobin vasodilates the human circulation. Nat Med. 2003;9:1498–505.
14. Stamler JS, Meissner G. Physiology of nitric oxide in skeletal muscle. Physiol Rev. 2001;81:209–37.
15. Secomb TW, Alberding JP, Hsu R, Dewhirst MW, Pries AR. Angiogenesis: an adaptive dynamic biological patterning problem. PLoS Comput Biol. 2013;9:e1002983.
16. Sprague RS, Hanson MS, Achilleus D, Bowles EA, Stephenson AH, Sridharan M, Adderley S, Procknow J, Ellsworth ML. Rabbit erythrocytes release ATP and dilate skeletal muscle arterioles in the presence of reduced oxygen tension. Pharmacol Rep. 2009;61:183–90.
17. Arciero JC, Carlson BE, Secomb TW. Theoretical model of metabolic blood flow regulation: roles of ATP release by red blood cells and conducted responses. Am J Physiol Heart Circ Physiol. 2008;295(4):H1562–71.
18. Koller A, Sun D, Kaley G. Role of shear stress and endothelial prostaglandins in flow- and viscosity-induced dilation of arterioles in vitro. Circ Res. 1993;72:1276–84.
19. Pries AR, Kuebler WM, Habazettl H. Coronary microcirculation in ischemic heart disease. Curr Pharm Des. 2018;24:2893–9.
20. Pries AR, Reglin B. Coronary microcirculatory pathophysiology: can we afford it to remain a black box? Eur Heart J. 2017;38:478–88.
21. Niccoli G, Burzotta F, Galiuto L, Crea F. Myocardial no-reflow in humans. J Am Coll Cardiol. 2009;54:281–92.
22. Crea F, Camici PG, Bairey Merz CN. Coronary microvascular dysfunction: an update. Eur Heart J. 2014;35:1101–11.
23. Camici PG, Crea F. Coronary microvascular dysfunction. N Engl J Med. 2007;356:830–40.
24. Bugiardini R, Bairey Merz CN. Angina with "normal" coronary arteries: a changing philosophy. JAMA. 2005;293:477–84.
25. Likoff W, Segal BL, Kasparian H. Paradox of normal selective coronary arteriograms in patients considered to have unmistakable coronary heart disease. N Engl J Med. 1967;276:1063–6.
26. Bugiardini R. Coronary microcirculation and ischemic heart disease, today. Curr Pharm Des. 2018;24:2891–2.
27. Cannon RO III, Camici PG, Epstein SE. Pathophysiological dilemma of syndrome X 11. Circulation. 1992;85:883–92.
28. Agrawal S, Mehta PK, Bairey Merz CN. Cardiac syndrome X: update 2014 1. Cardiol Clin. 2014;32:463–78.
29. Kaski JC, Aldama G, Cosin-Sales J. Cardiac syndrome X. Diagnosis, pathogenesis and management. Am J Cardiovasc Drugs. 2004;4:179–94.
30. Kaski JC, Rosano GM, Collins P, Nihoyannopoulos P, Maseri A, Poole-Wilson PA. Cardiac syndrome X: clinical characteristics and left ventricular function. Long-term follow-up study 13. J Am Coll Cardiol. 1995;25:807–14.
31. Murthy VL, Naya M, Taqueti VR, Foster CR, Gaber M, Hainer J, Dorbala S, Blankstein R, Rimoldi O, Camici PG, Di Carli MF. Effects of sex on coronary microvascular dysfunction and cardiac outcomes. Circulation. 2014;129:2518–27.

32. Bugiardini R, Manfrini O, Pizzi C, Fontana F, Morgagni G. Endothelial function predicts future development of coronary artery disease: a study of women with chest pain and normal coronary angiograms. Circulation. 2004;109:2518–23.
33. Bugiardini R. Women, 'non-specific' chest pain, and normal or near-normal coronary angiograms are not synonymous with favourable outcome. Eur Heart J. 2006;27:1387–9.
34. Kaski JC. Provocative tests for coronary artery spasm in MINOCA: necessary and safe? Eur Heart J. 2018;39:99–101.
35. Pasupathy S, Tavella R, Beltrame JF. Myocardial infarction with nonobstructive coronary arteries (MINOCA): the past, present, and future management. Circulation. 2017;135:1490–3.
36. Agewall S, Beltrame JF, Reynolds HR, Niessner A, Rosano G, Caforio AL, De CR, Zimarino M, Roffi M, Kjeldsen K, Atar D, Kaski JC, Sechtem U, Tornvall P. ESC working group position paper on myocardial infarction with non-obstructive coronary arteries. Eur Heart J. 2017;38:143–53.
37. Bugiardini R, Badimon L, Collins P, Erbel R, Fox K, Hamm C, Pinto F, Rosengren A, Stefanadis C, Wallentin L, Van de Werf F. Angina, "normal" coronary angiography, and vascular dysfunction: risk assessment strategies. PLoS Med. 2007;4:e12.
38. Marinescu MA, Loffler AI, Ouellette M, Smith L, Kramer CM, Bourque JM. Coronary microvascular dysfunction, microvascular angina, and treatment strategies 1. JACC Cardiovasc Imaging. 2015;8:210–20.
39. Verdant CL, De BD, Bruhn A, Clausi CM, Su F, Wang Z, Rodriguez H, Pries AR, Vincent JL. Evaluation of sublingual and gut mucosal microcirculation in sepsis: a quantitative analysis. Crit Care Med. 2009;37:2875–81.
40. Lipinska-Gediga M. Sepsis and septic shock-is a microcirculation a main player? Anaesthesiol Intensive Ther. 2016;48:261–5.
41. Potter EK, Hodgson L, Creagh-Brown B, Forni LG. Manipulating the microcirculation in sepsis - the impact of vasoactive medications on microcirculatory blood flow. A systematic review. Shock. 2019;52(1):5–12.
42. Pries AR, Cornelissen AJ, Sloot AA, Hinkeldey M, Dreher MR, Hopfner M, Dewhirst MW, Secomb TW. Structural adaptation and heterogeneity of normal and tumor microvascular networks. PLoS Comput Biol. 2009;5:e1000394.
43. Secomb TW, Dewhirst MW, Pries AR. Structural adaptation of normal and tumour vascular networks. Basic Clin Pharmacol Toxicol. 2012;110:63–9.
44. Folkman J. Tumor angiogenesis: therapeutic implications. N Engl J Med. 1971;285:1182–6.

Chapter 4
Study of the Microcirculation Through Microscopic Techniques

Harry A. J. Struijker-Boudier

Introduction

The microcirculation has been focus of increasing research interest in recent years. Recent advances in technology to study the microcirculation have highlighted the crucial involvement of the microcirculation in many cardiovascular diseases, but also in other conditions such as cancer, diabetes, inflammatory diseases, sickle cell disease as well as neurological and psychiatric disorders.

This book reviews the role of the microcirculation in many of these clinical cases and the therapeutic considerations to target the microcirculation in these cases. The purpose of this chapter is to review techniques and methodological aspects with a particular focus on microscopic techniques.

Techniques to Study the Microcirculation

Table 4.1 summarizes the most important approaches to study the microcirculation in humans and animal models of disease. When applying strict anatomical criteria the study of isolated small arteries, having diameters in the range of 200–300 μm, cannot be regarded as a microcirculation study method. On the other hand, from a functional point of view they are part of the most distal section of the arterial system, the primary site for the control of vascular resistance and exchange processes.

In the past 30 years isolated small arteries have been used successfully in both experimental and clinical research to study mechanistic and therapeutic aspects of

H. A. J. Struijker-Boudier (✉)
Department of Pharmacology and Toxicology, Cardiovascular Research Institute Maastricht, Maastricht University, Maastricht, The Netherlands
e-mail: h.struijkerboudier@maastrichtuniversity.nl

M. Dorobantu, L. Badimon (eds.), *Microcirculation*,
https://doi.org/10.1007/978-3-030-28199-1_4

Table 4.1 Techniques to study the microcirculation

• Isolated small arteries
• Intravital microscopy/capillaroscopy
• Retinal imaging
• Orthogonal polarized light (OPL) video microscopy
• Sidestream dark-field (SDF) video microscopy
• Incident dark-field (IDF) imaging
• Laser Doppler flowmetry
• Optical coherence tomography (OCT)
• Photoacoustic tomography (PAT)
• Micro-computed tomography (MCT)
• Nuclear magnetic resonance (NMR) imaging

microcirculatory behavior in health and disease. Small arteries are usually obtained from surgical procedures or subcutaneous gluteal biopsies. Since this chapter focuses on microscopic techniques this small artery approach will not be further reviewed. The reader is referred to some excellent reviews by authorities in this area of research [1–3].

Direct (Intravital) Microscopy

Direct (intravital) microscopy has a long history. In the beginning of the seventeenth century Harvey postulated the existence of invisible "pores of the flesh" to support his hypothesis that blood passes through microscopic channels in circulating from artery to vein. A few years later Malpighi and Van Leeuwenhoek developed the first single lens microscopes to observe discrete capillaries connecting arteries and veins. Van Leeuwenhoek even succeeded to provide quantitative information on the size and spatial density of microcirculatory vessels and measured the velocity of red cells in these vessels [4]. After these original observations in the seventeenth century a wide variety of preparations have been developed for examining microcirculatory structure and function in specific organs. In experimental animals the rodent cremaster muscle, hamster cheeck pouch, cat mesentery and bat wing are among the most frequently studied preparations [4, 5].

Capillaroscopy in Humans

For obvious reasons the organ-related microcirculatory preparations in experimental animals mentioned above cannot be used in human studies. Studies of human microcirculation were for a long time limited to epiillumination of organs and tissues in which the microcirculation is very near the surface. The most relevant tissues in this respect have been the capillary nailfold and other skin regions and, of more recent date, the retina. We will first briefly discuss the clinical capillaroscopy of the nailfold and skin. We shall not discuss the retinal imaging in any detail since in Chap. 7 of this book A. Gallo and X. Girerd review this approach. Subsequently, the introduction and application of recent contrast enhancing imaging techniques, such as orthogonal polarization spectral (OPS) imaging and sidestream dark-field (SDF) video microscopy, will be discussed.

The early history of clinical capillaroscopy has been described in detail by Bollinger and Fagrell [6]. Briefly, after the original observations by Malpighi and Van Leeuwenhoek major progress was made in the first part of the twentieth century by August and Marie Krogh as well as Otfried Müller who made the first extensive drawings of the human skin capillaries on the basis of microscopic observations [7]. In the second half of the twentieth century major advances in electronic and digital technology led to highly sophisticated human capillaroscopy set-ups in various laboratories in the world. For details of these developments the reader is referred to the monograph by Bollinger and Faqrell [6] as well as the latest edition of the Handbook of the Microcirculation of the American Physiological Society [8].

Clinical capillaroscopy has contributed greatly to knowledge on microvascular abnormalities in various diseases, such as hypertension, arterial occlusive ischemia, diabetes and several hematological disorders. A loss of capillaries (rarefaction) now seems a hallmark of both hypertension and arterial occlusive ischemia [9–11]. In diabetes, the situation is more complex: on the one hand, proliferative growth of microvessels has been observed, but on the other hand the functionality of these vessels has been questioned [12].

A relatively new area of research that has not yet been investigated to its full extent is the potential role of capillary rarefaction in the treatment of cancer patients with anti-angiogenic drugs [13, 14].

Hand-Held Vital Microscopes

Intravital and capillary microscopy have played an important role in understanding microvascular physiology and pathophysiology, mostly in animal models and—to a limited degree—in humans. The introduction in the 1990s of hand-held vital microscopes (HVM) has given a boost to bedside observations and clinical studies. More than 400 studies have been published in the past two decades using HVM's [5, 15, 16]. The technology underlying imaging with hand-held microscopy has advanced considerably in recent years [5, 15]. These technologies allow a range of novel parameters to monitor in addition to the mostly structure-related parameters measured with more classical capillaroscopy techniques. The combination of HVM with Doppler-derived techniques, tissue spectrophotometry, transcutaneous pO2 electrodes and clinical biomarkers, such as lactate and venous-arterial CO2 gradients allow to obtain a complete picture of the microcirculation in critically ill patients [16].

HVM's allow to study the microcirculation of different organs and systems. Most applications have targeted the sublingual microcirculation. Three different HVM's have been introduced in the last two decades for directly observing the sublingual microcirculation [15]: the orthogonal polarized spectral (OPS), the side-stream dark field (SDF) and most recently the incident dark field (IDF) imaging techniques. The reader is referred to an excellent recent book [5] and review article [15] for detailed descriptions of the technologies underlying these innovative microscopic methods to assess the microcirculation in humans.

Conventional intravital microscopes for observing the microcirculation (see above) use transillumination to visualize the field of view. The light source in the more recent technologies illuminates from the side of the tissue at an angle that avoids surface reflections of the light entering the objective and thus allows to observe deeper structures in the microcirculation [5]. Initially, green light at a wavelength of 530 nm was used as an optical contrast agent for hemoglobin, which allows the observation of flow in the small vessels [17]. In the second generation SDF videomicroscopes a green LED was placed circularly at the tip of the image guide of the hand-held microscope [15]. The third generation of IDF imaging no longer uses a video sensor, but a computer-controlled sensor in combination with ultrashort illumination LED's. The image sensor, data acquisition, and illumination pulses are computer controlled in a synchronized manner [5, 15].

After an initial phase of technology development and testing of reproducibility and validity these novel vital microscopy techniques are now used more and more in clinical routine, in particular in the management of sepsis, shock and cardiac surgery [18]. A more generalized application in chronic cardiovascular diseases characterized by target organ damage can be expected with increased clinical experience using these advanced techniques. Already Ince and co-workers have given many examples of target organs that are suitable for such studies [5, 15].

Non-Microscopic Techniques

Although the study of the microcirculation has always depended heavily on the use of direct microscopic observations, more and more technologies have been developed to assess structural and functional properties of the microcirculation. Most of these are advanced perfusion imaging technologies, such as Laser Doppler flowmetry, optical or photoacoustic tomography, magnetic resonance imaging and angiography (see Table 4.1). Most of these technologies have not yet reached a scale to image very small arteries, arterioles or capillaries. However, since they measure perfusion they provide important information about the functional status of the microcirculation in important target organs, such as the heart, kidney and brain [11, 19].

Laser Doppler flowmetry is in use already for several decades to assess microvascular function by measuring the red cell flux in small-volume samples of body and organ surfaces, e.g. the skin. The quantity measured by laser Doppler is usually referred to as perfusion, defined as the product of local speed and concentration of blood cells, and the laser Doppler perfusion monitor records the integrated perfusion within the sampling volume. Because the laser Doppler flowmeter operates on the basis of characterizing a shift in frequency from a particular reference, it is important that the reference source is both highly stable and of single frequency [19].

More recent technological innovations since the 1990s have significantly advanced the range of applications of laser Doppler microvascular imaging. These innovations involve advances in laser beam technology, fast full-field signal analysis and improved laser speckle contrast analysis. Since it is beyond the scope of this chapter to review non-microscopic techniques, the reader is referred to an excellent recent comprehensive book on these non-microscopic techniques [5].

Other relatively new approaches to microcirculation imaging have been based on various tomography methods, e.g. optical coherence (OCT), photoacoustic (PAT) or micro-computed tomography (MCT, see Table 4.1). Again, these methods are primarily focused on flow measurements within the microcirculation, but allow a deeper penetration than the more classical microscopic or Doppler-based techniques. The basic principle behind the tomography technologies is that they measure the magnitude and echo-time delay of backscattered light with a very high sensitivity, which was first described by Isaac Newton. For further technical details and applications the reader is referred to the previously mentioned detailed book on microcirculation imaging by non-microscopic techniques [5].

Finally, nuclear magnetic resonance has developed in the past three decades as a technique to detect flow of all velocity regimens going from fast flow in larger arteries down to microscopic transport on a cellular level. During the past three decades it has developed into a technique with wide applications in the medical world. It can generate diagnostic quality images of blood vessels and is now standard procedure to diagnose stenoses, aneurysms and the mechanics of the vessel wall. NMR has found wide applications in both the heart and brain microcirculation. In the heart it is particularly used in relation to the study of microvascular reperfusion following an acute myocardial infarction. NMR can obtain data about microvascular flow, regional myocardial wall motion, and viability in one single examination and without the administration of a pharmacological challenge [19]. In the brain NMR is now an important tool in assessing brain damage following a stroke or in dementia patients [20].

Conclusions

The microcirculation is the primary site of target organ damage in many (cardiovascular) diseases. Appreciation of the importance of the microcirculation has been hampered for a long time by the perceived lack of appropriate techniques for its study. The classical direct microscopic techniques have revealed much about structure and function of the microcirculation, particularly in experimental animals. Their clinical applicability has been relatively limited. However, major advances in retinal imaging (the topic of Chap. 7 in this book) now allows comprehensive studies on the epidemiology, pathophysiology and treatment of microvascular damage in (cardiovascular) disease. Novel hand-held video-based techniques have widened the possibilities for microvascular assessment in other tissues or organs than the eye. Finally, a range of non-microscopic techniques have shown dramatic improvements in terms of technical quality and availability for clinical use.

References

1. Mulvany MJ, Aalkjaer C. Structure and function of small arteries. Physiol Rev. 1990;70:921–61.
2. Rizzoni D, Agabiti-Rosei C, Agabiti-Rosei E. Hemodynamic consequences of changes in microvascular structure. Am J Hypertens. 2017;30:939–46.
3. Schiffrin EL. Remodeling of resistance arteries in essential hypertension. Am J Hypertens. 2004;17:1192–200.
4. Johnson P. Overview of the microcirculation. In: Tuma RF, Duran WN, Ley K, editors. Handbook of physiology: microcirculation. Amsterdam: Elsevier; 2008.
5. Leahy MJ. Microcirculation imaging. Weinheim: Wiley Blackwell; 2012.
6. Bollinger A, Fagrell B. Clinical capillaroscopy. Toronto: Hogrefe and Huber; 1990.
7. Müller O. Die Kapillaren der menschlichen Körperoberfläche in gesunden und kranken Tagen. Stuttgart: Enke; 1922.
8. Tuma RF, Duran WN, Ley K. Handbook of physiology: microcirculation. Amsterdam: Elsevier; 2008.
9. Levy BI, Ambrosio G, Pries AR, Struijker-Boudier H. Microcirculation in hypertension: a new target for treatment? Circulation. 2001;104:735–40.
10. Serne EH, Gans RO, Ter Maarten JC, Tangelder GJ, Donker AJ, Stehouwer CD. Impaired capillary recruitment in essential hypertension is caused by both functional and structural capillary rarefaction. Hypertension. 2001;38:238–42.
11. Levy BI, Schiffrin EL, Mourad JJ, Agostini D, Vicaut E, Safar ME, Struijker-Boudier HA. Impaired tissue perfusion: a pathology common to hypertension, obesity and diabetes mellitus. Circulation. 2008;118:968–76.
12. Strain WD, Adingupu DD, Shore AC. Microcirculation on a large scale: techniques, tactics and relevance of studying the microcirculation in larger population samples. Microcirculation. 2011;19:37–46.
13. Mourad JJ, Levy BI. Mechanisms of anti-angiogenic drug induced hypertension. Curr Hypertens Rep. 2011;13:289–93.
14. Le Noble FA, Stassen FR, Hacking WJ, Struijker-Boudier H. Angiogenesis and hypertension. J Hypertens. 1998;16:1563–72.
15. Ocak I, Kara A, Ince C. Monitoring microcirculation. Best Pract Res Clin Anaesthesiol. 2016;30:407–18.
16. Kara A, Akin S, Ince C. Monitoring microcirculation in critical illness. Curr Opin Crit Care. 2016;22:444–52.
17. Slaaf DW, Tangelder GJ, Reneman RS. A versatile incident illuminator for intravital microscopy. Int J Microcirc Clin Exp. 1987;6:391–7.
18. Henzler D, Scheffler M, Westheider A, Köhler T. Microcirculation measurements: barriers for use in clinical routine. Clin Hemorheol Microcric. 2017;67:505–9.

19. Struijker-Boudier HA, Rosei AE, Bruneval P, Camici PG, Christ F, Henrion D, Levy BI, Pries A, Vanoverschelde JH. Evaluation of the microcirculation in hypertension and cardiovascular disease. Eur Heart J. 2007;28:2834–40.
20. De Roos A, van der Grond J, Mitchell G, Westenberg J. Magnetic resonance imaging of cardiovascular function and the brain: is dementia a cardiovascular driven disease? Circulation. 2017;135:2178–95.

Chapter 5
Platelet Function and Coronary Microvascular Dysfunction

Sandrine Horman, Melanie Dechamps, Marie Octave, Sophie Lepropre, Luc Bertrand, and Christophe Beauloye

Introduction

The ability of platelets to activate and aggregate to form blood clots in response to endothelial injury is well established. They are therefore critical contributors to ischaemia in atherothrombosis [1]. However, their role in cardiovascular disease is not limited to end-stage thrombosis in large vessels [2]. Abundant experimental evidence has established that activated platelets are also important mediators of microvascular thrombosis and promote the inflammatory response during ischaemia-reperfusion (IR) injury [3–5]. While platelets do not physically interact with the healthy endothelium, they can bind to the wall of hypoxic microvessels and release a plethora of inflammatory mediators that further enhance the activation of the endothelial monolayer and the recruitment of circulating leukocytes

S. Horman (✉) · M. Octave · S. Lepropre · L. Bertrand
Université catholique de Louvain (UCLouvain), Institut de Recherche Expérimentale et Clinique (IREC), Pôle de Recherche Cardiovasculaire, Brussels, Belgium
e-mail: Sandrine.Horman@uclouvain.be; Marie.Octave@uclouvain.be; Sophie.Lepropre@uclouvain.be; Luc.Bertrand@uclouvain.be

M. Dechamps
Université catholique de Louvain (UCLouvain), Institut de Recherche Expérimentale et Clinique (IREC), Pôle de Recherche Cardiovasculaire, Brussels, Belgium

Cliniques Universitaires Saint-Luc, Cardiac Intensive Care Unit, Brussels, Belgium
e-mail: Melanie.Dechamps@uclouvain.be

C. Beauloye
Université catholique de Louvain (UCLouvain), Institut de Recherche Expérimentale et Clinique (IREC), Pôle de Recherche Cardiovasculaire, Brussels, Belgium

Cliniques Universitaires Saint-Luc, Division of Cardiology, Brussels, Belgium
e-mail: Christophe.Beauloye@uclouvain.be

M. Dorobantu, L. Badimon (eds.), *Microcirculation*,
https://doi.org/10.1007/978-3-030-28199-1_5

(monocytes, neutrophils, T-cells) [2]. In addition, deposition of platelets to the dysfunctional endothelium can lead to vasoconstriction which accelerates microvascular occlusion, thereby impairing tissue perfusion [3]. In this chapter, we discuss the role of platelets in promoting microvascular dysfunction and inflammation during IR injury. Focus is placed on the cross-talk between platelets and other cell types (endothelial cells [ECs] and leukocytes) via platelet adhesion receptors and platelet-derived proinflammatory mediators. We also consider new paradoxical functionalities of platelets promoting cardiac recovery after myocardial infarction (MI).

Thrombus Formation in Coronary Arteries and Microvessels

Coronary Artery Disease and Plaque Rupture

Atherosclerotic plaques forming inside the vessel's intima layer lead to endothelial dysfunction which is the first trigger for coronary artery disease. An increased blood level of plasma lipids, especially low-density lipoproteins (LDL) [6–8], in combination with other risk factors including hypertension, diabetes mellitus, smoking and male gender [9] induce vascular damage. The binding of LDL to intimal proteoglycans is an important step for disease initiation [10]. Once sequestered in the intimal microenvironment, LDL particles may undergo extensive oxidation, aggregation/fusion or enzymatic fragmentation which may potentially contribute to their enhanced pro-atherogenic properties [11–13]. Modified LDL particles activate ECs, inducing the expression of adhesion receptors and disrupting intercellular junctions. These modifications potentiate the recruitment and infiltration of leukocytes (monocytes and lymphocytes) into the subendothelial space [7, 14]. Once in the intima, monocytes differentiate into macrophages which express scavenger receptors (SRAI and SRAII, CD36, LOX-1 or CXCL16), leading to the internalization and cytosolic accumulation of cholesterol molecules and cholesterol esters from modified LDL particles [15, 16]. Such macrophage-derived cells, called foam cells, release a multitude of inflammatory cytokines, chemokines, growth factors, metalloproteinases (MMPs) and reactive oxygen species (ROS) that perpetuate inflammation [17]. Apoptosis and secondary necrosis of foam cells and smooth muscle cells (SMCs) are an important cause of necrotic core development [18, 19]. The necrotic core material may act as a nucleus for calcium deposits in the vascular wall [20]. In vulnerable plaques, the lipid-rich atheromatous core is hypocellular and devoid of supporting extracellular matrix proteins due to reduced SMC amounts combined with high levels of MMPs [21, 22]. These plaques are at high risk of rupture. With plaque rupture, thin collagen cap and the highly thrombogenic lipid core are exposed to circulating platelets which initiate thrombotic occlusion of the coronary vessel leading to myocardial ischaemia and infarction [22].

Atherothrombosis: Platelet Recruitment, Activation and Aggregation

The mechanisms leading to platelet activation following plaque rupture closely resemble physiological haemostasis and can be divided into three main steps: (1) platelet rolling and adhesion on the subendothelium, (2) recruitment and activation of circulating platelets through the secretion of secondary platelet agonists and (3) platelet aggregation. Under elevated shear stress (e.g. found in coronary vessels), platelet tethering to the subendothelium is mediated by the interaction of platelet glycoprotein (GP) Ib-IX-V and the von Willebrand factor (vWF) bound to the exposed collagen. Platelets attached to vWF roll along the vessel wall following blood flow [23]. Stable attachment is provided by binding to other receptors, especially GPVI that binds collagen and induces a strong and sustained platelet stimulation [24]. Platelet-collagen interaction can shift αIIbβ3 and α2bβ1 integrins from a low to a high affinity state. While α2bβ1 binds directly to collagen, αIIbβ3 promotes irreversible adhesion by binding to vWF [25]. The stable integrin-dependent adhesion of platelets leads to further platelet activation, morphological changes via actin cytoskeleton remodelling, and release from three different platelet granules (α-, dense, and lysosomal) of a broad range of biomolecules which comprise over 300 distinct proteins, nucleotides (ADP, ATP), and neurotransmitters [26, 27]. These molecules act in both autocrine and paracrine manners to amplify platelet activation and consolidate the thrombotic process. In addition, degranulation alters the composition of the plasma membrane and results in surface exposure of P-selectin and formation of thromboxane A_2 (TxA_2) from arachidonic acid. TxA_2 binding to specific receptors (largely distributed in platelets and vascular cells) enhances platelet activation and vasoconstriction. Finally, the interaction of circulating platelets with adherent platelets proceeds via the extracellular region of αIIbβ3 expressing a high-affinity binding site for fibrinogen and allowing aggregation via the formation of stable bridges between platelets [28].

Platelets in Ischaemia-Reperfusion and No-Reflow

After MI, reperfusion therapy aiming to dissolve the thrombus inside the coronary artery is critical for the recovery of cardiac function. However, the abrupt restoration of blood supply following ischaemia is characterized by a significant burst of ROS production by ECs and macrophages, the release of various cytokines and chemokines, leukocyte recruitment and activation, vasoconstriction and embolization of thrombotic platelet-rich aggregates which are responsible for luminal obstruction of the microvasculature [3, 4, 29, 30]. This tissue hypo-perfusion at the level of myocardial and coronary microcirculation is characterized as no-reflow and

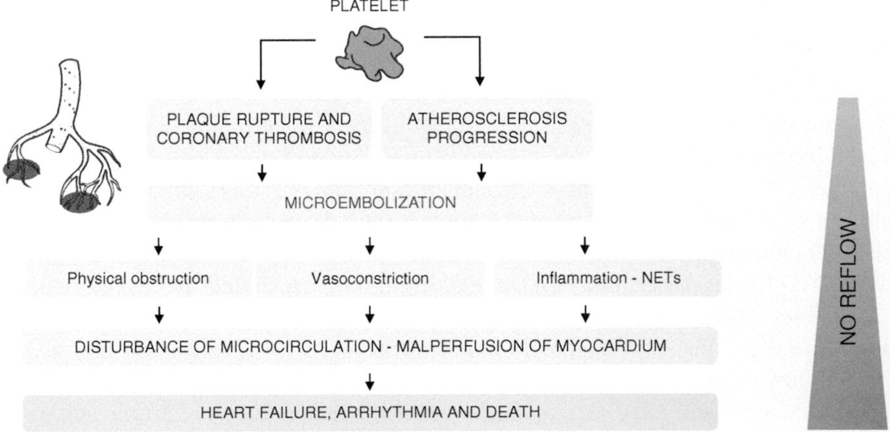

Fig. 5.1 Role of platelets in no-reflow. No-reflow refers to a state of myocardial tissue hypoperfusion after re-establishment of patency of an occluded epicardial coronary artery by reperfusion therapy. No-reflow is associated with a high risk of heart failure, arrhythmia and death and its aetiology is microvascular embolization by thrombotic and atherosclerotic debris. Activated platelets release vasoconstrictors and inflammatory mediators which promote the formation of microvascular thrombi responsible for no-reflow

is associated with a high risk of heart failure, arrhythmias and mortality [31] (Fig. 5.1). Platelets have a central role in the pathophysiology of no-reflow, notably via their capacity to adhere to ischaemic ECs and to cells of the innate and adaptative immune system.

Crosstalk Between Platelets, Endothelial Cells and Leukocytes During IR injury

Platelet-Endothelium Interaction

Healthy arterial ECs limit thrombosis by releasing nitric oxide (NO) and prostacyclins [32, 33]. ECs also express the exonucleotidases CD39 and CD73, that hydrolyze ATP and ADP (both platelet agonists) to AMP and ultimately to the platelet antagonist adenosine [34]. Upon ischaemic conditions and oxygen deprivation, the normal EC function is dysregulated. ECs switch to anaerobic glycolysis, accumulating metabolic intermediates and ROS. The excess generation of ROS results in the loss of NO availability. In addition, oxidative stress and proinflammatory cytokines downregulate CD39, promoting ADP accumulation and lowering AMP levels [35]. NO and adenosine depletion combined with the accumulation of proinflammatory mediators also increase expression of adhesion molecules, leading to enhanced crosstalk between platelets and ECs [36]. Hence, endothelial disruption is not a prerequisite to commit platelet attachment to the vasculature.

The Adhesion Molecules

Different surface molecules have been involved in the platelet-EC interaction during acute IR. They comprise P-selectin, GPIb-IX-V, αIIbβ3, intercellular adhesion molecule-1 (ICAM-1) and vitronectin [2, 37] (Fig. 5.2).

P-selectin is a glycoprotein stored in granules of platelets and in Weibel-Palade Bodies of ECs, and exposed at cell surface upon activation. Endothelial P-selectin has been demonstrated to mediate platelet rolling in inflammatory processes via the binding of P-selectin glycoprotein ligand-1 (PSGL-1) expressed on platelet surface [38]. PSGL-1 is also responsible for leukocyte adhesion to the vessel wall and for the formation of platelet-neutrophil aggregates at sites of endothelial injury [39]. Accordingly, anti-PSGL-1 antibodies markedly inhibited platelet-leukocyte interaction and the effect of platelets on neutrophil intravascular migration, both in vitro and in vivo, in a model of limbal microvessel injury [38].

Platelet attachment to intact but dysfunctional endothelium also involves GPIb-IX-V. The main ligand of GPIbα is vWF but this receptor has also been identified as counter-receptor for P-selectin [40]. GPIbα blockade has been reported to decrease infarct volumes and improve neurological functional outcomes in a model of transient middle cerebral artery occlusion [41–43], a protective effect attributed to a reduction in microvascular obstruction [44]. Furthermore, GPIbα can facilitate leukocyte recruitment via the leukocyte-expressed integrin Mac-1 [45].

The tight platelet adhesion on the inflamed endothelium is achieved via αIIbβ3 and intracellular adhesion molecule-1 (ICAM-1) (37). The latter plays a crucial role as it strongly binds to fibrinogen-platelet αIIbβ3 complexes [46, 47], extending the role of the integrin αIIbβ3 beyond platelet-platelet aggregation. In addition to interacting with ICAM-1, αIIbβ3-fibrinogen interacts with $\alpha_V\beta_3$, an integrin upregulated upon endothelial activation [48]. Interestingly, αIIbβ3 antagonists have been used in

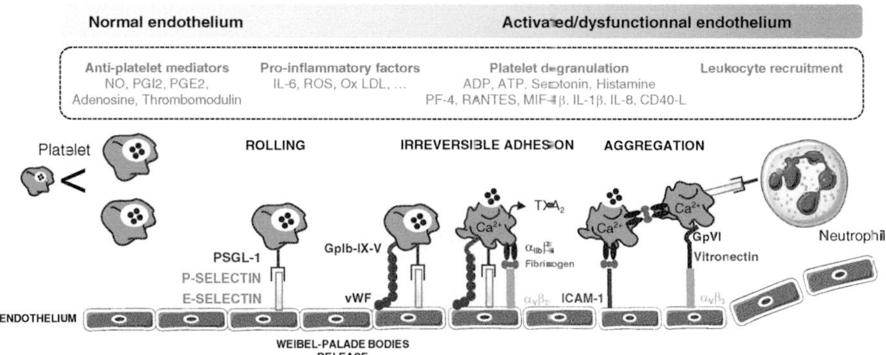

Fig. 5.2 Crosstalk between platelets and activated endothelial cells. Different surface molecules have been involved in the platelet-endothelium interaction: P-selectin, GPIb-IX-V, αIIbβ3, intercellular adhesion molecule-1 (ICAM-1) and vitronectin. "Servier Medical Art" was used for the illustration

the context of no-reflow and their infusion improves myocardial perfusion, involving the presence of microvascular platelet thrombi in this phenomenon [49]. In addition, αIIbβ3 inhibitors prevent the shedding of cell differentiation 40 ligand (CD40L) from platelet surface, thereby attenuating the inflammatory process [50]. Lastly, another mechanism involved in platelet-endothelium interaction is mediated by the binding of vitronectin to platelet GPVI [51]. Vitronectin is a plasma glycoprotein that binds to upregulated endothelial molecules, including the urokinase plasminogen receptor and various integrins such as $\alpha_V\beta_3$ [52].

Once deposited in the microvasculature, platelets participate to thrombo-inflammation via multiple mechanisms including (1) amplification of coagulation cascade leading to thrombin and fibrin generation, (2) secretion of a variety of pro-inflammatory and vasoconstricting molecules which further exacerbate the physical obstruction of microvessels and (3) interaction with neutrophils and generation of neutrophil extracellular traps (NETs) serving as a prothrombogenic matrix inciting platelet aggregation and growth of microvascular thrombi.

Cooperation of Platelets and the Coagulation Pathway

The classic blood clotting cascade can be triggered via either the tissue factor (TF) pathway or the contact pathway. Intravascular TF is present on microparticles (MPs) and exosomes (Es) produced by activated platelets. Initially, it lays in an encrypted silent form that needs to be activated by redox modifications involving the disulfide isomerases (PDI, ERp5, ERp57) that are secreted by platelets and activated ECs [53]. The contact pathway also clearly participates in thrombosis and can be triggered by inorganic polyphosphates (PolyP) abundantly present in platelet dense granules [54, 55]. PolyP enhance the amplification steps of the coagulation cascade via the binding of multiple coagulation enzymes [56]. Furthermore, activated platelets interact with the coagulation pathway by various other mechanisms [57]. They secrete (anti)coagulation factors (prothrombin, FV, FXIII, fibrinogen, antithrombin, various serpins, etc) and expose phosphatidylserine (PS) on cell surface. PS exposure is triggered by strong agonists via prolonged elevated cytosolic calcium. PS-containing membranes have a high affinity for coagulation factors such as the tenase and prothrombinase complexes and their binding at platelet surface enhances their activity. Thus, platelets support local thrombin and fibrin formation [58]. Under flow conditions, thrombin initially binds to PS-exposing platelets via protease-activated receptors (PAR1 and PAR4), and then relocalizes to the newly-formed fibrin fibers which confine the protease to the thrombus proximity [59]. Early findings suggest that fibrin-bound thrombin is protected from inactivation by antithrombin [60]. Platelets also bind coagulation factors via the glycoprotein complexes GPIb-V-IX, integrin αIIbβ3 and GPVI. The platelet GPIb-V-IX complex interacts with thrombin, which potentiates platelet activation through protease-activated receptors (PAR) [61]. The integrin αIIbβ3 binds fibrinogen and induces outside-in signalling which is required for the retraction of the platelet-fibrin thrombus [62]. Finally, GPVI has been recently identified as a receptor for fibrin. GPVI-fibrin interaction leads to formation of a GPVI signalosome involved in the continued growth of platelet-fibrin thrombus, independently of αIIbβ3 [63]. Altogether, this indicates that platelets and the coagulation system are interconnected processes and interact in multifaceted ways, not only during the phases of thrombus formation, but also in specific areas within a formed thrombus. Accordingly, strong evidence suggests that the thrombus is composed of a heterogeneous population of activated platelets forming a very hierarchical structure with distinct regions defined by the level of platelet activation and packing density which depend on the nature of the agonist and its distribution [64].

Proinflammatory Mediators

Platelet activation results in the release of multiple proteins and other biomolecules that can influence the function of endothelial or circulating cells [26]. Many of these molecules are preformed and stored in granules and notably include chemokines, growth factors, fibrinolytic proteins, coagulation factors, adhesion molecules, nucleotides, ions and agonists. Others are synthesized by platelets (TxA_2, ROS, IL-1β) or shed from the cell surface (sCD40L, sP-selectin) upon activation [65]. Some of these mediators induce the expression of adhesion molecules on the endothelial surface, enhance neutrophil recruitment at the site of injury, and promote the formation of platelet-leukocyte aggregates [2]. When attached to platelets, the leukocytes can achieve a more activated state and so, are able to produce more ROS than their platelet-free counterparts [66]. As it is recognized that the oxidative burst increases cell permeability, platelets can indirectly contribute to endothelial barrier dysfunction via their interaction with leukocytes [67]. However, the role of platelets in vascular integrity remains unclear. Indeed, some reports suggest that platelets can exert opposing effects on endothelial permeability, notably in the tumour microvasculature [68]. This controversy probably reflects the diversity of mediators that can be released by platelets in different models of thromboinflammation.

Platelets also contain microRNAs (miRNAs) retained from megakaryocyte-derived mRNAs [69]. Recent advances in platelet biology demonstrate that activated platelets release MPs or Es containing abundant amounts of miRNAs. They can be internalised and modulate gene expression and function of recipient cells, e.g. ECs, leukocytes or macrophages [70, 71]. Therefore, the horizontal transfer of platelet miRNAs represents a novel form of cell-cell communication, which may participate in the inflammatory process.

Platelets and Neutrophil Extracellular Traps

As mentioned above, monocytes and neutrophils recruitment is supported by activated platelets via the granule release of chemokines and expression of adhesion receptors such as P-selectin [36]. One way neutrophils may promote thrombus stability is by producing neutrophil extracellular traps (NETs) [72], a process that is enhanced by activated platelets presenting high mobility group box 1 (HMGB1) protein to neutrophils [73]. NETs are extracellular DNA fibers coated with histones and proteases and catapulted out of neutrophils. They are known for their antimicrobial function but recent evidence indicates that NETs may have a role in non-infectious diseases including atherosclerosis and thrombosis [74]. Mechanistically, NETs provide a scaffold for platelet adhesion and concentrate effector proteins involved in thrombosis and fibrin generation. The interaction with platelets can be mediated via vWF and fibrinogen immobilized on NETs, or alternatively by direct binding to DNA and histones [72]. NETs can also initiate fibrin formation more directly by activating the contact pathway of coagulation which is initiated by the activation of factor XII to factor XIIa [75]. Finally, NETs also promote a strong procoagulant response by forming a catalytic platform that stimulates the proteolytic activity of neutrophil elastase which induces the degradation and inactivation of natural anticoagulants such as thrombomodulin or TF pathway inhibitor (TFPI) [76] (Fig. 5.3).

Recent studies have demonstrated that, in a rat experimental model of IR, both platelets and NET-mediated microthrombosis contribute essentially to no-reflow [77]. Accordingly, a reperfusion strategy based on deoxyribonuclease I (DNaseI)

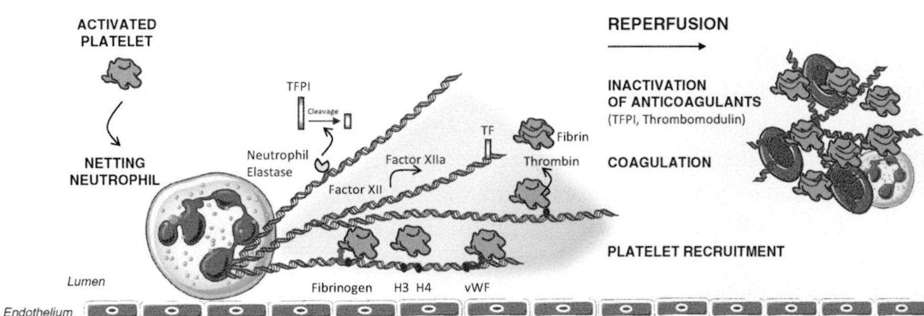

Fig. 5.3 Role of platelets and Neutrophil extracellular traps in IR-induced microvascular thrombosis. Neutrophil extracellular traps (NETs) provide a scaffold for platelet adhesion and concentrate effector proteins involved in thrombosis and fibrin generation. The interaction with platelets can be mediated via von Willebrand factor (vWF) and fibrinogen immobilized on NETs, or alternatively by direct binding to DNA or histones. NETs can also initiate fibrin formation more directly by activating the contact pathway of coagulation which is initiated by the activation of factor XII to factor XIIa. Finally, NETs also promote the degradation and inactivation of natural anticoagulants such as thrombomodulin or tissue factor pathway inhibitor (TFPI); *NE* Neutrophil elastase. "Servier Medical Art" was used for the illustration

used in combination with recombinant tissue-type plasminogen activator (rt-PA), a thrombolytic agent, has proved to be capable of attenuating significantly myocardial IR-induced no-reflow, suggesting that this combination might be a promising therapeutic option [77].

Double-Edged Sword Functionality of Platelets in IR Cardiac Injury

Resolution of Cardiac Inflammation

While platelets and their secreted cargo are widely accepted as crucial players in the inflammation-associated injury inflicted on the myocardium during IR, a growing body of evidence implicates them in inflammation resolution via the release ofpro-resolving mediators such as lipoxin A4, maresin 1, and annexin A1 [78, 79]. Interestingly, it has been shown that maresin-1 can decrease the level of proinflammatory mediators in platelet releasates [80]. The mechanisms underlying this differential secretory pattern need to be further characterized.

Cardiomyocyte Survival and Fibrotic Remodelling After Myocardial Infarction

A recent study shows that platelets and their secretome can exert a cardioprotective activity on ventricular cardiomyocytes during myocardial IR injury, independently of their role in coronary thrombosis. This protective effect requires α-granule components such as stromal cell-derived factor-1α (SDF-1α) and transforming-growth factor-β1 (TGF-β1), and is significantly attenuated in the presence of specific platelet antagonists [81]. Following MI, fibrotic scarring in the left ventricular (LV) necrotic area can trigger deleterious LV remodelling, when distending forces cause excessive volume and pressure load on non-infarcted areas. Myofibroblasts (MFs) are crucial components of this fibrotic response. Indeed, multiple regulators of the myodifferentiation process, including TGF-β1 [82], serotonin [83] and thrombospondin-1 (TSP-1) [84] are present in platelet granules. In addition, numerous miRNAs are enriched in platelet MPs/Es and can promote (miRNA-21 and miRNA-199) or attenuate (miRNA-29 and miRNA-101) the fibrotic response in cardiac tissue [85]. The high heterogeneity of the platelet secretome and MPs/Es challenges the clear characterization of platelet contribution in the cardiac repair process. Further studies using conditional (PF4/GPIba-Cre) transgenic mice with specific platelet defects will be required to assess the complex role of platelet secretome in the post-MI fibrotic remodelling.

Conclusion

The central role played by platelets and platelet-derived mediators in promoting microvascular thrombus formation during IR injury is increasingly well recognized. The underlying mechanisms involve endothelial activation, release of proinflammatory factors, vasoconstriction, leukocyte recruitment and NETosis (Fig. 5.3). All these events can—in turn—increase further platelet activation, leading to a vicious cycle that exacerbates tissue malperfusion and cardiac injury. Beyond thrombosis-mediated ischaemic damage, platelets may also exert additional "non-classical" functions within the infarcted myocardium, in particular through the release of bioactive cargo that can paradoxically facilitate cardiac repair processes. Therefore, considering the high functional diversity of the platelet secretome, much more attention should be paid to the efficacy of antiplatelet therapies in the management of cardiac recovery after MI.

Acknowledgments The authors thank Evangelos P. Daskalopoulos for his careful proofreading of the manuscript. Authors are supported by grants from the *Fonds National de la Recherche Scientifique et Médicale (FNRS)*, Belgium, and the *Action de Recherche Concertée de la Communauté Wallonie-Bruxelles* (ARC 16/21), Belgium, and by unrestricted grants from Bayer and AstraZeneca. S.H. is Research Associate and L.B. is Senior Research Associate of *FNRS*, Belgium; M.D. is supported by the *Fonds de Recherche Clinique (Cliniques Universitaires Saint-Luc, Belgium)*; M.O. is supported by *the Fonds pour la Recherche dans l'Industrie et l'Agriculture (FRIA),* Belgium. S.L. was supported by *FNRS*, Belgium; C.B. was a clinical Master specialist at *FNRS*, Belgium.

References

1. van der Meijden PEJ, Heemskerk JWM. Platelet biology and functions: new concepts and clinical perspectives. Nat Rev Cardiol. 2019;16(3):166–79.
2. Maiocchi S, Alwis I, Wu MCL, Yuan Y, Jackson SP. Thromboinflammatory functions of platelets in ischemia-reperfusion injury and its dysregulation in diabetes. Semin Thromb Hemost. 2018;44(2):102–13.
3. Gawaz M. Role of platelets in coronary thrombosis and reperfusion of ischemic myocardium. Cardiovasc Res. 2004;61(3):498–511.
4. Kalogeris T, Baines CP, Krenz M, Korthuis RJ. Cell biology of ischemia/reperfusion injury. Int Rev Cell Mol Biol. 2012;298:229–317.
5. Pachel C, Mathes D, Arias-Loza AP, Heitzmann W, Nordbeck P, Deppermann C, et al. Inhibition of platelet GPVI protects against myocardial ischemia-reperfusion injury. Arterioscler Thromb Vasc Biol. 2016;36(4):629–35.
6. Badimon L, Vilahur G, Padro T. Lipoproteins, platelets and atherothrombosis. Rev Esp Cardiol. 2009;62(10):1161–78.
7. Libby P, Ridker PM, Hansson GK. Progress and challenges in translating the biology of atherosclerosis. Nature. 2011;473(7347):317–25.
8. Soehnlein O, Swirski FK. Hypercholesterolemia links hematopoiesis with atherosclerosis. Trends Endocrinol Metab. 2013;24(3):129–36.
9. Lim SS, Vos T, Flaxman AD, Danaei G, Shibuya K, Adair-Rohani H, et al. A comparative risk assessment of burden of disease and injury attributable to 67 risk factors and risk factor

clusters in 21 regions, 1990-2010: a systematic analysis for the global burden of disease study 2010. Lancet. 2012;380(9859):2224–60.
10. Skalen K, Gustafsson M, Rydberg EK, Hulten LM, Wiklund O, Innerarity TL, et al. Subendothelial retention of atherogenic lipoproteins in early atherosclerosis. Nature. 2002;417(6890):750–4.
11. Napoli C, D'Armiento FP, Mancini FP, Postiglione A, Witztum JL, Palumbo G, et al. Fatty streak formation occurs in human fetal aortas and is greatly enhanced by maternal hypercholesterolemia. Intimal accumulation of low density lipoprotein and its oxidation precede monocyte recruitment into early atherosclerotic lesions. J Clin Invest. 1997;100(11):2680–90.
12. Llorente-Cortes V, Badimon L. LDL receptor-related protein and the vascular wall: implications for atherothrombosis. Arterioscler Thromb Vasc Biol. 2005;25(3):497–504.
13. Badimon L, Martinez-Gonzalez J, Llorente-Cortes V, Rodriguez C, Padro T. Cell biology and lipoproteins in atherosclerosis. Curr Mol Med. 2006;6(5):439–56.
14. Sima AV, Stancu CS, Simionescu M. Vascular endothelium in atherosclerosis. Cell Tissue Res. 2009;335(1):191–203.
15. Collot-Teixeira S, Martin J, McDermott-Roe C, Poston R, McGregor JL. CD36 and macrophages in atherosclerosis. Cardiovasc Res. 2007;75(3):468–77.
16. Chistiakov DA, Melnichenko AA, Myasoedova VA, Grechko AV, Orekhov AN. Mechanisms of foam cell formation in atherosclerosis. J Mol Med (Berl). 2017;95(11):1153–65.
17. Chistiakov DA, Grechko AV, Myasoedova VA, Melnichenko AA, Orekhov AN. The role of monocytosis and neutrophilia in atherosclerosis. J Cell Mol Med. 2018;22(3):1366–82.
18. Moore KJ, Tabas I. Macrophages in the pathogenesis of atherosclerosis. Cell. 2011;145(3):341–55.
19. Clarke MC, Bennett MR. Cause or consequence: what does macrophage apoptosis do in atherosclerosis? Arterioscler Thromb Vasc Biol. 2009;29(2):153–5.
20. Otsuka F, Sakakura K, Yahagi K, Joner M, Virmani R. Has our understanding of calcification in human coronary atherosclerosis progressed? Arterioscler Thromb Vasc Biol. 2014;34(4):724–36.
21. Kolodgie FD, Burke AP, Farb A, Gold HK, Yuan J, Narula J, et al. The thin-cap fibroatheroma: a type of vulnerable plaque: the major precursor lesion to acute coronary syndromes. Curr Opin Cardiol. 2001;16(5):285–92.
22. Bentzon JF, Otsuka F, Virmani R, Falk E. Mechanisms of plaque formation and rupture. Circ Res. 2014;114(12):1852–66.
23. Bergmeier W, Chauhan AK, Wagner DD. Glycoprotein Ibalpha and von Willebrand factor in primary platelet adhesion and thrombus formation: lessons from mutant mice. Thromb Haemost. 2008;99(2):264–70.
24. Massberg S, Gawaz M, Gruner S, Schulte V, Konrad I, Zohlnhofer D, et al. A crucial role of glycoprotein VI for platelet recruitment to the injured arterial wall in vivo. J Exp Med. 2003;197(1):41–9.
25. Singbartl K, Forlow SB, Ley K. Platelet, but not endothelial, P-selectin is critical for neutrophil-mediated acute postischemic renal failure. FASEB J. 2001;15(13):2337–44.
26. Senzel L, Gnatenko DV, Bahou WF. The platelet proteome. Curr Opin Hematol. 2009;16(5):329–33.
27. Onselaer MB, Oury C, Hunter RW, Eeckhoudt S, Barile N, Lecut C, et al. The Ca(2+)/calmodulin-dependent kinase kinase beta-AMP-activated protein kinase-alpha1 pathway regulates phosphorylation of cytoskeletal targets in thrombin-stimulated human platelets. J Thromb Haemost. 2014;12(6):973–86.
28. Nesbitt WS, Westein E, Tovar-Lopez FJ, Tolouei E, Mitchell A, Fu J, et al. A shear gradient-dependent platelet aggregation mechanism drives thrombus formation. Nat Med. 2009;15(6):665–73.
29. Schofield ZV, Woodruff TM, Halai R, Wu MC, Cooper MA. Neutrophils--a key component of ischemia-reperfusion injury. Shock. 2013;40(6):463–70.
30. Granger DN, Kvietys PR. Reperfusion injury and reactive oxygen species: the evolution of a concept. Redox Biol. 2015;6:524–51.

31. Bouleti C, Mewton N, Germain S. The no-reflow phenomenon: state of the art. Arch Cardiovasc Dis. 2015;108(12):661–74.
32. Freedman JE, Ting B, Hankin B, Loscalzo J, Keaney JF Jr, Vita JA. Impaired platelet production of nitric oxide predicts presence of acute coronary syndromes. Circulation. 1998;98(15):1481–6.
33. Freedman JE, Loscalzo J, Barnard MR, Alpert C, Keaney JF, Michelson AD. Nitric oxide released from activated platelets inhibits platelet recruitment. J Clin Invest. 1997;100(2):350–6.
34. Johnston-Cox HA, Koupenova M, Ravid K. A2 adenosine receptors and vascular pathologies. Arterioscler Thromb Vasc Biol. 2012;32(4):870–8.
35. Robson SC, Sevigny J, Zimmermann H. The E-NTPDase family of ectonucleotidases: structure function relationships and pathophysiological significance. Purinergic Signal. 2006;2(2):409–30.
36. Stokes KY, Granger DN. Platelets: a critical link between inflammation and microvascular dysfunction. J Physiol. 2012;590(5):1023–34.
37. May AE, Seizer P, Gawaz M. Platelets: inflammatory firebugs of vascular walls. Arterioscler Thromb Vasc Biol. 2008;28(3):s5–10.
38. Lam FW, Burns AR, Smith CW, Rumbaut RE. Platelets enhance neutrophil transendothelial migration via P-selectin glycoprotein ligand-1. Am J Physiol Heart Circ Physiol. 2011;300(2):H468–75.
39. Kaplan ZS, Zarpellon A, Alwis I, Yuan Y, McFadyen J, Ghasemzadeh M, et al. Thrombin-dependent intravascular leukocyte trafficking regulated by fibrin and the platelet receptors GPIb and PAR4. Nat Commun. 2015;6:7835.
40. Theilmeier G, Michiels C, Spaepen E, Vreys I, Collen D, Vermylen J, et al. Endothelial von Willebrand factor recruits platelets to atherosclerosis-prone sites in response to hypercholesterolemia. Blood. 2002;99(12):4486–93.
41. De Meyer SF, Schwarz T, Schatzberg D, Wagner DD. Platelet glycoprotein Ibalpha is an important mediator of ischemic stroke in mice. Exp Transl Stroke Med. 2011;3:9.
42. Kraft P, Schuhmann MK, Fluri F, Lorenz K, Zernecke A, Stoll G, et al. Efficacy and safety of platelet glycoprotein receptor blockade in aged and comorbid mice with acute experimental stroke. Stroke. 2015;46(12):3502–6.
43. Li TT, Fan ML, Hou SX, Li XY, Barry DM, Jin H, et al. A novel snake venom-derived GPIb antagonist, anfibatide, protects mice from acute experimental ischaemic stroke and reperfusion injury. Br J Pharmacol. 2015;172(15):3904–16.
44. Pham M, Helluy X, Kleinschnitz C, Kraft P, Bartsch AJ, Jakob P, et al. Sustained reperfusion after blockade of glycoprotein-receptor-Ib in focal cerebral ischemia: an MRI study at 17.6 tesla. PLoS One. 2011;6(4):e18386.
45. Wang Y, Sakuma M, Chen Z, Ustinov V, Shi C, Croce K, et al. Leukocyte engagement of platelet glycoprotein Ibalpha via the integrin Mac-1 is critical for the biological response to vascular injury. Circulation. 2005;112(19):2993–3000.
46. Bombeli T, Schwartz BR, Harlan JM. Adhesion of activated platelets to endothelial cells: evidence for a GPIIbIIIa-dependent bridging mechanism and novel roles for endothelial intercellular adhesion molecule 1 (ICAM-1), alphavbeta3 integrin, and GPIbalpha. J Exp Med. 1998;187(3):329–39.
47. Massberg S, Enders G, Matos FC, Tomic LI, Leiderer R, Eisenmenger S, et al. Fibrinogen deposition at the postischemic vessel wall promotes platelet adhesion during ischemia-reperfusion in vivo. Blood. 1999;94(11):3829–38.
48. Gawaz M, Brand K, Dickfeld T, Pogatsa-Murray G, Page S, Bogner C, et al. Platelets induce alterations of chemotactic and adhesive properties of endothelial cells mediated through an interleukin-1-dependent mechanism. Implications for atherogenesis. Atherosclerosis. 2000;148(1):75–85.
49. Monassier JP. Reperfusion injury in acute myocardial infarction: from bench to cath lab. Part II: clinical issues and therapeutic options. Arch Cardiovasc Dis. 2008;101(9):565–75.
50. Nannizzi-Alaimo L, Alves VL, Phillips DR. Inhibitory effects of glycoprotein IIb/IIIa antagonists and aspirin on the release of soluble CD40 ligand during platelet stimulation. Circulation. 2003;107(8):1123–8.

51. Schonberger T, Ziegler M, Borst O, Konrad I, Nieswandt B, Massberg S, et al. The dimeric platelet collagen receptor GPVI-Fc reduces platelet adhesion to activated endothelium and preserves myocardial function after transient ischemia in mice. Am J Physiol Cell Physiol. 2012;303(7):C757–66.
52. Madsen CD, Sidenius N. The interaction between urokinase receptor and vitronectin in cell adhesion and signalling. Eur J Cell Biol. 2008;87(8–9):617–29.
53. Muller I, Klocke A, Alex M, Kotzsch M, Luther T, Morgenstern E, et al. Intravascular tissue factor initiates coagulation via circulating microvesicles and platelets. FASEB J. 2003;17(3):476–8.
54. Muller F, Mutch NJ, Schenk WA, Smith SA, Esterl L, Spronk HM, et al. Platelet polyphosphates are proinflammatory and procoagulant mediators in vivo. Cell. 2009;139(6):1143–56.
55. Hassanian SM, Avan A, Ardeshirylajimi A. Inorganic polyphosphate: a key modulator of inflammation. J Thromb Haemost. 2017;15(2):213–8.
56. Travers RJ, Smith SA, Morrissey JH. Polyphosphate, platelets, and coagulation. Int J Lab Hematol. 2015;37(Suppl 1):31–5.
57. Swieringa F, Spronk HMH, Heemskerk JWM, van der Meijden PEJ. Integrating platelet and coagulation activation in fibrin clot formation. Res Pract Thromb Haemost. 2018;2(3):450–60.
58. Monroe DM, Hoffman M, Roberts HR. Platelets and thrombin generation. Arterioscler Thromb Vasc Biol. 2002;22(9):1381–9.
59. Berny MA, Munnix IC, Auger JM, Schols SE, Cosemans JM, Panizzi P, et al. Spatial distribution of factor Xa, thrombin, and fibrin(ogen) on thrombi at venous shear. PLoS One. 2010;5(4):e10415.
60. Weitz JI, Hudoba M, Massel D, Maraganore J, Hirsh J. Clot-bound thrombin is protected from inhibition by heparin-antithrombin III but is susceptible to inactivation by antithrombin III-independent inhibitors. J Clin Invest. 1990;86(2):385–91.
61. De Candia E, Hall SW, Rutella S, Landolfi R, Andrews RK, De Cristofaro R. Binding of thrombin to glycoprotein Ib accelerates the hydrolysis of par-1 on intact platelets. J Biol Chem. 2001;276(7):4692–8.
62. de Witt SM, Verdoold R, Cosemans JM, Heemskerk JW. Insights into platelet-based control of coagulation. Thromb Res. 2014;133(Suppl 2):S139–48.
63. Alshehri OM, Hughes CE, Montague S, Watson SK, Frampton J, Bender M, et al. Fibrin activates GPVI in human and mouse platelets. Blood. 2015;126(13):1601–8.
64. Stalker TJ, Traxler EA, Wu J, Wannemacher KM, Cermignano SL, Voronov R, et al. Hierarchical organization in the hemostatic response and its relationship to the platelet-signaling network. Blood. 2013;121(10):1875–85.
65. Badimon L, Padro T, Vilahur G. Atherosclerosis, platelets and thrombosis in acute ischaemic heart disease. Eur Heart J Acute Cardiovasc Care. 2012;1(1):60–74.
66. Nagata K, Tsuji T, Todoroki N, Katagiri Y, Tanoue K, Yamazaki H, et al. Activated platelets induce superoxide anion release by monocytes and neutrophils through P-selectin (CD62). J Immunol. 1993;151(6):3267–73.
67. He P, Zhang H, Zhu L, Jiang Y, Zhou X. Leukocyte-platelet aggregate adhesion and vascular permeability in intact microvessels: role of activated endothelial cells. Am J Physiol Heart Circ Physiol. 2006;291(2):H591–9.
68. Demers M, Ho-Tin-Noe B, Schatzberg D, Yang JJ, Wagner DD. Increased efficacy of breast cancer chemotherapy in thrombocytopenic mice. Cancer Res. 2011;71(5):1540–9.
69. Xia L, Zeng Z, Tang WH. The role of platelet microparticle associated microRNAs in cellular crosstalk. Front Cardiovasc Med. 2018;5:29.
70. Laffont B, Corduan A, Ple H, Duchez AC, Cloutier N, Boilard E, et al. Activated platelets can deliver mRNA regulatory Ago2∗microRNA complexes to endothelial cells via microparticles. Blood. 2013;122(2):253–61.
71. Laffont B, Corduan A, Rousseau M, Duchez AC, Lee CH, Boilard E, et al. Platelet microparticles reprogram macrophage gene expression and function. Thromb Haemost. 2016;115(2):311–23.
72. Fuchs TA, Brill A, Duerschmied D, Schatzberg D, Monestier M, Myers DD Jr, et al. Extracellular DNA traps promote thrombosis. Proc Natl Acad Sci U S A. 2010;107(36):15880–5.

73. Maugeri N, Campana L, Gavina M, Covino C, De Metrio M, Panciroli C, et al. Activated platelets present high mobility group box 1 to neutrophils, inducing autophagy and promoting the extrusion of neutrophil extracellular traps. J Thromb Haemost. 2014;12(12):2074–88.
74. Jorch SK, Kubes P. An emerging role for neutrophil extracellular traps in noninfectious disease. Nat Med. 2017;23(3):279–87.
75. von Bruhl ML, Stark K, Steinhart A, Chandraratne S, Konrad I, Lorenz M, et al. Monocytes, neutrophils, and platelets cooperate to initiate and propagate venous thrombosis in mice in vivo. J Exp Med. 2012;209(4):819–35.
76. Massberg S, Grahl L, von Bruehl ML, Manukyan D, Pfeiler S, Goosmann C, et al. Reciprocal coupling of coagulation and innate immunity via neutrophil serine proteases. Nat Med. 2010;16(8):887–96.
77. Ge L, Zhou X, Ji WJ, Lu RY, Zhang Y, Zhang YD, et al. Neutrophil extracellular traps in ischemia-reperfusion injury-induced myocardial no-reflow: therapeutic potential of DNase-based reperfusion strategy. Am J Physiol Heart Circ Physiol. 2015;308(5):H500–9.
78. Basil MC, Levy BD. Specialized pro-resolving mediators: endogenous regulators of infection and inflammation. Nat Rev Immunol. 2016;16(1):51–67.
79. Abdulnour RE, Dalli J, Colby JK, Krishnamoorthy N, Timmons JY, Tan SH, et al. Maresin 1 biosynthesis during platelet-neutrophil interactions is organ-protective. Proc Natl Acad Sci U S A. 2014;111(46):16526–31.
80. Lannan KL, Spinelli SL, Blumberg N, Phipps RP. Maresin 1 induces a novel pro-resolving phenotype in human platelets. J Thromb Haemost. 2017;15(4):802–13.
81. Walsh TG, Poole AW. Platelets protect cardiomyocytes from ischaemic damage. TH Open. 2017;1(1):e24–32.
82. Meyer A, Wang W, Qu J, Croft L, Degen JL, Coller BS, et al. Platelet TGF-beta1 contributions to plasma TGF-beta1, cardiac fibrosis, and systolic dysfunction in a mouse model of pressure overload. Blood. 2012;119(4):1064–74.
83. Yabanoglu S, Akkiki M, Seguelas MH, Mialet-Perez J, Parini A, Pizzinat N. Platelet derived serotonin drives the activation of rat cardiac fibroblasts by 5-HT2A receptors. J Mol Cell Cardiol. 2009;46(4):518–25.
84. Frangogiannis NG, Ren G, Dewald O, Zymek P, Haudek S, Koerting A, et al. Critical role of endogenous thrombospondin-1 in preventing expansion of healing myocardial infarcts. Circulation. 2005;111(22):2935–42.
85. Wang H, Cai J. The role of microRNAs in heart failure. Biochim Biophys Acta Mol basis Dis. 2017;1863(8):2019–30.

Chapter 6
The Role of Perivascular Adipose Tissue in Microvascular Function and Coronary Atherosclerosis

Alexios S. Antonopoulos, Paraskevi Papanikolaou, and Dimitris Tousoulis

Introduction

The widespread adoption of Western dietary habits and the lack of physical activity in modern societies have major implications for obesity-related vascular disease development and the risk of coronary artery disease (CAD) [1]. It is estimated that approximately ~20% of cardiovascular deaths in the U.S. are partly attributed to obesity [2, 3]. The perils of abdominal adiposity for cardiometabolic health are well known [4]. Expansion of visceral adiposity clusters with systemic insulin resistance, dyslipidemia, increased levels of proinflammatory mediators, while at molecular level adipose tissue is characterized by adverse changes in its secretomic profile, which cumulatively favor vascular dysfunction and arterial hypertension development [5].

Clinical studies over the last decade have also highlighted the importance of ectopic adiposity for cardiovascular disease risk [6]. More recently, studies have demonstrated that next to fat mass, fat phenotype *per se* is crucial in mediating adiposity-related cardiovascular hazards [7]. Along these observations, perivascular adipose tissue (PVAT) has recently been at the centerstage as a major determinant of vascular health and disease [8]. Robust evidence suggests that PVAT regulates vascular biology by receiving paracrine signals from the vascular wall and responding by secreting a wide range of vasoactive adipocytokines that affect vascular function and atherosclerosis development [9, 10]. PVAT can affect microvascular function and vascular tone via secretion of vasodilatory or vasoconstrictive substances [9, 10].

Microvascular function is an independent predictor of cardiovascular events in both healthy individuals and high-risk subjects. Moreover, microvascular function

A. S. Antonopoulos · P. Papanikolaou · D. Tousoulis (✉)
1st Department Cardiology, Hippokration Hospital, Medical School, National and Kapodistrian University of Athens, Athens, Greece

M. Dorobantu, L. Badimon (eds.), *Microcirculation*,
https://doi.org/10.1007/978-3-030-28199-1_6

is implicated in the pathogenesis of angina in patients with non-obstructive epicardial disease. Given the well-established links between PVAT and microvascular function, the noninvasive imaging of coronary PVAT has gained attention [11, 12] as a promising biomarker in microvascular disease and coronary atherosclerosis. Clinical studies using computed tomography (CT) imaging have provided important insights into the role of PVAT in vascular disease development [11], microvascular angina [13] and plaque rupture [14]. Additionally, CRISP-CT study [15] has recently demonstrated that phenotyping of coronary PVAT by CT imaging offers incremental prognostic and risk reclassification information for cardiovascular disease development.

In this review article, we summarize the existing knowledge on PVAT and vascular biology and provide an overview of the current concepts on the links between PVAT, angina and coronary atherosclerosis. The results of recent studies supporting the use of imaging biomarkers of PVAT for cardiovascular risk stratification are also discussed.

Cardiac Adiposity: Epicardial and Perivascular Adipose Tissue

Cardiac adiposity refers to the distinct types of fatty tissue located around and in proximity with the heart [16]. Cardiac adiposity is typically classified according to its anatomic location and consists of: (a) intramyocardial fat, which penetrates myocardium, located as fatty islets among cardiomyocytes, (b) epicardial adipose tissue, which is located between the myocardium and the pericardium, and includes also PVAT of coronary arteries, and (c) pericardial adipose tissue, which is the intrathoracic fat located outside the pericardium, commonly called also paracardial adipose tissue [16]. Epicardial (and pericoronary) adipose tissue has evolved from brown adipose tissue during embryogenesis and is more closely related to visceral than subcutaneous fat [17]. The physiology of epicardial adipose tissue and human myocardium are strongly inter-related as they share the same coronary blood supply. In the adult heart, fully differentiated epicardial adipose tissue can typically be found in the atrioventricular and interventricular grooves extending to the cardiac apex [16]. Smaller amounts of adipose tissue are also located subepicardially in the free walls of the atria and around the two appendages [18]. A state of chronic positive energy balance results in obesity and fat expansion, and adipose tissue progressively fills the space between the ventricles, sometimes covering the entire epicardial surface. Small islets of adipose tissue also extend from the epicardial surface into the myocardium, often following the adventitia of the coronary artery branches [16]. Epicardial fat located over both ventricles accounts for approximately 20% of total ventricular mass. Although left ventricular mass far exceeds that of the right ventricle, the absolute amount of epicardial fat tissue is similar in the right and left ventricles. As a result, the ratio of fat to myocardium weight for the right side of the heart is more than three times that of the left side [19].

Perivascular adipose tissue: PVAT, which reflects approximately 3% of the total body adipose tissue, microscopically contains adipocytes, stromal cells, mainly fibroblasts and vasa vasorum [20]. There is no obvious anatomical barrier between PVAT and vascular wall [21] or with the surrounding fat and therefore a widely accepted definition of PVAT does not exist. There is probably a continuum of changes in adipose tissue biology with decreasing distance from the vascular wall [14]. In rodents, PVAT characteristics resemble more those of brown adipose tissue, as defined by the presence of abundant vasculature and adipocytes with small lipid droplets and numerous mitochondria [22]. In humans, PVAT shares similarities with visceral adipose tissue, but its exact morphology and biological phenotype is dictated by local regulatory mechanisms and the interactions with the underling vessel [23]. PVAT is abundant around the aorta and virtually absent from cerebral vasculature and microvasculature, while the coronary arteries are embedded in PVAT. The evolutionary preservation of pericoronary fat could serve in the mechanical protection of epicardial coronary arteries [16]. The traditional beliefs on the roles of epicardial and pericoronary adipose tissue on cardiovascular health are summarized in Fig. 6.1. The role of PVAT in coronary vascular biology seems to involve much more than the simple cushioning of vessels [20]. The observation that myocardial bridges, i.e. coronary segments that have an intramyocardial course and are not covered by PVAT, do not develop atherosclerosis led to the concept of the causal role of PVAT in atherosclerosis. We now appreciate that the relationship between PVAT and coronary atherosclerosis is much more complex, and involves a bidirectional communication between the two, whereby changes in vascular biology directly affect PVAT phenotype and vice versa [14, 24, 25].

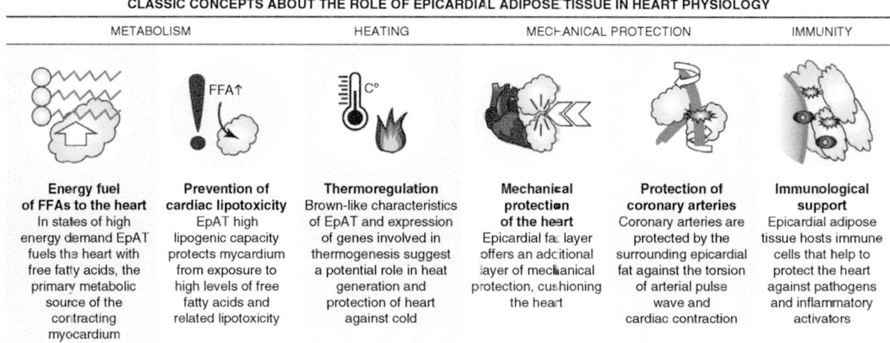

CLASSIC CONCEPTS ABOUT THE ROLE OF EPICARDIAL ADIPOSE TISSUE IN HEART PHYSIOLOGY
METABOLISM
HEATING
MECHANICAL PROTECTION
IMMUNITY
FFA↑
C°
Energy fuel of FFAs to the heart
In states of high energy demand EpAT fuels the heart with free fatty acids, the primary metabolic source of the contracting myocardium
Prevention of cardiac lipotoxicity
EpAT high lipogenic capacity protects mycardium from exposure to high levels of free fatty acids and related lipotoxicity
Thermoregulation
Brown-like characteristics of EpAT and expression of genes involved in thermogenesis suggest a potential role in heat generation and protection of heart against cold
Mechanical protection of the heart
Epicardial fat layer offers an additional layer of mechanical protection, cushioning the heart
Protection of coronary arteries
Coronary arteries are protected by the surrounding epicardial fat against the torsion of arterial pulse wave and cardiac contraction
Immunological support
Epicardial adipose tissue hosts immune cells that help to protect the heart against pathogens and inflammatory activators

Fig. 6.1 The classic concepts about the role of epicardial adipose tissue in heart physiology. Reproduced with permission from Antonopoulos et al. [16]

The Role of PVAT in Vascular Biology: Evidence from Basic Science Studies

The pivotal role of PVAT in the regulation of vascular biology is supported by ample translational and experimental evidence [26]. While remote adipose tissue depots (e.g. subcutaneous or abdominal visceral adipose tissue) can affect the cardiovascular system only in an endocrine manner (i.e. by releasing bioactive adipocytokines into blood circulation), PVAT can directly affect vascular function via paracrine or vasocrine routes. This is facilitated by the absence of any fascia separating PVAT from the vascular wall [27]. Thus PVAT-secreted adipokines can diffuse directly to the vascular wall and influence vascular biology and phenotype (Table 6.1). The net effect of PVAT on vascular function depends on the balance between vaso-protective and deleterious adipokines in PVAT secretome [25], which is in turn determined by both systemic (e.g., insulin resistance, obesity, hypertension, smoking) and local factors.

PVAT (like any other human adipose tissue depot) secretes a wide variety of adipocytokines with both beneficial (e.g., adiponectin, hydrogen sulphide and omentin) and detrimental (e.g. tumor necrosis factor-alpha (TNF-a), interleukin-6, and resistin) effects on the vasculature [28]. In disease states, such as in obesity and diabetes mellitus, PVAT secretome is shifted towards a pro-inflammatory and vaso-

Table 6.1 Perivascular adipose tissue secretome and effects on vascular physiology

Promoting vascular dysfunction	Function
TNF-a	Pro-inflammatory, pro-oxidant effects and IR induction
IL-1b	Pro-inflammatory effects
IL-6	Pro-inflammatory effects
MCP-1	Migration and infiltration of monocytes
Angiotensin II	Pro-inflammatory, pro-atherosclerotic effects
Leptin	Chronic hyperleptinemia induces vasoconstriction
Omentin	Induces oxidative stress and pro-inflammatory effects
Resistin	Induction of IR, inflammation, and oxidative stress
ROS/H_2O_2	Vasoconstriction and endothelial dysfunction
Maintaining vascular health	
IL-10	Anti-inflammatory effects
IL-19	Anti-inflammatory effects
ADRF	Anti-contractile effects
Adiponectin	Insulin-sensitizing, antioxidant and anti-inflammatory effects
Methyl palmitate	Vasodilatory effects via Kv channels on VSMCs
Hydrogen sulphide	Anti-inflammatory, vasodilatory effect

ADRF adipocyte derived relaxing factor, *IL* interleukin, *MCP-1* monocyte chemoattractant protein-1, *TNF-a* tumor necrosis factor-a, *IR* insulin resistance

constrictive adipokine profile [29]. PVAT dysfunction has been suggested as the mechanistic link between obesity and atherosclerosis and may contribute to or modulate hypertension development, although a direct causal role has not yet been established [30].

Importantly, next to the direct effect of PVAT on human vessels, in our recent studies with human adipose tissue we have provided strong translational evidence for an "inside-out signaling" from the vascular wall to PVAT [14, 24, 25, 31–33]. Thus, vascular inflammation (e.g. via interleukin-6 or TNF-a) [14] or vascular redox state (via secretion of lipid peroxidation products such as 4-hydroxynonenal) [25] can affect PVAT biology in a process labelled 'inside-out signaling'. PVAT then responds by respective changes in its secretome that signals back to the vascular wall to promote vascular health or dysfunction (i.e. via 'outside-in signaling'). These concepts are summarized in Fig. 6.2.

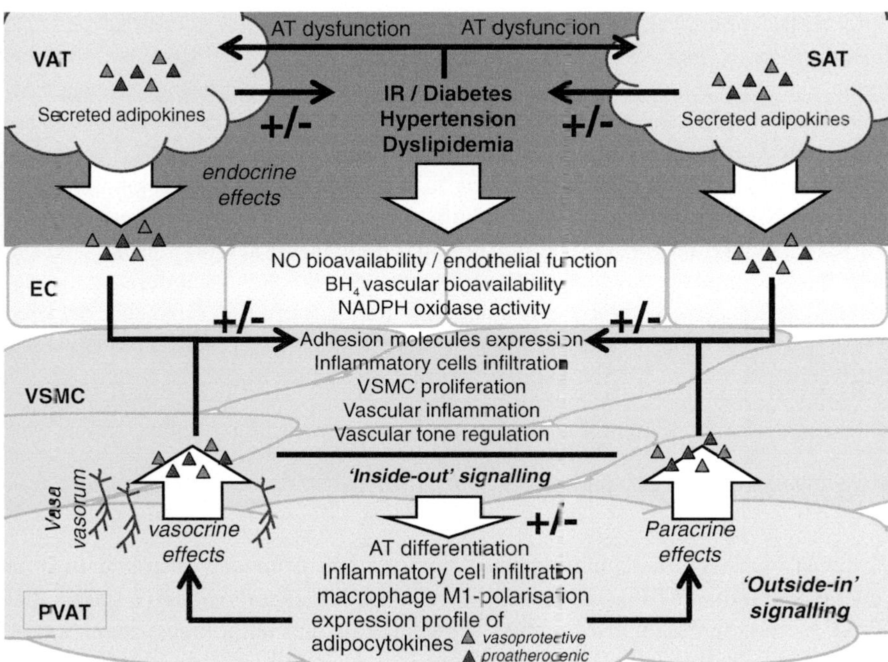

Fig. 6.2 The cross-talk of remote and local adipose tissue depots with the vascular wall. Cardiovascular risk factors promote the dysfunctional adipose tissue (AT) phenotype. Secreted adipokines into systemic circulation are involved in the pathogenesis of insulin resistance (IR), diabetes, arterial hypertension and dyslipidemia and have endocrine effects on vascular wall. Perivascular AT (PVAT) can also affect vascular wall biology by secretion of adipokines which act on endothelium or VSMC in a paracrine or vasocrine manner ('outside-to-inside' signalling). The net balance of proatherogenic vs. vasoprotective adipokines determines the net effect of AT on vascular wall and the development of atherosclerosis. Importantly, under conditions of increased inflammation and oxidative stress the vascular wall can also signal back to surrounding PVAT altering its biology ('inside-to-outside' signalling). *BH4* tetrahydrobiopterin, *NO* nitric oxide

PVAT and Regulation of Vascular Redox State

In our recent studies we have provided evidence on how vascular redox dictates PVAT biology and vice-versa [24, 25, 33]. By using a model of ex-vivo co-incubations of human arteries with perivascular adipocytes, we demonstrated that vascular oxidative stress and increased release of lipid peroxidation products, such as 4-hydroxynonenal, act as messengers to the surrounding adipocytes and activate PPAR-γ/ adiponectin axis. Increased adiponectin expression serves as a defense mechanism to lower vascular oxidative stress by inducing vascular AMP-activated protein kinase/protein kinase B (Akt)-signaling and inhibiting activation and translocation of Rac1 as well as the phosphorylation of p47phox, which are all key steps in the activation of NADPH oxidase. Adiponectin also acts on human vessels to restore nitric oxide bioavailability [34]. In humans vessels this is mediated via the effects of both circulating and PVAT-secreted adiponectin on vascular tetrahydrobiopterin (BH_4) bioavailability and Akt-induced eNOS phosphorylation at Ser1177, leading to both increased eNOS coupling and activity [8, 24]. Reduced NADPH oxidase activity also indirectly favors eNOS coupling by increasing vascular BH_4 bioavailability [35]. Such interactions between fat and the cardiovascular system are not unique to vessels and PVAT. In addition, we have described a similar cross-talk between PPAR-gamma/adiponectin axis in epicardial fat and AMP-kinase/Rac1–regulated NADPH oxidase activity in human cardiomyocytes [25]. These findings suggest that the adipose tissue surrounding human vessels or cardiac muscle responds to signals received from these organs and activates local defense mechanisms that regulate vascular redox state. Key messages in this cross-talk between PVAT and the vascular wall are products of lipid oxidation (e.g. 4-hydroxynonenal), natriuretic peptides [25, 33] and possibly other molecules too.

PVAT Effects on Microvascular Function

The role of PVAT in regulating vascular tone has been demonstrated in both rodents and humans [36]. Ex-vivo vasomotor studies in animals have shown that PVAT secretome is rich in vasoactive molecules such as adipokines, chemokines, nitric oxide, hydrogen sulfide and palmitic acid methyl ester and other not yet identified substances such as the adipocyte–derived relaxing factor (ADRF) [37]. The vasodilatory effects of PVAT on resistance vessels is partly mediated by the voltage gated potassium channels of vascular smooth muscle cells (VSMC) [38]. This effect has been attributed to the secretion of ADRF, although it is not fully clarified whether ADRF constitutes a novel independent moiety or a combination of PVAT secreted products with known vasodilatory effects [21]. For example, adiponectin has well-documented beneficial effects on vascular NO bioavailability via Akt-signaling (discussed also in the previous section) [8]. Furthermore hydrogen sulphide elicits vasodilatory effects on PVAT by opening the

KCNQ-type Kv and K_{ATP} channels in VSMC [39] The regulation of vascular superoxide generation by PVAT-secreted adipokines could also indirectly affect vascular tone since redox-sensitive intracellular pathways are involved in calcium handling and relaxation [40]. Ghrelin secretion by PVAT is another moiety that enhances NO bioavailability by stimulating its production. This is supported by observations in endothelial cell cultures, showing that ghrelin directly activates endothelial NO synthase through the phosphatidylinositol 3-kinase pathway, without concurrently activating mitogen-activated protein kinase–dependent production of endothelil-1 [41]. Adipose-tissue derived leptin may also be involved in the regulation of coronary microvascular function [32], although its exact role in vasomotor function is less well clear. For example, leptin at physiological concentrations activates the Akt-signaling cascade in endothelial cells, which in turn induces eNOS activity via phosphorylation at Ser1177, thereby leading to enhanced NO-dependent vasorelaxation [42]. On the other hand, leptin can also act in the brain to activate sympathetic nerve system, thereby leading to elevated blood pressure by inducing vasoconstriction and sodium retention [43]. Thus chronic hyperleptinemia causes sustained, unopposed activation of sympathetic nerve system, the result of which is arterial hypertension [44]. Apart from the endothelium and sympathetic nerve system, leptin also acts directly on VSMC to modulate vascular tone, by reducing calcium release [45]. As discussed next the anti-contractile effect of PVAT is abolished in disease states, such as metabolic syndrome, obesity, and arterial hypertension [46].

PVAT Inflammation and Coronary Vasospasm

Vasospastic angina, which was previously referred to as Prinzmetal or variant angina, is a clinical entity characterized by episodes of rest angina that promptly respond to short-acting nitrates and are attributable to coronary artery vasospasm [47] more frequently observed in Caucasians and Asians [48]. The pathophysiology of vasospastic angina is not fully understood but may relate to endothelial and VSMC dysfunction, altered myocardial metabolic demand, autonomic nervous system, and inflammation [49]. Recent evidence suggests that the hypercontractility of coronary VSMC is the major cause of vasospastic angina, whereas the role of endothelial dysfunction is minimal [50]. The most important step leading to VSCM contraction is the phosphorylation of myosin's light chain (MLC) by Ca^{2+}/calmodulin-activated MLC kinase (MLCK). Rho kinase regulates the receptor-mediated sensitization of the MLC phosphorylation and is involved in the GTP-enhanced Ca^{2+} sensitivity of VSMC contraction. Recent evidence demonstrates that pro-inflammatory cytokines released by PVAT could have a pivotal role in the pathophysiology of vasospastic angina [51]. Kandabashi et al. [52] demonstrated that the adventitial expression of interleukin-1b, an inflammatory cytokine, could cause coronary artery spasm of intact endothelium in a porcine model. In the same study it was shown that, Rho-kinase was up regulated at the site of vasospasm and played a key role in inducing VSMC hypercontraction [52]. Ohyama et al. [53] have also demonstrated that PVAT inflammation as assessed by 18F-fluorodeoxyglucose (^{18F}FDG) positron emission tomography/computed tomography (PET/CT) imaging is involved in in-vivo hypercontracting responses of the left anterior descending artery of pigs that had previously undergone stent implantation [53].

PVAT Dysfunction in Obesity

Dysfunctional PVAT may have a pivotal role in mediating obesity-related vascular disease. Mice on a high fat diet for 2 weeks exhibited significant up-regulation of pro-inflammatory leptin and macrophage inflammatory protein (MIP)-1α and down-regulation of PPAR-γ/ adiponectin axis in PVAT [54]. Similar were the findings of another study on mice on a high fat diet, which reported upregulation of the pro-inflammatory adipokines leptin, interleukin-6, TNF-α, and interferon-γ and reduction in the expression of interleukin−10 and adiponectin [55]. The temporal sequence of this events is not fully known. For example, it remains unclarified whether these changes are the result of vascular inflammation or a response of PVAT to excess energy intake and obesity development, subsequently inducing vascular dysfunction.

Nonetheless, evidence suggests that adipocyte hypertrophy in obesity leads to tissue hypoxia via a reduction of capillary density and angiogenic capacity of PVAT [56], and these changes could initiate pro-inflammatory responses in PVAT. The hypoxic conditions favor the production of inflammatory chemokines and cytokines, triggering the accumulation of macrophages and other immune cells (such as CD4+ and CD8+ T cells, natural killer T cells and mast cells) in adipose tissue that perpetuate the inflammatory process [57]. In this pro-inflammatory milieu and obesity-related adipose tissue dysfunction, resident adipose tissue macrophages change their polarization status from an M2 (anti-inflammatory) to an M1 (pro-inflammatory) phenotype [58]. Classically activated macrophages contribute to adipose tissue inflammation and the expression of proinflammatory cytokines in obesity [59]. In human obesity, pericoronary adipose tissue contains a higher ratio of M1/M2 polarized macrophages compared to non-obese individuals [60]. On the other hand, it has been also shown that vascular wall inflammation elicits a pro-inflammatory phenotype in fat too. For example, endovascular wire-injury in rats leads to rapid pro-inflammatory alterations in PVAT [61]. Also, we have recently demonstrated that if human vessels pre-stimulated with angiotensin to induce release of pro-inflammatory cytokines are co-incubated with human adipocytes this leads to a loss of adipocyte differentiation and inhibition of intracellular lipid accumulation [14]. These findings suggest that PVAT surrounding inflamed vessels quickly changes its phenotype towards one characterized by small adipocytes and low levels of intracellular lipid content.

In obesity, local PVAT hypoxia as a result of adipocyte hypertrophy and adipose tissue inflammation may also abolish the protective anti-contractile properties of PVAT and favour vasoconstriction [10]. The molecular mechanisms responsible for the loss of PVAT vasodilatory properties in obesity include reduced NO bioavailability. Decreased eNOS expression has been reported in the mesenteric PVAT of a rat obesity model [62]. In addition, PVAT dysfunction of mice fed a high fat diet results in lower NO bioavailability due to eNOS uncoupling and reduced eNOS phosphorylation at serine 1177 residue in murine mesenteric arteries [63]. Also, obesity-related vascular dysfunction leads to reduced adiponectin biosynthesis globally in adipose tissue [64], adversely affecting eNOS and NO bioavailability [65]. Changes in the secretion of vasoactive factors by PVAT could also underlie obesity-related vascular dysfunction. Gao et al. demonstrated that the anticontractile effect of PVAT was lost in an animal model of obesity despite higher amounts of perivascular fat [66]. Similarly, New Zealand obese (NZO) mice, which have a severe metabolic syndrome and a higher amount of perivascular fat with less potent anticontractile effects [66]. In these NZO mice, obesity-induced PVAT inflammation led to the loss of PVAT anticontractile properties, leading to increased vascular oxidative stress, the remodeling of hypertrophic resistance artery and endothelial dysfunction via eNOS uncoupling [67]. Studies in obese Ossabaw pigs have reported increased epicardial PVAT leptin via a PKC-beta dependent pathway [68], as well as an alteration of 186 proteins in the proteomic profile of coronary PVAT which are linked to pro-contractile effects via changes Ca^{2+} handling via $Ca_V1.2$ channels, H_2O_2-sensitive K^+ channels, and Rho-dependent signaling pathway in VSMCs [69].

Perivascular Adipose Tissue and Coronary Artery Disease: Evidence from Clinical Studies

While there is ample evidence on the mechanisms of obesity-related PVAT dysfunction in animal studies, it remains less well-known whether PVAT dysfunction has any role in human microvascular disease or coronary epicardial atherosclerosis. The reason for this is that until recently we have been lacking proper tools to study human PVAT. However recent advances in the field of non-invasive imaging have provided insights into the association of coronary PVAT with human vascular disease.

Epicardial Adipose Tissue as a Disease Marker

Initial evidence on this links between cardiac adiposity and human coronary artery disease was provided by studies assessing epicardial adiposity either by echocardiography (measured as epicardial fat pad thickness) or epicardial fat volume by CT imaging. Epicardial fat thickness is reportedly increased in patients with CAD compared to healthy controls, and in patients with unstable angina as compared to patients with stable angina or atypical chest pain [70]. Epicardial fat thickness has ben also associated with subclinical markers of atherosclerosis, such as increased carotid intima media thickness, carotid artery stiffness [71] and myocardial diastolic dysfunction [72]. In patients with CAD, echocardiographic epicardial fat thickness has been linked with coronary atherosclerosis burden as assessed by the Gensini score [73, 74]. Nonetheless this relationship between epicardial adiposity and CAD is not consistent in all studies [75, 76].

In autopsy studies epicardial adipose tissue weight is positively associated to myocardial mass in normal and hypertrophied hearts [75], while in clinical cohorts epicardial adiposity is associated with left ventricular mass and right ventricular chamber size [77], atrial enlargement [75] and inversely correlated with cardiac index [78]. In two large population-based cohorts, the Multi-Ethnic Study of Atherosclerosis and the Framingham Heart study, epicardial fat volume (measured as the sum of epicardial and pericardial adipose tissue) by CT imaging was an independent predictor of cardiovascular disease development [6]. Despite these findings, the association between epicardial adiposity and cardiovascular disease may be U- or J-shaped. For example, advanced heart failure there is increased natriuretic-peptide mediated lipolytic signaling and epicardial fat mass regression and therefore low epicardial fat mass is a marker of advanced disease in these patients [79].

Perivascular Adipose Tissue Imaging in Microvascular Angina

Given the ample evidence on the role of PVAT in vasomotor function, a recent study examined the role of PVAT inflammation in patients with vasospastic angina using ^{18F}FDG PET/CT. In this study, Ohyama et al. [13] prospectively examined 27 consecutive patients with vasospastic angina documented by acetylcholine-induced diffuse spasm in the left anterior descending artery (LAD), and 13 subjects with suspected angina but without organic coronary lesions or coronary spasm. Using CCTA and ^{18F}FDG PET imaging, coronary PVAT volume and coronary perivascular FDG uptake in the LAD were determined [13]. The study demonstrated that coronary perivascular FDG uptake was significantly increased in patients with vasospastic angina. Also, the extent of coronary PVAT volume and coronary perivascular FDG uptake were significantly increased in patients with vasospastic angina, suggesting that PVAT inflammation and/or expansion are involved in the pathogenesis of vasospastic angina [13]. Interestingly, these inflammatory changes in PVAT (i.e. perivascular FDG uptake) were reduced after appropriate medical treatment [13]. The findings of this study have provided the first clinical evidence that the inflammation of PVAT could be a major substrate for vasospastic angina development and can be altered with medical treatment.

Perivascular Adipose Tissue and Coronary Atherosclerosis

In contrary to epicardial fat, the imaging of PVAT is technically challenging. Initial studies in the field using manual contouring of epicardial adipose tissue in proximity with coronary vessels, demonstrated that PVAT volume is positively correlated with atherosclerotic plaque burden [11]. Another study co-registered information by CT imaging with data from invasive coronary angiography and intravascular ultrasound, which was used to identify fibrous plaque, lipid-rich plaque or normal coronaries. In a total of 60 coronary segments from 29 patients the mean CT attenuation of PVAT was significantly lower around normal compared to atherosclerotic coronary segments. The authors concluded that differences in the subtypes or activity of PVAT could be linked with atherogenesis and plaque stability [80].

However in our recent translational studies [24, 25, 33] we have provided evidence that contrary to the traditional concept of PVAT as the cause of atherosclerosis, 'inside-out' signaling takes place too. Thus vascular inflammation leads to changes in PVAT, i.e. reduction in adipocyte size and intracellular lipid content [14]. This means a shift in the lipid:aqueous phase of PVAT which can be effectively tracked by CT imaging. To achieve this, we recently developed a new CTA-based methodology to quantify phenotypic changes in PVAT induced by vascular inflammation [14]. A novel imaging biomarker, the perivascular fat attenuation index (FAI), captures coronary inflammation by mapping spatial changes of perivascular fat attenuation on coronary CT angiography (CCTA). In that original study that included validation against tissue histology, gene expression and ^{18F}FDG PET/CT, we demonstrated that perivascular FAI can be used as a biomarker of coronary inflammation [14]. The gradients of perivascular FAI were increased in patients with obstructive CAD compared to healthy controls. FAI was also independently, positively correlated with atherosclerotic plaque burden in the tracked coronary arteries, but not with coronary calcium, an index of plaque stability [14].

Perivascular Adipose Tissue and Plaque Rupture

The links between PVAT and vascular biology suggest that the study of PVAT could be useful also in patients with acute coronary syndromes or to detect vulnerable plaques at risk for rupture. It is well known that visual CT imaging appearance of fat changes as the result of local inflammation (e.g. retroperitoneum or abdominal fat). A similar visual finding can be observed in pericoronary fat around dissected coronary segments. A recent study in patients with a first acute coronary syndrome that underwent CCTA also reported that the CT attenuation of PVAT was increased around culprit lesions compared with non-culprit lesions of patients with acute coronary syndromes and the lesions of stable, matched controls [12].

By using CCTA, we have recently demonstrated that perivascular FAI is increased around culprit lesions of ACS patients compared to either non-culprit lesions or previously stented, stable coronary lesions and had excellent diagnostic value for discriminating between stable and unstable plaques (AUC = 0.91, 95%CI: 0.80–1.00) [14]. More importantly, perivascular FAI followed variations in coronary inflammation after the plaque rupture event and returned to baseline values within 4–6 weeks after the acute coronary event.

The ability to noninvasively quantify coronary inflammation and identify vulnerable coronary lesions by CCTA is an important step forward. Whilst ^{18F}FDG-PET/CT is the gold-standard modality to assess vascular inflammation in-vivo, it cannot be used to study coronary inflammation given the noise by the high uptake of the radiotracer by the underlying myocardium. Others PET tracers such as ^{18}NaF could be useful, but still PET imaging has limitations related to its clinical availability, high costs and radiation exposure. The method for FAI calculation and representative images of FAI mapping around stable and unstable plaques are provided in Fig. 6.3.

Perivascular Adipose Tissue Imaging for Cardiovascular Risk Stratification

Following the development of FAI and its first clinical application, the predictive value of this biomarker has been recently investigated in two large clinical cohorts. The Cardiovascular RISk Prediction using Computed Tomography (CRISP-CT) study included the post-hoc analysis of outcome data gathered prospectively from two independent cohorts of consecutive patients undergoing coronary CTA in

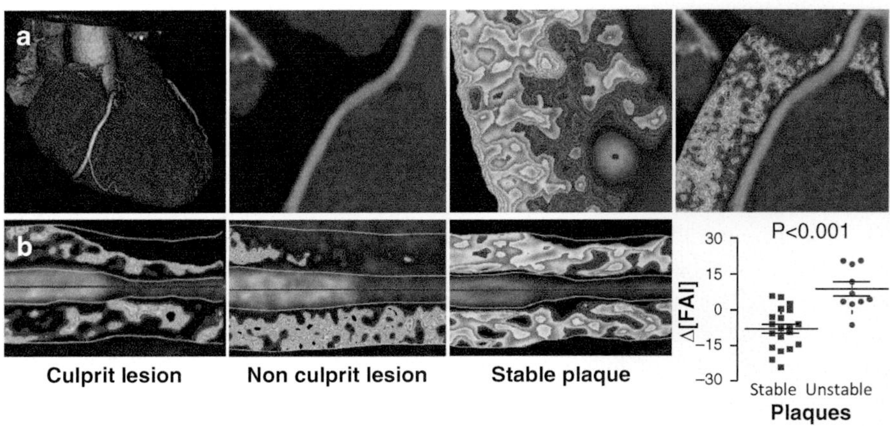

Fig. 6.3 Example of perivascular Fat Attenuation Index (FAI) mapping of human coronaries for the detection of coronary inflammation by standard coronary CTA (**a**); representative examples of the appearance of culprit, non-culprit and stable lesions and classification accuracy of FAI (**b**). Reproduced with permission from Antonopoulos et al. [14]

Erlangen, Germany (derivation cohort) and Cleveland, USA (validation cohort) [15]. Perivascular FAI from standard CTA was measured around all three major coronary arteries with the primary objective being to assess its predictive value for all-cause mortality and cardiac mortality (Fig. 6.4). In both cohorts, high FAI values in the perivascular fat of all three coronary vessels were strongly inter-related and associated with a significantly higher adjusted risk for all-cause and cardiac specific mortality [15]. Perivascular FAI around the right coronary artery was independently associated with a hazard ratio (HR) for cardiac mortality of 2.15 (95%CI: 1.33–1.48; $p = 0.0017$) in the derivation cohort, and 2.06 (95%CI: 1.50–2.83, $p < 0.0001$) in the validation cohort. A cut-off of −70.1HU in perivascular FAI was associated

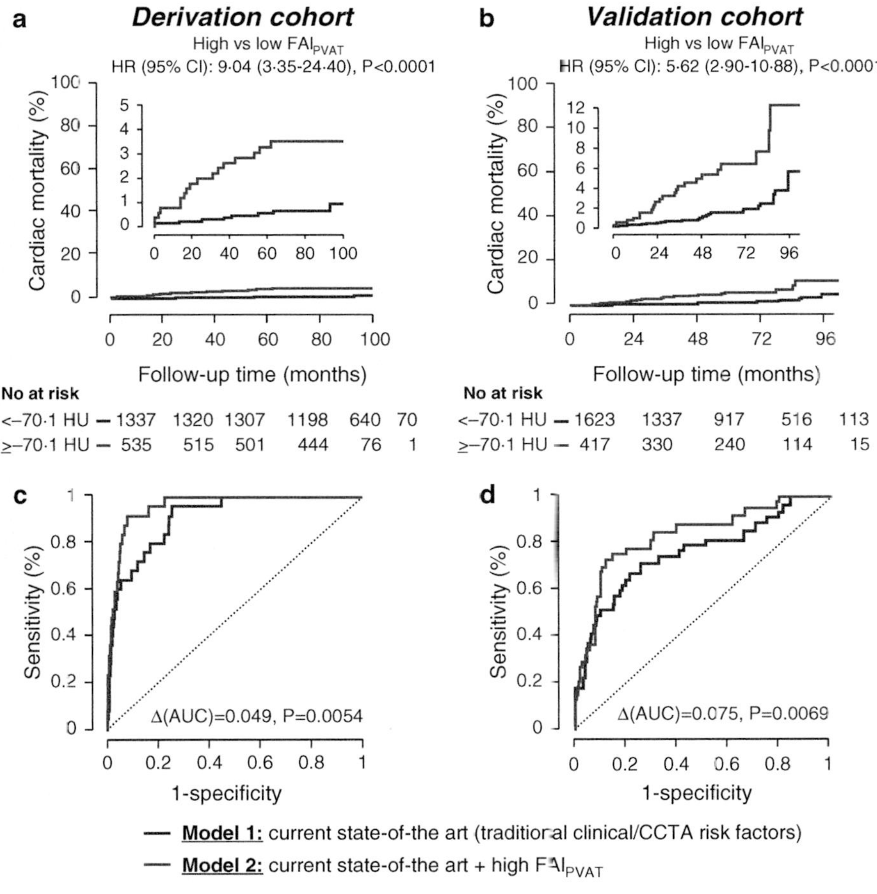

Fig. 6.4 Prognostic value of perivascular Fat Attenuation Index (FAI). Kaplan-Meier curves for cardiac mortality according to baseline FAI in the derivation (**a**) and validation cohort (**b**) from a total of 3912 individuals undergoing diagnostic coronary computed tomography angiography (CCTA) in the CRISP-CT study. Improvement in model's performance by adding FAI on top of traditional risk factors, the extent of coronary atherosclerosis, calcium score and the presence of high-risk plaque features (**c**, **d**). Reproduced with permission from Oikonomou et al. [15]

with steep increase in cardiac mortality (HR = 9.04, 95%CI: 3.35–24.40, $p < 0.0001$ in the derivation cohort and HR = 5.62, 95%CI: 2.90–10.88, $p < 0.0001$ in the validation cohort) [15]. CRISP-CT study used data from two large and diverse real-life prospective cohorts of patients undergoing clinically indicated coronary CTA provided first robust evidence that PVAT imaging by CTA can offers independent predictive and risk discrimination information for future cardiac events. In total, our findings suggest that PVAT imaging could be a useful biomarker for the detection of vulnerable atherosclerotic plaques leading to acute coronary syndromes and offers complementary biological information to the traditional anatomical high-risk plaque features of CCTA (i.e. positive remodeling, napkin ring sign, low-attenuation plaque and spotty calcification).

Conclusion

The role of perivascular adipose tissue (PVAT) in the regulation of vascular biology is now a well-established concept supported by ample evidence from animal and translational studies. Contrary to the traditional notion of PVAT as the cause of vascular dysfunction we now appreciate that there is a bidirectional communication between PVAT and the vascular wall, playing a role in diverse aspects of vascular disease from endothelial dysfunction and vasospastic angina to atherosclerosis development and plaque rupture. Recent advances in the field of cardiovascular imaging allow detailed phenotyping of human coronary PVAT. Coronary CT angiography imaging and use of perivascular Fat Attenuation Index has emerged as powerful noninvasive biomarker to characterize PVAT and risk stratify patients for the cardiovascular disease risk. Further research in the field is expected to show whether targeting of PVAT could be also used to prevent or modify the course of coronary artery disease.

Conflict of Interests None.

Sources of Funding None declared.

References

1. Kissebah AH, Krakower GR. Regional adiposity and morbidity. Physiol Rev. 1994;74(4):761–811.
2. Gesta S, Tseng YH, Kahn CR. Developmental origin of fat: tracking obesity to its source. Cell. 2007;131(2):242–56.
3. Bastien M, et al. Overview of epidemiology and contribution of obesity to cardiovascular disease. Prog Cardiovasc Dis. 2014;56(4):369–81.
4. Nazare JA, et al. Usefulness of measuring both body mass index and waist circumference for the estimation of visceral adiposity and related cardiometabolic risk profile (from the INSPIRE ME IAA study). Am J Cardiol. 2015;115(3):307–15.

5. Subirana I, et al. Prediction of coronary disease incidence by biomarkers of inflammation, oxidation, and metabolism. Sci Rep. 2018;8(1):3191.
6. Antonopoulos AS, Tousoulis D. The molecular mechanisms of obesity paradox. Cardiovasc Res. 2017;113(9):1074–86.
7. Cirulli ET, et al. Profound perturbation of the metabolome in obesity is associated with health risk. Cell Metab. 2019;29(2):488–500.e2.
8. Margaritis M, et al. Interactions between vascular wall and perivascular adipose tissue reveal novel roles for adiponectin in the regulation of endothelial nitric oxide synthase function in human vessels. Circulation. 2013;127(22):2209–21.
9. Guzik TJ, et al. Perivascular adipose tissue as a messenger of the brain-vessel axis: role in vascular inflammation and dysfunction. J Physiol Pharmacol. 2007;58(4):591–610.
10. Greenstein AS, et al. Local inflammation and hypoxia abolish the protective anticontractile properties of perivascular fat in obese patients. Circulation. 2009;119(12):1661–70.
11. Mahabadi AA, et al. Association of pericoronary fat volume with atherosclerotic plaque burden in the underlying coronary artery: a segment analysis. Atherosclerosis. 2010;211(1):195–9.
12. Goeller M, et al. Pericoronary adipose tissue computed tomography attenuation and high-risk plaque characteristics in acute coronary syndrome compared with stable coronary artery disease. JAMA Cardiol. 2018;3(9):858–63.
13. Ohyama K, et al. Coronary adventitial and perivascular adipose tissue inflammation in patients with vasospastic angina. J Am Coll Cardiol. 2018;71(4):414–25.
14. Antonopoulos AS, et al. Detecting human coronary inflammation by imaging perivascular fat. Sci Transl Med. 2017;9(398):eaal2658.
15. Oikonomou EK, et al. Non-invasive detection of coronary inflammation using computed tomography and prediction of residual cardiovascular risk (the CRISP CT study): a post-hoc analysis of prospective outcome data. Lancet. 2018;392(10151):929–39.
16. Antonopoulos AS, Antoniades C. The role of epicardial adipose tissue in cardiac biology: classic concepts and emerging roles. J Physiol. 2017;595(12):3907–17.
17. Sharma AM. Adipose tissue: a mediator of cardiovascular risk. Int J Obes Relat Metab Disord. 2002;26(Suppl 4):S5–7.
18. Marchington JM, Mattacks CA, Pond CM. Adipose tissue in the mammalian heart and pericardium: structure, foetal development and biochemical properties. Comp Biochem Physiol B. 1989;94(2):225–32.
19. Iacobellis G, et al. Epicardial fat from echocardiography: a new method for visceral adipose tissue prediction. Obes Res. 2003;11(2):304–10.
20. Szasz T, Bomfim GF, Webb RC. The influence of perivascular adipose tissue on vascular homeostasis. Vasc Health Risk Manag. 2013;9:105–16.
21. Siegel-Axel DI, Haring HU. Perivascular adipose tissue: an unique fat compartment relevant for the cardiometabolic syndrome. Rev Endocr Metab Disord. 2016;17(1):51–60.
22. Saely CH, Geiger K, Drexel H. Brown versus white adipose tissue: a mini-review. Gerontology. 2012;58(1):15–23.
23. Gil-Ortega M, et al. Regional differences in perivascular adipose tissue impacting vascular homeostasis. Trends Endocrinol Metab. 2015;26(7):367–75.
24. Antonopoulos AS, et al. Adiponectin as a link between type 2 diabetes and vascular NADPH oxidase activity in the human arterial wall: the regulatory role of perivascular adipose tissue. Diabetes. 2015;64(6):2207–19.
25. Antonopoulos AS, et al. Mutual regulation of epicardial adipose tissue and myocardial redox state by PPAR-gamma/adiponectin signalling. Circ Res. 2016;118(5):842–55.
26. Aghamohammadzadeh R, et al. Perivascular adipose tissue from human systemic and coronary vessels: the emergence of a new pharmacotherapeutic target. Br J Pharmacol. 2012;165(3):670–82.
27. Akoumianakis I, Antoniades C. The interplay between adipose tissue and the cardiovascular system: is fat always bad? Cardiovasc Res. 2017;113(9):999–1008.
28. Rajsheker S, et al. Crosstalk between perivascular adipose tissue and blood vessels. Curr Opin Pharmacol. 2010;10(2):191–6.

29. Emilova R, et al. Diabetes converts arterial regulation by perivascular adipose tissue from relaxation into H(2)O(2)-mediated contraction. Physiol Res. 2016;65(5):799–807.
30. Kagota S, et al. Time-dependent differences in the influence of perivascular adipose tissue on vasomotor functions in metabolic syndrome. Metab Syndr Relat Disord. 2017;15(5):233–9.
31. Antonopoulos AS, Antoniades C. Perivascular fat attenuation index by computed tomography as a metric of coronary inflammation. J Am Coll Cardiol. 2018;71(23):2708–9.
32. Antonopoulos AS, Antoniades C, Tousoulis D. Unravelling the "adipokine paradox": when the classic proatherogenic adipokine leptin is deemed the beneficial one. Int J Cardiol. 2015;197:125–7.
33. Antonopoulos AS, et al. Reciprocal effects of systemic inflammation and brain natriuretic peptide on adiponectin biosynthesis in adipose tissue of patients with ischemic heart disease. Arterioscler Thromb Vasc Biol. 2014;34(9):2151–9.
34. Lee S, et al. Exercise training improves endothelial function via adiponectin-dependent and independent pathways in type 2 diabetic mice. Am J Physiol Heart Circ Physiol. 2011;301(2):H306–14.
35. Antonopoulos AS, et al. Novel therapeutic strategies targeting vascular redox in human atherosclerosis. Recent Pat Cardiovasc Drug Discov. 2009;4(2):76–87.
36. Axelsson J, et al. Adipose tissue and its relation to inflammation: the role of adipokines. J Ren Nutr. 2005;15(1):131–6.
37. Lau DC, et al. Adipokines: molecular links between obesity and atheroslcerosis. Am J Physiol Heart Circ Physiol. 2005;288(5):H2031–41.
38. Zavaritskaya O, et al. Role of KCNQ channels in skeletal muscle arteries and periadventitial vascular dysfunction. Hypertension. 2013;61(1):151–9.
39. Kohn C, et al. Hydrogen sulfide: potent regulator of vascular tone and stimulator of angiogenesis. Int J Biomed Sci. 2012;8(2):81–6.
40. Ardanaz N, Pagano PJ. Hydrogen peroxide as a paracrine vascular mediator: regulation and signaling leading to dysfunction. Exp Biol Med (Maywood). 2006;231(3):237–51.
41. Xu X, et al. Molecular mechanisms of ghrelin-mediated endothelial nitric oxide synthase activation. Endocrinology. 2008;149(8):4183–92.
42. Beltowski J. Leptin and the regulation of endothelial function in physiological and pathological conditions. Clin Exp Pharmacol Physiol. 2012;39(2):168–78.
43. Haynes WG, et al. Receptor-mediated regional sympathetic nerve activation by leptin. J Clin Invest. 1997;100(2):270–8.
44. Rahmouni K, et al. Role of selective leptin resistance in diet-induced obesity hypertension. Diabetes. 2005;54(7):2012–8.
45. Belin de Chantemele EJ, et al. Impact of leptin-mediated sympatho-activation on cardiovascular function in obese mice. Hypertension. 2011;58(2):271–9.
46. Lu C, et al. Alterations in perivascular adipose tissue structure and function in hypertension. Eur J Pharmacol. 2011;656(1-3):68–73.
47. Prinzmetal M, et al. Angina pectoris. I. A variant form of angina pectoris; preliminary report. Am J Med. 1959;27:375–88.
48. Ong P, et al. Coronary artery spasm as a frequent cause of acute coronary syndrome: the CASPAR (coronary artery spasm in patients with acute coronary syndrome) study. J Am Coll Cardiol. 2008;52(7):523–7.
49. Li J, Zhang H, Zhang C. Role of inflammation in the regulation of coronary blood flow in ischemia and reperfusion: mechanisms and therapeutic implications. J Mol Cell Cardiol. 2012;52(4):865–72.
50. Shimokawa H. 2014 Williams Harvey Lecture: importance of coronary vasomotion abnormalities-from bench to bedside. Eur Heart J. 2014;35(45):3180–93.
51. Brown NK, et al. Perivascular adipose tissue in vascular function and disease: a review of current research and animal models. Arterioscler Thromb Vasc Biol. 2014;34(8):1621–30.
52. Kandabashi T, et al. Inhibition of myosin phosphatase by upregulated rho-kinase plays a key role for coronary artery spasm in a porcine model with interleukin-1beta. Circulation. 2000;101(11):1319–23.

53. Ohyama K, et al. Association of Coronary Perivascular Adipose Tissue Inflammation and Drug-Eluting Stent-Induced Coronary Hyperconstricting Responses in pigs: (18) F-Fluorodeoxyglucose positron emission tomography imaging study. Arterioscler Thromb Vasc Biol. 2017;37(9):1757–64.
54. Cheang WS, et al. The peroxisome proliferator-activated receptors in cardiovascular diseases: experimental benefits and clinical challenges. Br J Pharmacol. 2015;172(23):5512–22.
55. Ketonen J, et al. Periadventitial adipose tissue promotes endothelial dysfunction via oxidative stress in diet-induced obese C57Bl/6 mice. Circ J. 2010;74(7):1479–87.
56. Pasarica M, et al. Adipose tissue collagen VI in obesity. J Clin Endocrinol Metab. 2009;94(12):5155–62.
57. Greenstein AJ, et al. Prevalence of adverse intraoperative events during obesity surgery and their sequelae. J Am Coll Surg. 2012;215(2):271–7.e3.
58. Lumeng CN, Bodzin JL, Saltiel AR. Obesity induces a phenotypic switch in adipose tissue macrophage polarization. J Clin Invest. 2007;117(1):175–84.
59. Mosser DM, Edwards JP. Exploring the full spectrum of macrophage activation. Nat Rev Immunol. 2008;8(12):958–69.
60. Gurses KM, et al. Netrin-1 is associated with macrophage infiltration and polarization in human epicardial adipose tissue in coronary artery disease. J Cardiol. 2017;69(6):851–8.
61. Takaoka M, et al. Endovascular injury induces rapid phenotypic changes in perivascular adipose tissue. Arterioscler Thromb Vasc Biol. 2010;30(8):1576–82.
62. Bussey CE, et al. Obesity-related perivascular adipose tissue damage is reversed by sustained weight loss in the rat. Arterioscler Thromb Vasc Biol. 2016;36(7):1377–85.
63. Gil-Ortega M, et al. Imbalance between pro and anti-oxidant mechanisms in perivascular adipose tissue aggravates long-term high-fat diet-derived endothelial dysfunction. PLoS One. 2014;9(4):e95312.
64. Antoniades C, et al. Adiponectin: from obesity to cardiovascular disease. Obes Rev. 2009;10(3):269–79.
65. Wang Y, et al. Childhood obesity prevention programs: comparative effectiveness review and meta-analysis. Rockville: Agency for Healthcare Research and Quality; 2013.
66. Fesus G, et al. Adiponectin is a novel humoral vasodilator. Cardiovasc Res. 2007;75(4):719–27.
67. Marchesi C, et al. Endothelial nitric oxide synthase uncoupling and perivascular adipose oxidative stress and inflammation contribute to vascular dysfunction in a rodent model of metabolic syndrome. Hypertension. 2009;54(6):1384–92.
68. Payne GA, et al. Epicardial perivascular adipose-derived leptin exacerbates coronary endothelial dysfunction in metabolic syndrome via a protein kinase C-beta pathway. Arterioscler Thromb Vasc Biol. 2010;30(9):1711–7.
69. Owen MK, et al. Perivascular adipose tissue potentiates contraction of coronary vascular smooth muscle: influence of obesity. Circulation. 2013;128(1):9–18.
70. Sarin S, et al. Clinical significance of epicardial fat measured using cardiac multislice computed tomography. Am J Cardiol. 2008;102(6):767–71.
71. Natale F, et al. Visceral adiposity and arterial stiffness: echocardiographic epicardial fat thickness reflects, better than waist circumference, carotid arterial stiffness in a large population of hypertensives. Eur J Echocardiogr. 2009;10(4):549–55.
72. Adolph TE, et al. Adipokines and non-alcoholic fatty liver disease: multiple interactions. Int J Mol Sci. 2017;18:8.
73. J. P. Morgan 32nd annual healthcare conference. J Diabetes. 2014;6(4):275–6.
74. Jeong JW, et al. Echocardiographic epicardial fat thickness and coronary artery disease. Circ J. 2007;71(4):536–9.
75. Summaries for patients. The obesity paradox in type 2 diabetes mellitus. Ann Intern Med. 2015;162(9):I–26.
76. Silaghi A, et al. Epicardial adipose tissue extent: relationship with age, body fat distribution, and coronaropathy. Obesity (Silver Spring). 2008;16(11):2424–30.
77. Iacobellis G, et al. Relation between epicardial adipose tissue and left ventricular mass. Am J Cardiol. 2004;94(8):1084–7.

78. Retraction note to: the 'obesity paradox' and survival after colorectal cancer: true or false? Cancer Causes Control. 2015;26(8):1203.
79. Antonopoulos AS, Antoniades C. Cardiac magnetic resonance imaging of epicardial and intramyocardial adiposity as an early sign of myocardial disease. Circ Cardiovasc Imaging. 2018;11(8):e008083.
80. Marwan M, et al. CT attenuation of pericoronary adipose tissue in normal versus atherosclerotic coronary segments as defined by intravascular ultrasound. J Comput Assist Tomogr. 2017;41(5):762–7.

Chapter 7
Myocardial Infarction with Non-obstructive Coronary Artery Disease

Giampaolo Niccoli, Giancarla Scalone, and Filippo Crea

Clinical Case

A 65 years old female patient with systolic hypertension, dyslipidemia, history of transient ischemic attack and diagnosis of Patent Foramen Ovale (PFO) subjected to a percutaneous closure procedure with Amplatzer device 1 year ago, was referred to our Hospital for No-ST segment elevation myocardial infarction (NSTEMI). The electrocardiogram (ECG) showed diffuse repolarization abnormalities (Fig. 7.1), and the peak of high sensible (HS) Troponine T was 0.168 ng/mL. Trans-thoracic echocardiogram revealed a slightly hypertrophic left ventricle (LV), with normal volumes and preserved global and regional function, and Amplatzer device localized in the atrial septum. The contrast echocardiography did not show passage of microbubbles from the right to the left atrium both at rest and after the Valsalva maneuver, rulling out the hypothesis of acute myocardial infarction (AMI) caused by embolization. Coronary angiography did not point out the presence of significant coronary stenosis, while intra-coronary ergonovine administration (up to 50 μg) caused diffuse ST-segment depression at ECG and symptoms, in absence of epicardic coronary spasm (Fig. 7.2, panel A and B). For this reason, the diagnosis of MI and non-obstructive coronary arteries (MINOCA) due to coronary microvascular spasm (CMS) was done. The medical therapy was optimized with the add of calcium blockers and the patient was discharged without symptoms 7 day after. She remained asymptomatic until 4 years later, when she was admitted at our Hospital for sinus nodal disease and underwent to the procedure of pacemaker implantation.

G. Niccoli · G. Scalone · F. Crea (✉)
Fondazione Policlinico Universitario A. Gemelli IRCCS, Rome, Italy

Department of Cardiovascular Sciences, Catholic University of the Sacred Heart, Rome, Italy
e-mail: filippo.crea@unicatt.it

M. Dorobantu, L. Badimon (eds.), *Microcirculation*,
https://doi.org/10.1007/978-3-030-28199-1_7

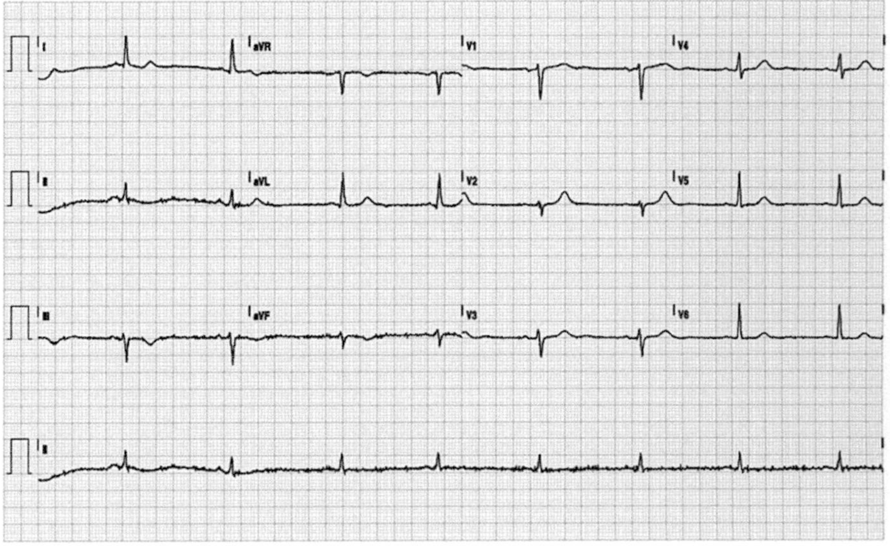

Fig. 7.1 ECG of the patient, showing a diffuse repolarization abnormalities

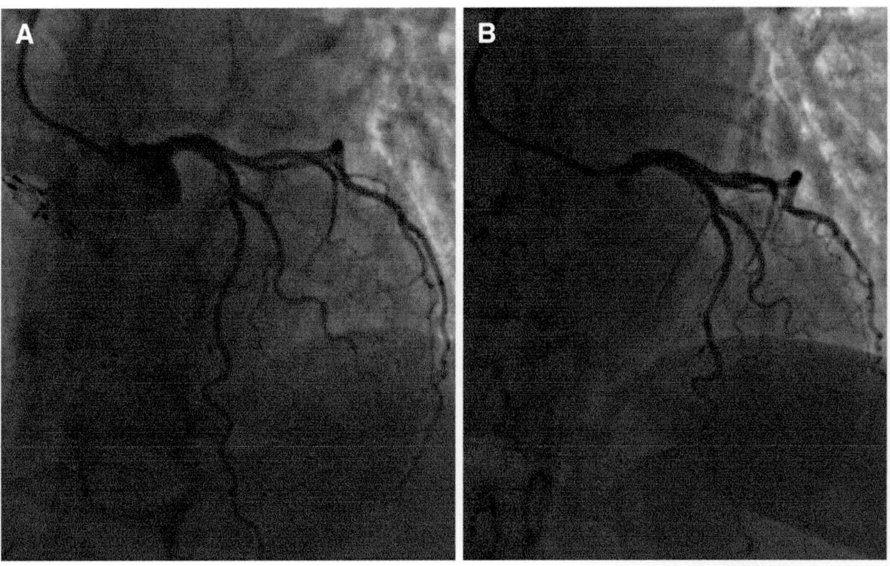

Fig. 7.2 Coronary-angiography at baseline (panel **A**) and after ergonovine intra-coronary administration (up to 50 μg) (panel **B**)

Introduction

MINOCA is a syndrome with different causes, characterized by clinical evidence of MI with normal or near-normal coronary arteries on angiography [1, 2] (Table 7.1). Data from large MI registries suggest a prevalence between 5% and 25% [3], but the most recent study, in a contemporary cohort of patients, reported a prevalence of 8.8%, which appears to reflect daily clinical experience [4]. Of note, the prognosis of MINOCA is not as benign as reported by early cohort studies and as commonly assumed by physicians [4]. Moreover, a recent retrospective analysis of patients enrolled in the ACUITY trial showed that, compared with NSTEMI patients and obstructive coronary arteries disease (CAD), patients with MINOCA had a higher adjusted risk of mortality at 1 year, driven by a greater non-cardiac mortality [4]. Recently, compared to patients with obstructive CAD, those with MINOCA showed both physical and mental distress from 6 weeks to 3 months after the acute event and, in some perspectives, even lower scores especially in the mental component of quality of life [5]. MINOCA patients represent a conundrum given the very many possible aetiologies and pathogenic mechanisms associated with this syndrome [6]. For this reason, the key principle in the management of this syndrome is clarify the underlying individual mechanisms to achieve patient-specific treatments.

Clinical history, ECG, cardiac enzymes, echocardiography, coronary angiography and left ventricular (LV) angiography, represent the first level diagnostic investigations to identify the causes of MINOCA. In particular, regional wall motion abnormalities at LV angiography limited to a single epicardial coronary artery territory identify an "epicardial pattern", whereas regional wall motion abnormalities extended beyond a single epicardial coronary artery territory identifiy a "microvascular pattern" [1]. In this context, the most common causes of MINOCA that the clinicians must consider are: coronary plaque disease, coronary dissection, coronary artery spasm (CAS), CMS, Takotsubo Syndrome (TTS), myocarditis, coronary thromboembolism, other forms of type-2 MI and MINOCA of uncertain aetiology [7] (Fig. 7.3 and Table 7.2).

Table 7.1 Diagnostic criteria for MINOCA

The diagnosis of MINOCA is made immediately upon coronary angiography in a patient presenting with features consistent with an AMI, as detailed by the following criteria:
Universal AMI criteria [13]
Non obstructive coronary arteries on angiography, defined as no coronary artery stenosis ≥50% in any potential IRA
No clinically overt specific cause for the acute presentation

AMI acute myocardial infarction, *IRA* infarct related artery, *MINOCA* myocardial infarction without non obstructive coronary artery disease

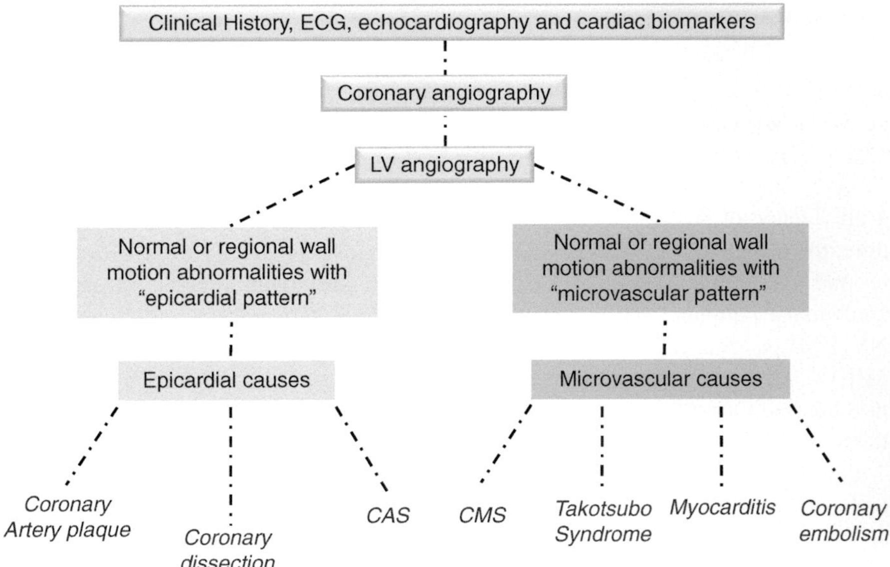

Fig. 7.3 Clinical history, ECG, cardiac enzymes, echocardiography, coronary angiography and left ventricular (LV) angiography, represent the first level diagnostic investigations to identify the causes of myocardial infarction without obstructive coronary artery obstruction (MINOCA). In particular, regional wall motion abnormalities at LV angiography limited to a single epicardial coronary artery territory identify an "epicardial pattern", whereas regional wall motion abnormalities extended beyond a single epicardial coronary artery territory identify a "microvascular pattern". The most common epicardial causes of MINOCA are represented by: coronary plaque disease, coronary dissection and coronary artery spasm (CAS). The principal microvascular causes of MINOCA are: coronary microvascular spasm (CMS), Takotsubo Syndrome, myocarditis, coronary embolism

Epicardial Causes of MINOCA

Coronary Plaque Disease

Plaque rupture (PR) and erosion (PE) are comprised within type-1 AMI in the Universal Definition of MI, even when no thrombus can be found [8]. Of note, MINOCA comprises 5–20% of all type-1 AMI cases [7].

Two independent studies using intravascular ultrasound (IVUS) identified PR and PE in 40% of patients with MINOCA [7, 8]. Higher resolution intracoronary images, like optical coherence tomography (OCT), would likely show an even higher prevalence of PR and PE but this technique has not been routinely applied in controlled studies within the MINOCA population. Calcified nodule with thrombus has also been suggested as a cause of AMI on intracoronary imaging [9]. PR or PE may occur in areas of the vessel appearing normal on conventional angiography or presenting some degree of atherosclerosis, even if minimal.

Table 7.2 Diagnostic tests, therapeutic treatments stratified for specific causes of MINOCA

Mechanism	Diagnosis	Therapy
Epicardic causes – Coronary artery disease – Coronary dissection – Coronary artery spasm	Intravascular imaging Intravascular imaging IC ergonovine or Ach test	PCI; anti-platelet therapy, statins, angiotensin-converting enzyme inhibitors/angiotensin receptor blockers, β-blocker treatment Conservative treatment (beta-blocker and single anti-platelet therapy) Calcium antagonist, nitrates, Rho-kinasi inhibitors
Microvascular causes – Microvascular coronary spasm – Takotsubo syndrome – PVB19 myocarditis – Coronary embolism	IC Ach test Ventriculography, echocardiography with adenosine, CMR CMR, EMB TTE, TOE, Bubble contrast echography	Rho-kinasi inhibitors? Heart failure treatment Heart failure treatment Trans-catheter device closure or surgical repair, anti-platelet therapy, anticoagulation
Miscellanea – Myocardial infarction type 2 – Uncertain aetiology	Identification the condition underlying the oxygen supply-demand mismatch Intra-vascular imaging, CMR	The condition underlying the oxygen supply–demand mismatch is to be reversed; aspirin and b-blockers Aspirin, statins, calcium channel blockers

Ach acethilcoline, *CMR* cardiac magnetic resonance, *EMB* endomyocardial biopsy, *IC* intracoronary, *IVUS* intravascular ultrasound, *OCT* optical coherence tomography, *PCI* percutaneous coronary intervention, *TOE* transesophageal echocardiography, *TTE* transthoracic echocardiography

Myonecrosis in MINOCA with PR and PE is mediated by thrombosis, thromboembolism, superimposed vasospasm, or a combination of these processes. The theory of spontaneous thrombolysis or autolysis of a coronary thrombosis has been proposed. Spontaneous thrombolysis is thought to be an endogenous protective mechanism against thrombus formation even in the presence of a PR [10]. In this context, cardiac magnetic resonance (CMR) imaging may show large areas of myocardial oedema with or without small areas of necrosis among patients with MINOCA and plaque disruption, suggesting that flow was compromised transiently in a larger vessel. However, the theory that spontaneous coronary thrombolysis rather than vasospasm leads to this appearance can neither be dismissed nor proved, and both may play a role. CMR imaging can shows a smaller, well-defined area of late gadolinium enhancement (LGE), subtended by a smaller vessel, suggesting that embolization of athero-thrombotic debris from the disruption site is the most likely mechanism of myonecrosis [11].

Thrombosis and/or thromboembolism almost certainly have a major role in pathogenesis of MINOCA with coronary plaque disease. Considering the limits of coronary angiography, the use of intra-vascular imaging (e.g. OCT and IVUS) seems mandatory.

From the prognostic point of view, the finding of PR on OCT was associated with major adverse cardiac events (MACEs) in a cohort of patients undergoing OCT for acute coronary syndrome (ACS) [1]. Overall, the risk of recurrent MI or death in MINOCA patients is about 2% up to 12 months [12, 13].

Dual antiplatelet therapy is recommended for 1 year followed by lifetime single antiplatelet therapy for patients with suspected or confirmed plaque disruption and MINOCA [14]. Because disruption occurs on a background of non-obstructive CAD, statin therapy is also recommended, even if only a minor degree of atherosclerosis is found.

Coronary Dissection

Spontaneous coronary dissection (SCAD) typically causes an AMI via luminal obstruction, although this may not always be apparent on coronary angiography, prompting a diagnosis of MINOCA [14]. Intramural haematoma of the coronary arteries without intimal tear presents similarly. Intracoronary imaging is crucial in making this diagnosis [14].

Findings can be graded into three types: (1) the classic description is of a longitudinal filling defect, representing the radiolucent intimal flap, there is often contrast staining of the arterial wall with appearance of a double lumen; (2) diffuse long smooth tubular lesions (due to intramural haematoma) with no visible dissection plane that can result in complete vessel occlusion, lesions are typically >30 mm in length with an abrupt change in vessel diameter between normal and diseased segments, there is no response to intracoronary nitrates and there are no atherosclerotic lesions in other coronary segments; (3) multiple focal tubular lesions due to intramural haematoma that mimic atherosclerosis.

The condition is more common among women. Indeed, it is estimated to be responsible for up to 25% of all ACS cases in women<50 years of age [15]. The reasons for the occurrence of coronary dissection are still unclear. However, in the majority of cases when screening is performed, fibromuscular dysplasia is present in other vascular beds [16]. Changes in the intima-media composition due to hormones, pregnancy and delivery have also been implicated. Regarding the prognosis, the in-hospital ad long-term survival has been shown to be excellent. However, the risk of recurrence of acute event has been reported to be high (27% at 5 years) [17]. At present, there is no effective treatment to reduce the long-term risk. A conservative approach is advocated because coronary intervention and stenting tend to cause propagation of the dissection and outcomes are acceptable with medical management [18]. Despite the lack of evidence, beta-blockers and single antiplatelet therapy are considered a cornerstone of medical treatment.

Recently, the SCAD registry reported that most patients (84.3%) received conservative treatment, others underwent percutaneous coronary intervention (PCI) (14.1%) and a minority had coronary artery bypass surgery (0.7%). The in-hospital major adverse event rate was 8.8%, including cardiac arrest (3.9%), cardiogenic shock (2.0%), recurrent MI (4.0%) and unplanned revascularisation (2.5%).

Importantly, the 34 patients (4.5%) with peri-partum SCAD had higher in-hospital major adverse events. The incidence of MACE at one month was 8.8%, consisting primarily of recurrent MI (6.1%), stroke/transient ischaemic attack (1.2%) and unplanned revascularisation (2.7%). Peri-partum SCAD and connective tissue disorder were independent predictors of 30-day MACE. Finally, acute in-hospital and one-month survival was good, with only one death (0.1%) reported [19].

Coronary Artery Spasm

The prevalence of CAS ranges between 3 and 95% of MINOCA patients; this wide difference depends on the stimuli used to trigger spasm, definitions of spasm and ethnic reasons [11]. In particular, in a recent study, provocative tests were positive in 46% of patients with MINOCA [20].

CAS usually occurs at a localized segment of an epicardial artery, but sometimes involves 2 or more segments of the same (multifocal spasm) or of different (multivessel spasm) coronary arteries, or may involve diffusely one or multiple coronary branches. CAS results from interaction of 2 components: (1) an usually localized, but sometimes diffuse, hyperreactivity of vascular smooth muscle cells (VSMCs), and (2) a transient vasoconstrictor stimulus acting on the hyperreactive VSMCs. The main cause of VSMCs hyperreactivity seems to be enhanced Rho kinase activity [7]. CAS can occur as vascular smooth muscle hyper-reactivity to endogenous vasospastic substances (as in vasospastic angina) but may also occur in the context of exogenous vasospastic agents (e.g. cocaine or metamphetamines) [21]. Patients with CAS typically refer angina at rest, during the night or early in the morning, associated with a transient ST segment elevation. In absence of ECG documentation, the diagnosis is based on an intracorororonary (IC) provocative test, whereas CAS is generally defined as reduction of at least 75% of the vessel caliber together with symptoms/signs of myocardial ischaemia [22]. The diagnostic test with IC ergonovine and Acetylcholine (Ach) have been shown to be safe and its positive result portends a worse prognosis with regard to both hard clinical endpoints (death from any cause, cardiac death, readmission for recurrent ACS) and quality of life (worse angina status). The negative prognostic value of positive provocative tests seems mainly related to the induction of epicardial spasm. Accordingly, a calcium antagonist dose reduction or discontinuation was associated with mortality, supporting the crucial role of epicardial spasm in the occurrence of fatal events in our patients. While the IC egonovine test is a well standardized procedure, the provocative test with IC Ach is performed in different ways in different countries [22–24] (Table 7.3).

The prognosis is variable. Apart from multivessel CAS, other independent predictors of cardiovascular outcome emerged from studies on the Japanese population: history of out-of-hospital cardiac arrest, smoking, angina at rest alone, organic coronary stenosis, ST-segment elevation during angina, and beta-blockers use [11, 25]. However, it is difficult to extrapolate these findings to Caucasian populations; indeed, while the prevalence of CAS is higher in the Japanese population, its outcome is better in the Caucasian population.

Table 7.3 Protocols of intra-coronary provocative tests with achetilcoline

Author (year)	IC route	Dosage	Administration modality	Mandatory pacing	Sides effects
Sueda (2008) [22]	Yes	20, 50 and 100 μg (LCA) or 20, 50 and 80 μg (RCA) in 5 mL NS[a]	Incremental doses over 20 s with at least a 3-min interval between each injection	Yes	NsVT (1.1%). shock (0.3%), cardiac tamponade (0.1%), PAF (17.1%)
Ong (2014) [23]	Yes	2, 20, 100, and 200 μg (LCA) or 80 μg (RCA)[b]	Incremental doses over 3 min	No/bailout	PAF (0.1%), NsVT (0.1%), bradycardia (0.6%), catheter-induced spasm (0.1%)
Wei (2012) [24]	Yes	0.182, 1.82 and 18.2 μg/mL in 2 mL NS[b]	Incremental doses over 3 min	No/bailout	CRT-SAEs: 0.2% (MI and coronary artery dissection)
[c]	Yes	20, 50, 100 μg in 2 mL NS[b]	Incremental doses over 3 min	No/bailout	Bradycardia (0.1%), NsVT (0.1%)

[a]Achetilcoline chloride (Neucholin-A, 30 mg/2 mL)
[b]Achetilcoline chloride (Miochol, 20 mg/2 mL)
[c]Unpublished data about IC Ach test protocol used in our Institute: a drug formulation employed for ocular disease is diluted as reported
Intracoronary nitrates are usually administered at the end of the protocol and a final coronary angiography after nitrates is performed
Ach achetilcoline, *CAS* coronary artery spasm, *CRT-SAEs* coronary reactivity testing related serious adverse events, *IC* intra-coronary, *LCA* left coronary artery, *MI* myocardial infarction, *NS* normal solution, *NsVT* nonsustained ventricular tachycardia, *PAF* paroxysmal atrial fibrillation, *RCA* right coronary artery

Non-specific vasodilators such nitrates and calcium channel blockers constitute the standard treatment. In case of refractory vasospastic angina (ranging from 10% to 20% of cases), fasudil has been found effective in Japanese patients, although these positive findings cannot be directly extrapolated to Caucasian patients. In selected cases, stent implantation or partial sympathetic denervation [25] can be employed. Utilization of implantable cardiac defibrillators are needed in patients at high risk of spasm-related cardiac death.

Microvascular Causes of MINOCA

Coronary Microvascular Spasm

CMS is characterized by transient myocardial ischaemia, as indicated by ST segment changes and angina, in the presence of non-obstructive coronary arteries. It may be considered the unstable counterpart of chronic microvascular angina [26]. Previous studies showed that about 25% of patients with MINOCA have evidence of CMS [26]. The diagnosis can be made when ergonovine or Ach test reproduces the symptoms usually experienced by the patients and triggered ischemic ECG changes (i.e. ST-segment depression or ST segment elevation of ≥0.1 mV or T-wave peaking in at least 2 contigous leads), in absence of epicardial spasm (>90% diameter reduction) [26].

Although previous studies pointed out excellent results with regard to mortality, angina seems to persist (ranging about 36%) in many patients even on calcium channel blockers [27]. In this case, Fasudil may be considered a possible alternative treatment. Finally, Arrebola-Moreno and Crea proposed that CMS may be able to cause perfusion and contractile abnormalities and cardiac troponin elevations, and therefore to have the potential to lead to adverse clinical outcomes during long-term follow up [28, 29].

Takotsubo Syndrome

TTS is estimated to represent approximately 1–3% of all and 5–6% of female patients presenting with suspected STEMI [30]. Recurrence rate of TTS is estimated to be 1.8% per-patient year [31] About 90% of TTS patients have been shown to be women with a mean age of 67–70 years and around 80% are older than 50 years. Women older than 55 years have a fivefold greater risk of developing TTS than women younger than 55 years and a tenfold greater risk than men. With growing awareness of TTS, male patients are diagnosed more often, especially after a physical triggering event [31]. Moreover, it has been reported that TTS seems to be uncommon in African–Americans and Hispanics while most of the cases reported in the United States have been Caucasians. Furthermore, patients of African-American descent seem to have more in-hospital complications such as respiratory failure, stroke and require more frequently mechanical ventilation compared to Caucasians and Hispanics [32]. With regard to ECG differences, it has been shown that QT prolongation as well as T-wave inversion are more often reported in African- American women with TTS [33]. Of note, regarding gender differences the TTS prevalence in men appears to be higher in Japan. The prevalence of TTS appears to be higher in patients with non-emotional triggers admitted to intensive care units. Moreover, it is likely that subclinical TTS cases remain undetected, especially in non-PCI [34].

TTS often presents as an ACS with ST segment changes. The transient nature of LV dysfunction has puzzled physicians worldwide. Clinical presentation is characterized by acute, reversible heart failure associated with myocardial stunning, in the absence of occlusive CAD.

The revised Mayo clinic diagnostic criteria include: (1) transient hypokinesis, akinesis, or dyskinesis of the LV mid segments with or without apical involvement; the regional wall motion abnormalities extend beyond a single epicardial vascular distribution; a stressful trigger is often, but not always present. (2) The absence of obstructive CAD or angiographic evidence of acute plaque rupture (though it is recognized that obstructive CAD may pre-date the Takotsubo event in some cases). (3) New electrocardiographic abnormalities (either ST-segment elevation and/or T-wave inversion) or modest elevation in cardiac troponin. (4) The absence of pheochromocytoma and myocarditis [35]. The Mayo Clinic Diagnostic Criteria are the most widely known, but exceptions to the rule [e.g. the presence of CAD] are poorly appreciated among physicians and cardiologists. More recently, other research groups have proposed slightly different criteria for TTS, i.e. the Japanese Guidelines, the Gothenburg criteria, the Johns Hopkins criteria, the Tako-tsubo Italian Network proposal, the criteria of the Heart Failure Association (HFA) TTS Taskforce of the European Society of Cardiology (ESC), as well as the criteria recommended by Madias [35]. Thus, there is a lack of a worldwide consensus. Based on current knowledge, new international diagnostic criteria (InterTAK Diagnostic Criteria, Table 7.4) have been recently developed for the diagnosis of TTS that may help to improve identification and stratification of TTS [36].

The pathophysiological mechanisms responsible for TTS are complex and may vary between patients. Although several mechanisms have been proposed (e.g. multivessel epicardial spasm, catecholamine-induced myocardial stunning, spontaneous coronary thrombus lysis, and acute microvascular spasm) the causes still remain debated. A previous study demonstrated that, irrespectively of its etiology, reversible coronary microvascular dysfunction is a common pathophysiological determinant of TTS [37]. Indeed, the extent of myocardial hypoperfusion at myocardial contrast echocardiography (MCE) was similar in patients with TTS and in patients with ST elevation MI, whereas a transient significant improvement of myocardial perfusion and of LV function during adenosine infusion was observed in the former only.

Left ventriculography after documentation of MINOCA allows the diagnosis of TTS. Although several anatomical TTS variants have been described, four major types can be differentiated based on the distribution of regional wall motion abnor-

Table 7.4 International Takotsubo diagnostic criteria (InterTAK diagnostic criteria)

1.	Patients show transient[a] left ventricular dysfunction (hypokinesia, akinesia, or dyskinesia) presenting as apical ballooning or midventricular, basal, or focal wall motion abnormalities. Right ventricular involvement can be present. Besides these regional wall motion patterns, transitions between all types can exist. The regional wall motion abnormality usually extends beyond a single epicardial vascular distribution; however, rare cases can exist where the regional wall motion abnormality is present in the subtended myocardial territory of a single coronary artery (focal TTS)[b]
2.	An emotional, physical, or combined trigger can precede the Takotsubo syndrome event, but this is not obligatory
3.	An emotional, physical, or combined trigger can precede the Takotsubo syndrome event, but this is not obligatory
4.	New ECG abnormalities are present (ST-segment elevation, ST-segment depression, T-wave inversion, and QTc prolongation); however, rare cases exist without any ECG changes
5.	Levels of cardiac biomarkers (troponin and creatine kinase) are moderately elevated in most cases; significant elevation of brain natriuretic peptide is common
6.	Significant coronary artery disease is not a contradiction in Takotsubo syndrome
7.	Patients have no evidence of infectious myocarditis
8.	Postmenopausal women are predominantly affected

[a]Wall motion abnormalities may remain for a prolonged period of time or documentation of recovery may not be possible. For example, death before evidence of recovery is captured
[b]Cardiac magnetic resonance imaging is recommended to exclude infectious myocarditis and diagnosis confirmation of Takotsubo syndrome

malities (Fig. 7.4) [38]. The most common TTS type and widely recognized form is the (1) apical ballooning type, also known as the typical TTS form, which occurs in the majority of cases [38]. Over the past years, atypical TTS types have been increasingly recognized [38]. These include the (2) midventricular, (3) basal, and (4) focal wall motion patterns. Recently, it has been demonstrated that patients suffering from atypical TTS have a different clinical phenotype [38]. These patients are younger, more often with neurologic comorbidities, lower brain natriuretic peptide values, a less impaired LVEF, and more frequent ST-segment depression compared

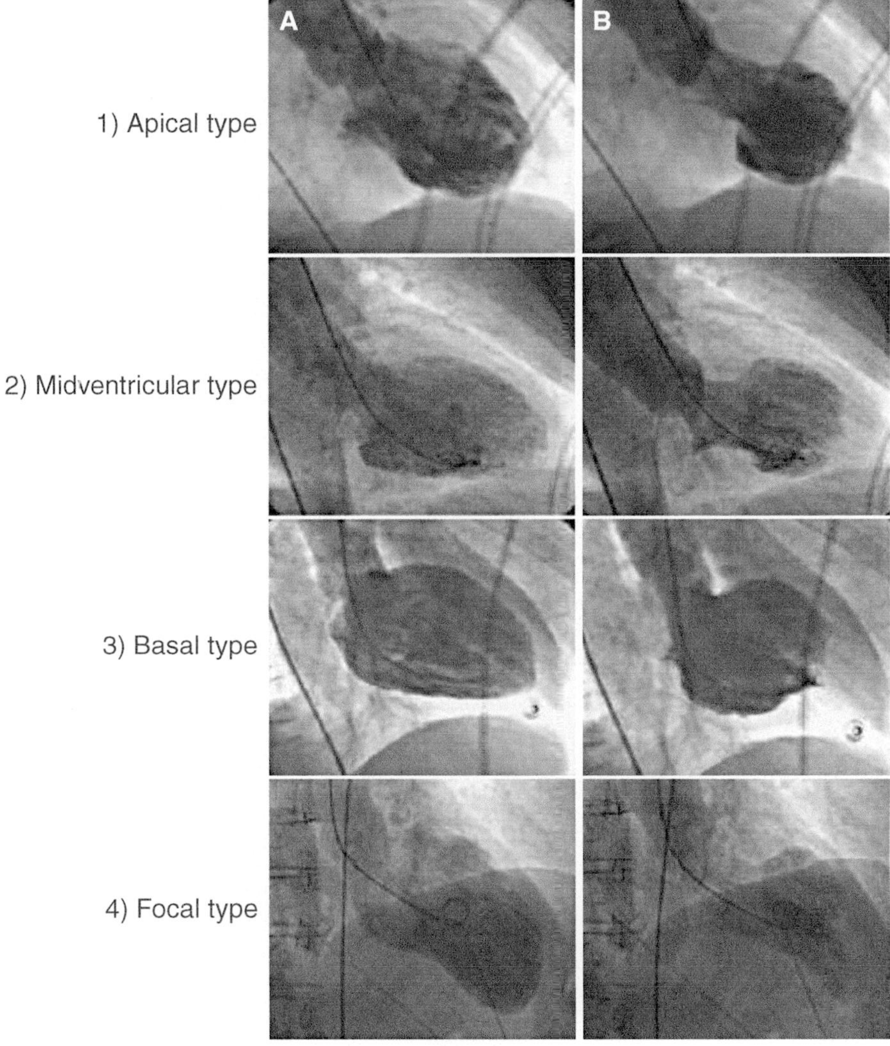

Fig. 7.4 The four different types of Takotsubo Syndrome during diastole (panel **A**) and systole (panel **B**): apical, midventricular, basal, and focal wall motion patterns

to typical TTS [38]. In-hospital complication rate is similar between typical and atypical types, while 1-year mortality is higher in typical TTS [38]. After adjustment for confounders, LVEF <45%, atrial fibrillation, neurologic disorders but not TTS phenotype were independent predictors of death. Beyond 1-year, long-term mortality is similar in typical and atypical TTS phenotypes, therefore, patients should be equally monitored and treated [38]. The basal phenotype has been reported to be associated with the presence of pheochromocytoma, epinephrine-induced TTS or subarachnoid haemorrhage consequently, these conditions should be considered in this particular setting [39]. Besides the four major TTS types, other morphological variants have been described including the biventricular (apical type and right ventricular involvement), isolated right ventricular, and global form [40]. Global hypokinesia as a manifestation of TTS is difficult to prove, given the very broad differential diagnoses including conditions such as tachycardia-induced cardiomyopathy. Right ventricular involvement is present in about one-third of TTS patients and may be a predictor for worse outcome [41]. The true prevalence of the isolated right ventricular form is unknown since little attention is paid to the right ventricle in daily clinical echo routine. Patients with recurrent TTS can demonstrate different wall motion patterns at each event suggesting that LV adrenergic receptor distribution does not explain different TTS types.

MCE with adenosine may confirm the diagnosis by showing reversible coronary microvascular constriction [42]. CMR with contrast medium shows the typical LV dysfunction associated with a hyperintense signal on T2 sequences without detectable myocardial necrosis after gadolinium administration [43].

Finally, F-18 fluorodeoxyglucose positron emission is providing encouraging results in the diagnosis of TTS [44].

Although TTS is generally considered a benign disease, contemporary observations show that rates of cardiogenic shock and death are comparable to ACS patients treated according to current guidelines.

While TTS is a reversible condition, hemodynamic and electrical instability during the acute phase expose patients to the risk of serious adverse in-hospital events which occur in approximately one-fifth of TTS patients. This substantial incidence of life-threatening complications requires close monitoring and early intervention in unstable TTS patients with risk stratification at diagnosis allowing triage to appropriate care. Parameters predicting adverse in-hospital outcome include: physical trigger, acute neurologic or psychiatric diseases, initial troponin >10 upper reference limit, and admission LVEF <45%. Furthermore, male patients have an up to three-fold increased rate of death and major adverse cardiac and cerebrovascular events (MACCE) and more often had an underlying critical illness, further contributing to the higher mortality [45]. Sobue et al. [46] demonstrated that physical triggers and male gender represent independent risk factors of in-hospital mortality in TTS. Data from the Tokyo Coronary Care Unit Network revealed that high values of BNP and white blood cell counts were also linked to higher rates of in-hospital complications [47]. Complications included cardiac death, pump failure (Killip grade ≥II), sustained ventricular tachycardia or ventricular fibrillation, and advanced atrio ventricular block. In the study by Takashio et al. [48] the magnitude and extent of ST-segment elevation with ECG were found to be independent predictors of in-hospital adverse events. However, those findings were not confirmed by others. Common in-hospital complications include cardiac arrhythmias, left ventricular outflow tract obstruction (LVOTO), cardiogenic shock, ventricular thrombus, pulmonary oedema, ventricular septal defect, and free wall rupture. In addition, to the demographic parameter of age ≥75, echocardiographic parameters that predict adverse in-hospital outcome (acute heart failure, cardiogenic shock, and in-hospital mortality) include LVEF, E/e' ratio, and reversible moderate to severe mitral regurgitation (MR). However, only reversible moderate to severe MR was an independent predictor when considering cardiogenic shock and death as the composite outcome in this study, in addition to heart rate [49]. Moreover, it has been demonstrated that high heart rate and low systolic blood pressure are associated with increased mortality in TTS [50]. Along with the Charlson comorbidity index and systolic pulmonary artery pressure, right ventricular involvement is an independent predictor of acute heart failure and of a composite endpoint including adverse events, such as acute heart failure, cardiogenic shock, and in-hospital mortality [50].

Data on long-term survival are scarce. In 2007, Elesber et al. [51] reported that long-term mortality did not differ between a TTS population and an age-, gender-, birth-, year-, and race-matched population.

While Sharkey et al. [52] found that all-cause mortality during follow up exceeded a matched general population with most deaths occurring in the first year. More recently, it has been reported that long-term mortality of patients with TTS is similar to patients with CAD [53]. TTS patient data from the Swedish Angiography and Angioplasty Registry (SCAAR) from 2009 to 2013 were compared to data from patients with and without CAD, and demonstrated that mortality rates for TTS were worse than in patients without CAD and comparable to those of patients with CAD [54]. In the largest TTS registry to date, death rates are estimated to be 5.6% and rate of MACCE 9.9% per-patient year, suggesting that TTS is not a benign disease. A recent study found that patients with the typical TTS type have a comparable outcome to patients presenting with the atypical type even after adjustment for confounders, suggesting that both patient groups should be equally monitored in the long-term [38]. On the other hand, 1-year mortality differs between the two groups, as it is driven by clinical factors including atrial fibrillation, LVEF on admission <45%, and neurologic disorders, rather than by TTS type [38]. In a smaller study, predictive factors of long-term mortality in TTS were male sex, Killip class III/IV, and diabetes mellitus [54].

The prognostic role of diabetes mellitus is controversial, as it is postulated that it may exert a protective effect in TTS, given that the prevalence of diabetes mellitus in TTS is lower than expected for an age and sex-matched population.

Patients who survive the initial event have a second event in approximately 5% of cases, mostly occurring 3 weeks to 3.8 years after the first event. Recurrent TTS afflicts men and women and may occur at any age including in childhood [36].

Some have postulated that an index TTS event may protect the affected LV regions from recurrent involvement through a mechanism akin to ischaemic 'preconditioning' [38]. However, detailed review of published cases and clinical experience suggest that there are frequent examples of recurrence in which the ballooning pattern is similar between episodes, thereby making this hypothesis unlikely.

Guidelines regarding TTS management are lacking as no prospective randomized clinical trials have been performed in this patient population. Therapeutic strategies are therefore based on clinical experience and expert consensus (evidence level C).

As TTS is clinically difficult to distinguish from ACS, upon first presentation patients should be transferred to a cardiology unit with imaging capabilities and a cardiac catheterization laboratory and receive guideline based treatment of ACS [38] in particular aspirin, heparin, and if required morphine and oxygen. Patients with cardiogenic shock or post cardiac arrest require intensive care. Electrocardiogram monitoring is essential as a prolonged QT-interval may trigger malignant ventricular arrhythmias (torsades de pointes) and AV-block may occur.

Takotsubo syndrome patients with cardiogenic shock, in particular those with apical ballooning should be promptly evaluated for the presence of LVOTO, which occurs in about 20% of cases. This should be performed during angiography with LV pressure recording during careful retraction of the pigtail catheter from the LV apex beyond the aortic valve. Similarly, a pressure gradient can be detected and quantified using Doppler echocardiography using continuous wave Doppler. Particularly, when using catecholamines serial Doppler studies should be considered to detect an evolving pressure gradient. In TTS patients treated with catecholamine drugs a 20% mortality has been reported; although this may represent a selection bias due to the initial presentation of the patients. Recently, it has been suggested that the Ca2þ-sensitizer levosimendan could be used safely and effectively in TTS as an alternative inotrope to catecholamine agents [38]. Furthermore, beta-blockers may improve LVOTO, but are contraindicated in acute and severe heart failure with low LVEF, hypotension, and in those with bradycardia. Although evidence is unproven, TTS patients with LVOTO may benefit from the If channel inhibitor ivabradine. As catecholamine levels are elevated in TTS, beta-blockers seem to be reasonable until full recovery of LVEF, but trials supporting this hypothesis are lacking. Animal experiments have shown that apical ballooning is attenuated after administration of drugs with both alpha and beta-adrenoceptor blocking properties. In an animal model, intravenous metoprolol improved epinephrine-induced apical ballooning [55]. However, due to the potential risk of pause-dependent torsades de pointes, beta-blockers should be used cautiously, especially in patients with bradycardia and QTc >500 ms. Angiotensinconverting-enzyme inhibitors (ACEi) or angiotensin II receptor blockers (ARB) may potentially facilitate LV recovery. Diuretics are recommended in patients with pulmonary oedema. In addition, nitroglycerin is useful to reduce LV and right ventricular filling pressures and afterload in the case of acute heart failure; however, the administration of nitroglycerin in the presence of LVOTO has been found to worsen the pressure gradient and therefore should be avoided in this scenario.

QT-interval prolonging drugs should be used cautiously in the acute phase because of the risk to induce torsades de pointes or ventricular tachycardia and fibrillation. Severe LV dysfunction with extended apical ballooning entails the risk of an LV thrombus and subsequent systemic embolism. Although evidence is lacking, anticoagulation with intravenous/subcutaneous heparin would appear to be appropriate in such patients and post-discharge oral anticoagulation or antiplatelet therapy may be considered on an individual, per-patient basis. As LV dysfunction and ECG abnormalities are reversible, an implantable cardioverter defibrillator for primary or secondary prevention is of uncertain value in TTS patients experiencing malignant ventricular arrhythmias.

In case of excessive prolongation of the QT interval or life-threatening ventricular arrhythmias a wearable defibrillator could be considered [38]. The residual risk of malignant arrhythmic events after recovery from TTS is unknown. A temporary trans-venous pacemaker is appropriate for those with haemodynamically significant bradycardia.

The use of ACEi or ARB was associated with improved survival at 1-year follow-up even after propensity matching. In contrast, there was no evidence of any survival benefit for the use of beta-blockers.

Moreover, one-third of patients experienced a TTS recurrence during beta-blockade suggesting that other receptors such as alpha-receptors, that are more prevalent in the coronary microcirculation, might be involved.

The prevalence of recurrent TTS is relatively low, consequently conducting randomised trials of pharmacological agents to prevent recurrence is challenging. Beta-blocker therapy after hospital discharge does not appear to prevent recurrence [31], whereas ACEi or ARB are associated with a lower prevalence of recurrence. The significance of this observation remains uncertain and requires validation in other cohorts.

If concomitant coronary atherosclerosis is present, aspirin and statins are appropriate. As TTS mainly occurs in postmenopausal women, oestrogen supplementation in those with recurrence is questionable.

Myocarditis

Myocarditis has a variable presentation including an ACS-like presentation in the presence/absence of ventricular dysfunction and without obstructive CAD. In patients with a classical myocarditis presentation, the specific diagnosis of myocarditis should be made before or at coronary angiography, but in many cases the diagnosis will not be clinically apparent and the working diagnosis of MINOCA should be made until specific testing is performed.

The prevalence of myocarditis among patients with a clinical diagnosis of MINOCA varies based on the populations studied, with a prevalence of 33% in a recent meta-analysis [56]. The most common cause of biopsy-proven myocarditis is viral infection, confirmed with polymerase chain reaction (PCR) assay of the pathogen DNA/RNA on endomyocardial biopsy (EMB). Adenoviruses, parvovirus B19 (PVB19), human herpesvirus 6 and Coxsackie virus are considered the most common causes of viral myocarditis [57]. Previous studies suggested that the clinical presentation is related to the type of virus [57]. In particular, PVB19 myocarditis may mimick MINOCA.

Endothelial cells represent PVB19-specific targets in PVB19-associated myocarditis, probably through blood group P antigen [58]. Thus, symptoms of chest pain and ST segment elevation at ECG in patients with viral myocarditis but no obstructive CAD, may be caused by intense coronary microvascular constriction, as a result of myocardial inflammation and/or PVB19 infection of vascular endothelial cells and microvascular dysfunction. Accordingly, Yilmaz et al. [58] demonstrated that, after administration of Ach, patients with myocarditis mimicking MINOCA showed a CAS at the distal segment of epicardial vessel, with probable extension at the microvascular level. In conclusion, the infection of coronary endothelial cells with PVB19 may cause a kind of "coronary vasculitis" which may constitute a major determinant of the clinical course and the myocardial spread of inflammation.

Other causes of myocarditis are immunomediated diseases, endocrine diseases, drugs and toxins [59].

Autoimmune myocarditis may occur with exclusive cardiac involvement or in the context of systemic autoimmune disorders, e.g. systemic lupus erythematosus and is infection-negative by PCR on EMB [59].

The initial investigation of suspected myocarditis should include CMR imaging. Although this non-invasive investigation compares favourably with the gold-standard technique of EMB [60], only EMB provides the opportunity of identifying the underlying cause for the myocarditis. CMR has been reported to detect 79% of EMB-confirmed myocarditis [61]. Furthermore, in the new ESC guidelines on Pericardial disease CMR is recommended for the confirmation of myocardial involvement (myocarditis) as a Class I recommendation [61].

The importance of diagnosing myocarditis in patients with MINOCA relates to its prognosis and treatment. Myocarditis resolve over a 2–4 weeks period in 50% of patients, but 12–25% may acutely deteriorate and either succumb to fulminant heart failure or progress onto end-stage dilated cardiomyopathy requiring heart transplantation [62]. Giant cell myocarditis is particularly associated with a poor prognosis [62]. Thus patients with myocarditis may require intravenous inotropic agents and/or mechanical circulatory support as a bridge to recovery or transplantation, and do not require anti-ischaemic therapies utilized in other causes of MINOCA.

The diagnosis of biopsy-proven infection-negative myocarditis is the basis for safe immunosuppression, that is indicated in specific autoimmune forms, such as in giant cell myocarditis, which is associated with a poor prognosis, cardiac sarcoidosis, eosinophilic myocarditis, as well as in lymphocitic forms refractory to standard therapy [62]. EMB also provides differential diagnosis with other causes of MINOCA, including Takotsubo cardiomyopathy.

Treatment of myocarditis mimicking MI and characterized by LV dysfunction is based on the use of beta-blockers and ACEI. In the last years, many trials have been designed in order to detect further therapeutic approach, with controversial results. A recent study demonstrated that, in the enteroviral and adenoviral myocarditis characterized by LV dysfunction, virus clearance obtained with the interferon-beta administration, seems be associated with a more favourable prognosis compared to those with virus persistence [63]. Actually, there are no effective treatments for PVB19 myocarditis.

Coronary Thromboembolism

Coronary embolism is included in microvascular causes of MINOCA as it usually involves microcirculation, although an angiographically visible embolization of epicardial coronary artery branches may occur. Of note, in this latter case, the coronary arteries are obviously not normal due to the evidence of either an abrupt vessel stump or thrombotic material inside epicardial coronary artery. Coronary thrombosis may arise from hereditary or acquired thrombotic disorders and coronary emboli may occur from coronary or systemic arterial thrombi.

Hereditary thrombophilia disorders include Factor V Leiden thrombophilia, Protein S and C deficiencies. Thrombophilia screening studies in patients with MINOCA have reported a 14% prevalence of these inherited disorders [64]. Acquired thrombophilia disorders should also be considered such as the antiphospholipid syndrome and myeloproliferative disorders, although these have not been systematically investigated in MINOCA.

Paradoxical embolism due to right-left shunts might be a rare cause of MINOCA. It can be related to a patent foramen ovale (PFO), a large atrial septal defect or a coronary arteriovenous fistula [65]. Of note, paradoxical embolism has been described relatively often as cause of systemic embolization, especially for cryptogenic stroke [65]. Coronary emboli may also occur in the context of the above thrombophilia disorders or other predisposing hypercoagulable states such as atrial fibrillation and valvular heart disease. Emboli may arise from non-thrombotic sources also including valvular vegetations, cardiac tumours (e.g. myxoma and papillary fibroelastoma), calcified valves, and iatrogenic air emboli.

The criteria for paradoxical embolism diagnosis include: evidence of arterial embolism in absence of a source in the left heart, source of embolism in the venous system, and communication between venous and arterial circulation [65]. Transthoracic, transesophageal, and bubble contrast- echocardiography are the cornerstone methods for detection of cardiac sources of embolism as causes of MINOCA. Moreover, Wöhrle et al. [66] demonstrated subclinical MI in 10.8% of patients with PFO undergoing CMR after a first cryptogenic cerebral ischemic event. Importantly, in patients in whom paradoxical embolism is suspected, coronary angiography needs to be carefully analyzed for the identification of amputation of distal coronary branches. Finally, left-side origin of coronary embolism should be also excluded.

Prognostic data of patients with paroxysmal embolism and MINOCA derive mostly from case reports and is mainly determined by the underlying cause which needs to be carefully identified as well as for cases caused by thrombus formation on left-side structures.

The standard treatment remains individualized and mostly focused on multiple factors including patient characteristics, time of presentation, and presence or absence of other embolic sites. Regarding atrial septal defect, paroxysmal embolism requires trans-catheter device closure or surgical repair [67, 68]. The options for secondary prevention of PFO induced cryptogenic embolism consist in the administration of antithrombotic medications or in percutaneous closure [67, 68]. Of note, the last studies showed that, among patients who had had a recent cryptogenic stroke attributed to PFO, the rate of stroke recurrence was lower among those assigned to PFO closure combined with antiplatelet therapy than among those assigned to antiplatelet therapy alone. However, PFO closure was associated with higher rates of device complications and atrial fibrillation [68].

Anticoagulant therapy may finally be appropriate for the prevention of embolic events in left-side origin coronary embolism.

Miscellanea

Other Forms of Type-2 MI

Type 2 AMI is defined as myocardial cell necrosis due to supply–demand mismatch, characterized by significant increase and/or decrease in troponins with at least one value above the 99th percentile of a normal reference population in the absence of evidence for coronary plaque rupture in addition to at least one of the other criteria for AMI [8]. Among patients with non-obstructive CAD, a profound supply–demand mismatch should be present to consider type-2 AMI. Therapeutically, the condition underlying the oxygen supply–demand mismatch is to be reversed if possible. Furthermore, aspirin and b-blockers may be useful and application of specific secondary prevention measures must be considered in the context of the specific insult.

MINOCA with Uncertain Aetiology

CMR imaging is a useful tool in MINOCA patients because it provides insights into potential causes and confirmation of the diagnosis of AMI. In particular, the presence and pattern of any LGE may point towards a vascular or non-vascular cause. However, 8–67% of patients with MINOCA have no evidence of LGE, myocardial oedema, or wall motion abnormalities on CMR [69].

A possible explanation could be that some patients with normal CMR may have too little myonecrosis to be detected. Alternatively, the normal CMR appearance might be the result of a broader spatial distribution of myonecrosis. That is, necrotic myocytes may be distributed over a larger area with no contiguous island of cell death of sufficient size to be detected by LGE imaging.

When CMR is normal and diagnostic evaluation as recommended herein does not reveal the mechanism of AMI, there is a diagnostic and therapeutic dilemma for clinicians. From first principles, vasospastic angina, coronary plaque disease, or thromboembolism may all potentially cause MINOCA with normal CMR imaging. In a series of patients with MINOCA who underwent both CMR and IVUS imaging, a subset of those with plaque disruption had a normal CMR (25%). If intracoronary imaging had not been performed during cardiac catheterization, this diagnosis would have been missed. Furthermore, MINOCA studies undertaking provocative spasm testing or assessing microvascular dysfunction have not routinely performed before CMR. However, epicardial CAS may produce transient trans-mural myocardial ischaemia that is associated with a small troponin rise [70] An alternative consideration is that the troponin rise is due to other causes such as pulmonary embolism or myocarditis.

Regarding the treatment, aspirin, statins and, in cases of vasospasm, calcium channel blockers as routine treatments could be proposed, since these would be of benefit for the potential underlying mechanisms of coronary plaque disease, coronary spasm, and thromboembolism.

Conclusions

MINOCA patients represent a conundrum given the very many possible aetiologies and pathogenic mechanisms associated with this syndrome. Clarify the underlying individual mechanisms is crucial to achieve patient-specific treatments.

References

1. Niccoli G, Scalone G, Crea F. Acute myocardial infarction with no obstructive coronary atherosclerosis: mechanisms and management. Eur Heart J. 2015;36:475–81.
2. Ibanez B, James S, Agewall S, Antunes MJ, Bucciarelli-Ducci C, Bueno H, Caforio ALP, Crea F, Goudevenos JA, Halvorsen S, Hindricks G, Kastrati A, Lenzen MJ, Prescott E, Roffi M, Valgimigli M, Varenhorst C, Vranckx P, Widimský P, ESC Scientific Document Group, ESC Scientific Document Group. 2017 ESC Guidelines for the management of acute myocardial infarction in patients presenting with ST-segment elevation: The Task Force for the management of acute myocardial infarction in patients presenting with ST-segment elevation of the European Society of Cardiology (ESC). Eur Heart J. 2018;39:119–77.
3. Gehrie ER, Reynolds HR, Chen AY, Neelon BH, Roe MT, Gibler WB, Ohman EM, Newby LK, Peterson ED, Hochman JS. Characterization and outcomes of women and men with non-ST-segment elevation myocardial infarction and nonobstructive coronary artery disease: results from the Can Rapid Risk Stratification of Unstable Angina Patients Suppress Adverse Outcomes with Early Implementation of the ACC/AHA Guidelines (CRUSADE) quality improvement initiative. Am Heart J. 2009;158:688–94.

4. Planer D, Mehran R, Ohman EM, White HD, Newman JD, Xu K, Stone GW. Prognosis of patients with non-ST-segment-elevation myocardial infarction and nonobstructive coronary artery disease: propensity-matched analysis from the Acute Catheterization and Urgent Intervention Triage Strategy Trial. Circ Cardiovasc Interv. 2014;7:285–93.
5. Daniel M, Agewall S, Caidahl K, Collste O, Ekenbäck C, Frick M, Y-Hassan S, Henareh L, Jernberg T, Malmqvist K, Schenck-Gustafsson K, Sörensson P, Sundin Ö, Hofman-Bang C, Tornvall P. Effect of myocardial infarction with nonobstructive coronary arteries on physical capacity and quality-of-life. Am J Cardiol. 2017;120:341–6.
6. Pasupathy S, Air T, Dreyer RP, Tavella R, Beltrame JF. Systematic review of patients presenting with suspected myocardial infarction and nonobstructive coronary arteries. Circulation. 2015;131:861–70.
7. Agewall S, Beltrame JF, Reynolds HR, Niessner A, Rosano G, Caforio AL, De Caterina R, Zimarino M, Roffi M, Kjeldsen K, Atar D, Kaski JC, Sechtem U, Tornvall P, WG on Cardiovascular Pharmacotherapy. ESC working group position paper on myocardial infarction with non-obstructive coronary arteries. Eur Heart J. 2017;38:143–53.
8. Thygesen K, Alpert JS, Jaffe AS, Simoons ML, Chaitman BR, White HD, Writing Group on the Joint ESC/ACCF/AHA/WHF Task Force for the Universal Definition of Myocardial Infarction, Thygesen K, Alpert JS, White HD, Jaffe AS, Katus HA, Apple FS, Lindahl B, Morrow DA, Chaitman BA, Clemmensen PM, Johanson P, Hod H, Underwood R, Bax JJ, Bonow RO, Pinto F, Gibbons RJ, Fox KA, Atar D, Newby LK, Galvani M, Hamm CW, Uretsky BF, Steg PG, Wijns W, Bassand JP, Menasché P, Ravkilde J, Ohman EM, Antman EM, Wallentin LC, Armstrong PW, Simoons ML, Januzzi JL, Nieminen MS, Gheorghiade M, Filippatos G, Luepker RV, Fortmann SP, Rosamond WD, Levy D, Wood D, Smith SC, Hu D, Lopez-Sendon JL, Robertson RM, Weaver D, Tendera M, Bove AA, Parkhomenko AN, Vasilieva EJ, Mendis S, ESC Committee for Practice Guidelines (CPG). Third universal definition of myocardial infarction. Eur Heart J. 2012;33:2551–67.
9. Ouldzein H, Elbaz M, Roncalli J, Cagnac R, Carrié D, Puel J, Alibelli-Chemarin MJ. Plaque rupture and morphological characteristics of the culprit lesion in acute coronary syndromes without significant angiographic lesion: analysis by intravascular ultrasound. Ann Cardiol Angeiol. 2012;61:20–6.
10. Jia H, Abtahian F, Aguirre AD, Lee S, Chia S, Lowe H, Kato K, Yonetsu T, Vergallo R, Hu S, Tian J, Lee H, Park SJ, Jang YS, Raffel OC, Mizuno K, Uemura S, Itoh T, Kakuta T, Choi SY, Dauerman HL, Prasad A, Toma C, McNulty I, Zhang S, Yu B, Fuster V, Narula J, Virmani R, Jang IK. In vivo diagnosis of plaque erosion and calcified nodule in patients with acute coronary syndrome by intravascular optical coherence tomography. J Am Coll Cardiol. 2013;62:1748–58.
11. Iqbal SN, Feit F, Mancini GB, Wood D, Patel R, Pena-Sing I, Attubato M, Yatskar L, Slater JN, Hochman JS, Reynolds HR. Characteristics of plaque disruption by intravascularultrasound in women presenting with myocardial infarction without obstructive coronary artery disease. Am Heart J. 2014;167:715–22.
12. Reynolds HR, Srichai MB, Iqbal SN, Slater JN, Mancini GB, Feit F, Pena-Sing I, Axel L, Attubato MJ, Yatskar L, Kalhorn RT, Wood DA, Lobach IV, Hochman JS. Mechanisms of myocardial infarction in women without angiographically obstructive coronary artery disease. Circulation. 2011;124:1414–25.
13. Patel MR, Chen AY, Peterson ED, Newby LK, Pollack CV Jr, Brindis RG, Gibson CM, Kleiman NS, Saucedo JF, Bhatt DL, Gibler WB, Ohman EM, Harrington RA, Roe MT. Prevalence, predictors, and outcomes of patients with non-ST-segment elevation myocardial infarction and insignificant coronary artery disease: results from the Can Rapid risk stratification of Unstable angina patients Suppress ADverse outcomes with Early implementation of the ACC/AHA Guidelines (CRUSADE) initiative. Am Heart J. 2006;152:641–7.
14. Roffi M, Patrono C, Collet JP, Mueller C, Valgimigli M, Andreotti F, Bax JJ, Borger MA, Brotons C, Chew DP, Gencer B, Hasenfuss G, Kjeldsen K, Lancellotti P, Landmesser U, Mehilli J, Mukherjee D, Storey RF, Windecker S, ESC Scientific Document Group. 2015

ESC Guidelines for the management of acute coronary syndromes in patients presenting without persistent ST-segment elevation: Task Force for the Management of Acute Coronary Syndromes in Patients Presenting without Persistent ST-Segment Elevation of the European Society of Cardiology (ESC). Eur Heart J. 2016;37:267–315.

15. Antonsen L, Thayssen P, Jensen LO. Large coronary intramural hematomas: a case series and focused literature review. Cardiovasc Revasc Med. 2015;16:116–23.
16. Saw J, Mancini GB, Humphries K, Fung A, Boone R, Starovoytov A, Aymong E. Angiographic appearance of spontaneous coronary artery dissection with intramural hematoma proven on intracoronary imaging. Catheter Cardiovasc Interv. 2016;87:E54–61.
17. Saw J, Aymong E, Mancini GB, Sedlak T, Starovoytov A, Ricci D. Nonatherosclerotic coronary artery disease in young women. Can J Cardiol. 2014;30:814–9.
18. Tweet MS, Hayes SN, Pitta SR, Simari RD, Lerman A, Lennon RJ, Gersh BJ, Khambatta S, Best PJ, Rihal CS, Gulati R. Clinical features, management, and prognosis of spontaneous coronary artery dissection. Circulation. 2012;126:579–88.
19. Jacqueline Saw Canadian SCAD Study ESC congress; 2018.
20. Montone RA, Niccoli G, Fracassi F, Russo M, Gurgoglione F, Cammà G, Lanza GA, Crea F. Patients with acute myocardial infarction and non-obstructive coronary arteries: safety and prognostic relevance of invasive coronary provocative tests. Eur Heart J. 2018;39:91–8.
21. Kaski JC, Crea F, Meran D, Rodriguez L, Araujo L, Chierchia S, Davies G, Maseri A. Local coronary supersensitivity to diverse vasoconstrictive stimuli in patients with variant angina. Circulation. 1986;74:1255–65.
22. Sueda S, Oshita A, Nomoto T, Izoe Y, Kohno H, Fukuda H, Mineoi K, Ochi T, Uraoka T. Recommendations for performing acetylcholine tests safely: STOP dangerous complications induced by acetylcholine tests (STOP DCIAT). J Cardiol. 2008;51:131–4.
23. Ong P, Athanasiadis A, Borgulya G, Vokshi I, Bastiaenen R, Kubik S, Hill S, Schäufele T, Mahrholdt H, Kaski JC, Sechtem U. Clinical usefulness, angiographic characteristics, and safety evaluation of intracoronary acetylcholine provocation testing among 921 consecutive white patients with unobstructed coronary arteries. Circulation. 2014;129:1723–30.
24. Wei J, Mehta PK, Johnson BD, Samuels B, Kar S, Anderson RD, Azarbal B, Petersen J, Sharaf B, Handberg E, Shufelt C, Kothawade K, Sopko G, Lerman A, Shaw L, Kelsey SF, Pepine CJ, Merz CN. Safety of coronary reactivity testing in women with no obstructive coronary artery disease: results from the NHLBI-sponsored WISE (Women's Ischemia Syndrome Evaluation) study. J Am Coll Cardiol Intv. 2012;5:646–53.
25. Lanza GA, Sestito A, Sgueglia GA, Infusino F, Manolfi M, Crea F, Maseri A. Current clinical features, diagnostic assessment and prognostic determinants of patients with variant angina. Int J Cardiol. 2007;118:41–7.
26. Mohri M, Koyanagi M, Egashira K, Tagawa H, Ichiki T, Shimokawa H, Takeshita A. Angina pectoris caused by coronary microvascular spasm. Lancet. 1998;351:1165–9.
27. Masumoto A, Mohri M, Takeshita A. Three-year follow-up of the Japanese patients with microvascular angina attributable to coronary microvascular spasm. Int J Cardiol. 2001;81:151–6.
28. Arrebola-Moreno AL, Arrebola JP, Moral-Ruiz A, Ramirez-Hernandez JA, Melgares-Moreno R, Kaski JC. Coronary microvascular spasm triggers transient ischemic left ventricular diastolic abnormalities in patients with chest pain and angiographically normal coronary arteries. Atherosclerosis. 2014;236:207–14.
29. Crea F, Bairey Merz CN, Beltrame JF, Kaski JC, Ogawa H, Ong P, Sechtem U, Shimokawa H, Camici PG, Coronary Vasomotion Disorders International Study Group (COVADIS). The parallel tales of microvascular angina and heart failure with preserved ejection fraction: a paradigm shift. Eur Heart J. 2017;38:473–7.
30. Redfors B, Vedad R, Angeras O, Ramunddal T, Petursson P, Haraldsson I, Ali A, Dworeck C, Odenstedt J, Ioaness D, Libungan B, Shao Y, Albertsson P, Stone GW, Omerovic E. Mortality in Takotsubo syndrome is similar to mortality in myocardial infarction—a report from the SWEDEHEART registry. Int J Cardiol. 2015;185:282–9.

31. Templin C, Ghadri JR, Diekmann J, Napp LC, Bataiosu DR, Jaguszewski M, Cammann VL, Sarcon A, Geyer V, Neumann CA, Seifert B, Hellermann J, Schwyzer M, Eisenhardt K, Jenewein J, Franke J, Katus HA, Burgdorf C, Schunkert H, Moeller C, Thiele H, Bauersachs J, Tschöpe C, Schultheiss H-P, Laney CA, Rajan L, Michels G, Pfister R, Ukena C, Böhm M, Erbel R, Cuneo A, Kuck K-H, Jacobshagen C, Hasenfuss G, Karakas M, Koenig W, Rottbauer W, Said SM, Braun-Dullaeus RC, Cuculi F, Banning A, Fischer TA, Vasankari T, Airaksinen KEJ, Fijalkowski M, Rynkiewicz A, Pawlak M, Opolski G, Dworakowski R, MacCarthy P, Kaiser C, Osswald S, Galiuto L, Crea F, Dichtl W, Franz WM, Empen K, Felix SB, Delmas C, Lairez O, Erne P, Bax JJ, Ford I, Ruschitzka F, Prasad A, Lüscher TF. Clinical features and outcomes of Takotsubo (stress) cardiomyopathy. N Engl J Med. 2015;373:929–38.
32. Franco E, Dias A, Koshkelashvili N, Pressman GS, Hebert K, Figueredo VM. Distinctive electrocardiographic features in African Americans diagnosed with Takotsubo cardiomyopathy. Ann Noninvasive Electrocardiol. 2016;21:486–92.
33. Qaqa A, Daoko J, Jallad N, Aburomeh O, Goldfarb I, Shamoon F. Takotsubo syndrome in African American vs. non-African American women. West J Emerg Med. 2011;12:218–23.
34. Park JH, Kang SJ, Song JK, Kim HK, Lim CM, Kang DH, Koh Y. Left ventricular apical ballooning due to severe physical stress in patients admitted to the medical ICU. Chest. 2005;128:296–302.
35. Madias JE. Why the current diagnostic criteria of Takotsubo syndrome are outmoded: a proposal for new criteria. Int J Cardiol. 2014;174:468–70.
36. Ghadri JR, Wittstein IS, Prasad A, Sharkey S, Dote K, Akashi YJ, Cammann VL, Crea F, Galiuto L, Desmet W, Yoshida T, Manfredini R, Eitel I, Kosuge M, Nef HM, Deshmukh A, Lerman A, Bossone E, Citro R, Ueyama T, Corrado D, Kurisu S, Ruschitzka F, Winchester D, Lyon AR, Omerovic E, Bax JJ, Meimoun P, Tarantini G, Rihal C, Y-Hassan S, Migliore F, Horowitz JD, Shimokawa H, Lüscher TF, Templin C. International expert consensus document on Takotsubo syndrome (part I): clinical characteristics, diagnostic criteria, and pathophysiology. Eur Heart J. 2018;39:2032–46.
37. Napp LC, Ghadri JR, Bauersachs J, Templin C. Acute coronary syndrome or Takotsubo cardiomyopathy: the suspect may not always be the culprit. Int J Cardiol. 2015;187:116–9.
38. Ghadri JR, Cammann VL, Napp LC, Jurisic S, Diekmann J, Bataiosu DR, Seifert B, Jaguszewski M, Sarcon A, Neumann CA, Geyer V, Prasad A, Bax JJ, Ruschitzka F, Luscher TF, Templin C, International Takotsubo Registry. Differences in the clinical profile and outcomes of typical and atypical Takotsubo syndrome: data from the International Takotsubo Registry. JAMA Cardiol. 2016;1:335–40.
39. Y-Hassan S. Clinical features and outcome of pheochromocytoma-induced Takotsubo syndrome: analysis of 80 published cases. Am J Cardiol. 2016;117:1836–44.
40. Elikowski W, Malek M, Lanocha M, Wroblewski D, Angerer D, Kurosz J, Rachuta K. [Reversible dilated cardiomyopathy as an atypical form of Takotsubo cardiomyopathy]. Pol Merkur Lekarski. 2013;34:219–23.
41. Eitel I, von Knobelsdorff-Brenkenhoff F, Bernhardt P, Carbone I, Muellerleile K, Aldrovandi A, Francone M, Desch S, Gutberlet M, Strohm O, Schuler G, Schulz-Menger J, Thiele H, Friedrich MG. Clinical characteristics and cardiovascular magnetic resonance findings in stress (Takotsubo) cardiomyopathy. JAMA. 2011;306:277–86.
42. Galiuto L, De Caterina AR, Porfidia A, Paraggio L, Barchetta S, Locorotondo G, Rebuzzi AG, Crea F. Reversible coronary microvascular dysfunction: a common pathogenetic mechanism in apical ballooning or Takotsubo syndrome. Eur Heart J. 2010;31:1319–27.
43. Collste O, Sörensson P, Frick M, Agewall S, Daniel M, Henareh L, Ekenbäck C, Eurenius L, Guiron C, Jernberg T, Hofman-Bang C, Malmqvist K, Nagy E, Arheden H, Tornvall P. Myocardial infarction with normal coronary arteries is common and associated with normal findings on cardiovascular magnetic resonance imaging: results from the Stockholm Myocardial Infarction with Normal Coronaries study. J Intern Med. 2013;273:189–96.
44. Cacciotti L, Passaseo I, Marazzi G, Camastra G, Campolongo G, Beni S, Lupparelli F, Ansalone G. Observational study on Takotsubo-like cardiomyopathy: clinical features, diagnosis, prognosis and follow-up. BMJ Open. 2012;5:e001165.

45. Brinjikji W, El-Sayed AM, Salka S. In-hospital mortality among patients with Takotsubo cardiomyopathy: a study of the National Inpatient Sample 2008 to 2009. Am Heart J. 2012;164:215–21.
46. Sobue Y, Watanabe E, Ichikawa T, Koshikawa M, Yamamoto M, Harada M, Ozaki Y. Physically triggered Takotsubo cardiomyopathy has a higher in-hospital mortality rate. Int J Cardiol. 2017;235:87–93.
47. Murakami T, Yoshikawa T, Maekawa Y, Ueda T, Isogai T, Konishi Y, Sakata K, Nagao K, Yamamoto T, Takayama M, Committee CCUNS. Characterization of predictors of in-hospital cardiac complications of Takotsubo cardiomyopathy: multi-center registry from Tokyo CCU Network. J Cardiol. 2014;63:269–73.
48. Takashio S, Yamamuro M, Kojima S, Izumiya Y, Kaikita K, Hokimoto S, Sugiyama S, Tsunoda R, Nakao K, Ogawa H. Usefulness of SUM of ST-segment elevation on electrocardiograms (limb leads) for predicting in-hospital complications in patients with stress (Takotsubo) cardiomyopathy. Am J Cardiol. 2012;109:1651–6.
49. Böhm M, Cammann VL, Ghadri JR, Ukena C, Gili S, Di Vece D, Kato K, Ding KJ, Szawan KA, Micek J, Jurisic S, D'Ascenzo F, Frangieh AH, Rechsteiner D, Seifert B, Ruschitzka F, Lüscher T, Templin C, InterTAK Collaborators. Interaction of systolic blood pressure and resting heart rate with clinical outcomes in Takotsubo syndrome: insights from the International Takotsubo Registry. Eur J Heart Fail. 2018;20:1021.
50. Citro R, Bossone E, Parodi G, Rigo F, Nardi F, Provenza G, Zito C, Novo G, Vitale G, Prota C, Silverio A, Vriz O, D'Andrea A, Antonini-Canterin F, Salerno-Uriarte J, Piscione F, Takotsubo Italian Network Investigators. Independent impact of RV involvement on in-hospital outcome of patients with Takotsubo syndrome. JACC Cardiovasc Imaging. 2016;9:894–5.
51. Elesber AA, Prasad A, Lennon RJ, Wright RS, Lerman A, Rihal CS. Four-year recurrence rate and prognosis of the apical ballooning syndrome. J Am Coll Cardiol. 2007;50:448–52.
52. Sharkey SW, Pink VR, Lesser JR, Garberich RF, Maron MS, Maron BJ. Clinical profile of patients with high-risk Tako-Tsubo cardiomyopathy. Am J Cardiol. 2015;116:765–72.
53. Stiermaier T, Moeller C, Oehler K, Desch S, Graf T, Eitel C, Vonthein R, Schuler G, Thiele H, Eitel I. Long-term excess mortality in Takotsubo cardiomyopathy: predictors, causes and clinical consequences. Eur J Heart Fail. 2016;18:650–6.
54. Tornvall P, Collste O, Ehrenborg E, Jarnbert-Petterson H. A case-control study of risk markers and mortality in Takotsubo stress cardiomyopathy. J Am Coll Cardiol. 2016;67:1931–6.
55. Izumi Y, Okatani H, Shiota M, Nakao T, Ise R, Kito G, Miura K, Iwao H. Effects of metoprolol on epinephrine-induced Takotsubo-like left ventricular dysfunction in non-human primates. Hypertens Res. 2009;32:339–46.
56. Tornvall P, Gerbaud E, Behaghel A, Chopard R, Collste O, Laraudogoitia E, Leurent G, Meneveau N, Montaudon M, Perez-David E, Sörensson P, Agewall S. A meta-analysis of individual data regarding prevalence and risk markers for myocarditis and infarction determined by cardiac magnetic resonance imaging in myocardial infarction with non-obstructive coronary artery disease. Atherosclerosis. 2015;241:87–91.
57. Mahrholdt H, Wagner A, Deluigi CC, Kispert E, Hager S, Meinhardt G, Vogelsberg H, Fritz P, Dippon J, Bock CT, Klingel K, Kandolf R, Sechtem U. Presentation, patterns of myocardial damage, and clinical course of viral myocarditis. Circulation. 2006;114:1581–90.
58. Yilmaz A, Mahrholdt H, Athanasiadis A, Vogelsberg H, Meinhardt G, Voehringer M, Kispert EM, Deluigi C, Baccouche H, Spodarev E, Klingel K, Kandolf R, Sechtem U. Coronary vasospasm as the underlying cause for chest pain in patients with PVB19 myocarditis. Heart. 2008;94:1456–63.
59. Caforio AL, Marcolongo R, Jahns R, Fu M, Felix SB, Iliceto S. Immune-mediated and autoimmune myocarditis: clinical presentation, diagnosis and management. Heart Fail Rev. 2013;18:715–32.
60. Caforio AL, Pankuweit S, Arbustini E, Basso C, Gimeno-Blanes J, Felix SB, Fu M, Heliö T, Heymans S, Jahns R, Klingel K, Linhart A, Maisch B, McKenna W, Mogensen J, Pinto YM, Ristic A, Schultheiss HP, Seggewiss H, Tavazzi L, Thiene G, Yilmaz A, Charron P, Elliott PM, European Society of Cardiology Working Group on Myocardial and Pericardial Diseases.

Current state of knowledge on aetiology, diagnosis, management and therapy of myocarditis. A position statement of the European Society of Cardiology Working Group on Myocardial and Pericardial Diseases. Eur Heart J. 2013;34:2636–48.
61. Leone O, Veinot JP, Angelini A, Baandrup UT, Basso C, Berry G, Bruneval P, Burke M, Butany J, Calabrese F, d'Amati G, Edwards WD, Fallon JT, Fishbein MC, Gallagher PJ, Halushka MK, McManus B, Pucci A, Rodriguez ER, Saffitz JE, Sheppard MN, Steenbergen C, Stone JR, Tan C, Thiene G, van der Wal AC, Winters GL. 2011 consensus statement on endomyocardial biopsy from the Association for European Cardiovascular Pathology and the Society for Cardiovascular Pathology. Cardiovasc Pathol. 2012;21:245–74.
62. Kindermann I, Kindermann M, Kandolf R, Klingel K, Bültmann B, Müller T, Lindinger A, Böhm M. Predictors of outcome in patients with suspected myocarditis. Circulation. 2008;118:639–48.
63. Kühl U, Lassner D, von Schlippenbach J, Poller W, Schultheiss HP. Interferon-beta improves survival in enterovirus-associated cardiomyopathy. J Am Coll Cardiol. 2012;60:1295–6.
64. Sastry S, Riding G, Morris J, Taberner D, Cherry N, Heagerty A, McCollum C. Young Adult Myocardial Infarction and Ischemic Stroke: the role of paradoxical embolism and thrombophilia (The YAMIS Study). J Am Coll Cardiol. 2006;48:686–91.
65. Srivastava TN, Payment MF. Images in clinical medicine. Paradoxical embolism thrombus in transit through a patent foramen ovale. N Engl J Med. 1997;337:681.
66. Wöhrle J, Kochs M, Hombach V, Merkle N. Prevalence of myocardial scar in patients with cryptogenic cerebral ischemic events and patent foramen ovale. JACC Cardiovasc Imaging. 2010;3:833–9.
67. Meier B, Kalesan B, Mattle HP, Khattab AA, Hildick-Smith D, Dudek D, Andersen G, Ibrahim R, Schuler G, Walton AS, Wahl A, Windecker S, Jüni P, PC Trial Investigators. Percutaneous closure of patent foramen ovale in cryptogenic embolism. N Engl J Med. 2013;368:1083–91.
68. Søndergaard L, Kasner SE, Rhodes JF, Andersen G, Iversen HK, Nielsen-Kudsk JE, Settergren M, Sjöstrand C, Roine RO, Hildick-Smith D, Spence JD, Thomassen L, Gore REDUCE Clinical Study Investigators. Patent foramen ovale closure or antiplatelet therapy for cryptogenic stroke. N Engl J Med. 2017;377:1033–42.
69. Baccouche H, Mahrholdt H, Meinhardt G, Merher R, Voehringer M, Hill S, Klingel K, Kandolf R, Sechtem U, Yilmaz A. Diagnostic synergy of non-invasive cardiovascular magnetic resonance and invasive endomyocardial biopsy in troponin-positive patients without coronary artery disease. Eur Heart J. 2009;30:2869–79.
70. Leurent G, Langella B, Fougerou C, Lentz PA, Larralde A, Bedossa M, Boulmier D, Le Breton H. Diagnostic contributions of cardiac magnetic resonance imaging in patients presenting with elevated troponin, acute chest pain syndrome and unobstructed coronary arteries. Arch Cardiovasc Dis. 2011;104:161–70.

Part II
Clinical Cases

Chapter 8
Role of Coronary Microcirculation in No-Reflow Phenomenon in Myocardial Infarction with ST Segment Elevation

Z. Vasiljevic-Pokrajcic, D. Trifunovic, G. Krljanac, and M. Zdravkovic

Case Presentation

A 45 years old male, heavy smoker, with BMI 24.2 kg/m^2, mild untreated hypertension, presented to the emergency department 4 h after initial chest pain, with significant ST segment elevation in anterior (anterolateral) leads consistent with acute myocardial infarction with ST segment elevation (STEMI) (Fig. 8.1). The greatest elevation of 11 mm was in V3 lead. He was given aspirin 300 mg po, clopidogrel 600 mg po and immediately referred to cath lab. Angiography revealed thrombotic occlusion of the proximal LAD and TIMI flow 0 (Fig. 8.2) with 70–90% stenosis of the right posterolateral branch and stenosis <50% in OM2.

Balloon predilatation of the culprit infarct lesion in the proximal LAD was done with 3.5 × 15 mm balloon at 8 ATM for 30 s, no indentation of the balloon was noted during the balloon inflation, and one bare metal stent (4.5 × 24 mm) was implanted on 18 ATM. However, a significant thrombus occurred on the distal edge of the stent. Accordingly, thrombus aspiration was done, 2 i.c. boluses of Tirofiban were given and the final result was optimized with in-stent postdilatation using 4.5 × 24 mm balloon, inflated on 14 ATM for 40 s. The final TIMI flow was 2 (Fig. 8.3). Immediately after pPCI transthoracic Doppler echocardiography revealed altered pattern of coronary flow through distal LAD: early systolic retrograde flow

Z. Vasiljevic-Pokrajcic (✉)
Faculty of Medicine, University of Belgrade, Belgrade, Serbia
e-mail: zoranav@eunet.rs

D. Trifunovic · G. Krljanac
Department of Cardiology, University Clinical Centre of Serbia, Faculty of Medicine, University of Belgrade, Belgrade, Serbia

M. Zdravkovic
University Clinical Hospital Centre Bezanijska Kosa, Faculty of Medicine, University of Belgrade, Belgrade, Serbia

M. Dorobantu, L. Badimon (eds.), *Microcirculation*,
https://doi.org/10.1007/978-3-030-28199-1_8

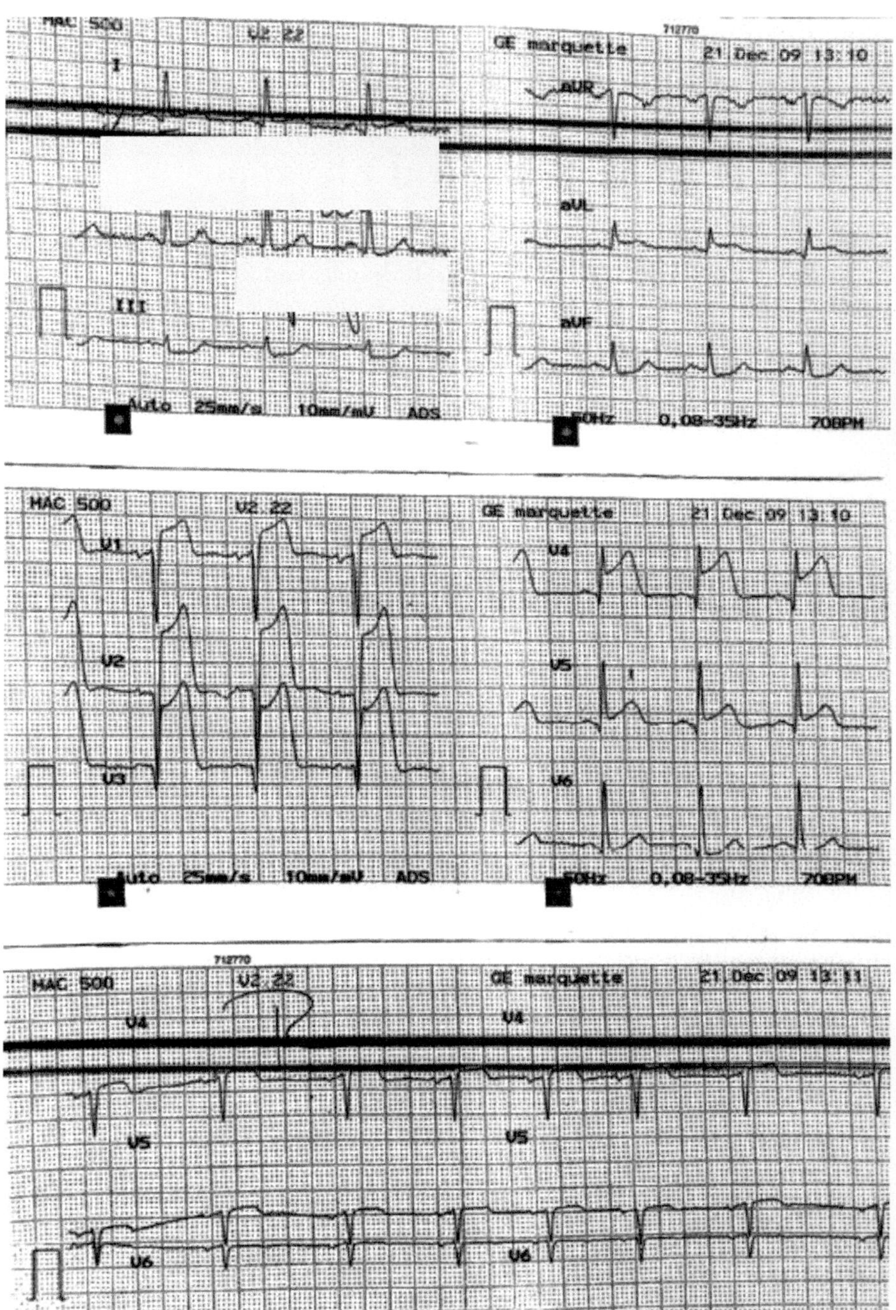

Fig. 8.1 ECG on admission: significant ST segment elevation in V1–V5, the greatest in V3

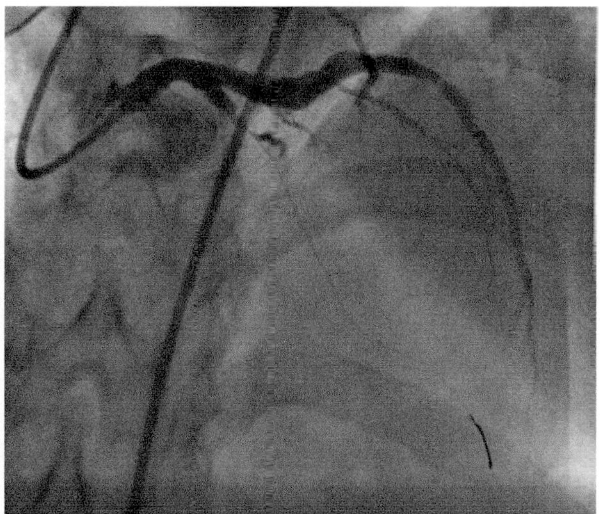

Fig. 8.2 Angiography revealed thrombotic occlusion of the proximal LAD and TIMI flow 0

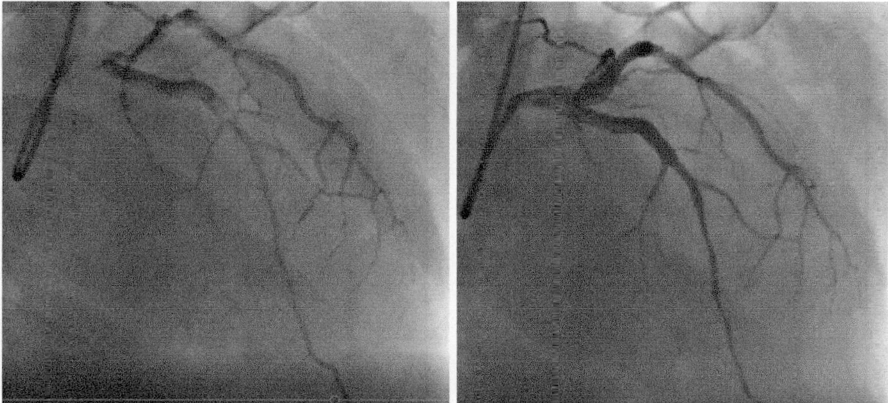

Fig. 8.3 Final angiography with stented LAD, slow-flow in LAD (TIMI flow 2)

(A) followed by low velocity anterograde systolic flow (B) and in diastole initial very short high velocity flow with steep deceleration (C) followed by the low flow velocity through the rest of diastole (D) (Fig. 8.4). This pattern was consistent with low flow/no-reflow. Echocardiography also revealed reduced left ventricular ejection fraction (LV EF) of 40% with akinesia of the medial and apical segments of septum, anterior wall and LV apex (Fig. 8.4). Patient was hemodynamically stable, tirofiban infusion was continued and he was back to the CCU. Control ECG after primary PCI revealed persistence of ST segment elevation with 36% reduction of ST segment elevation in V3 lead (from 11 mm to 4 mm) (Fig. 8.5).

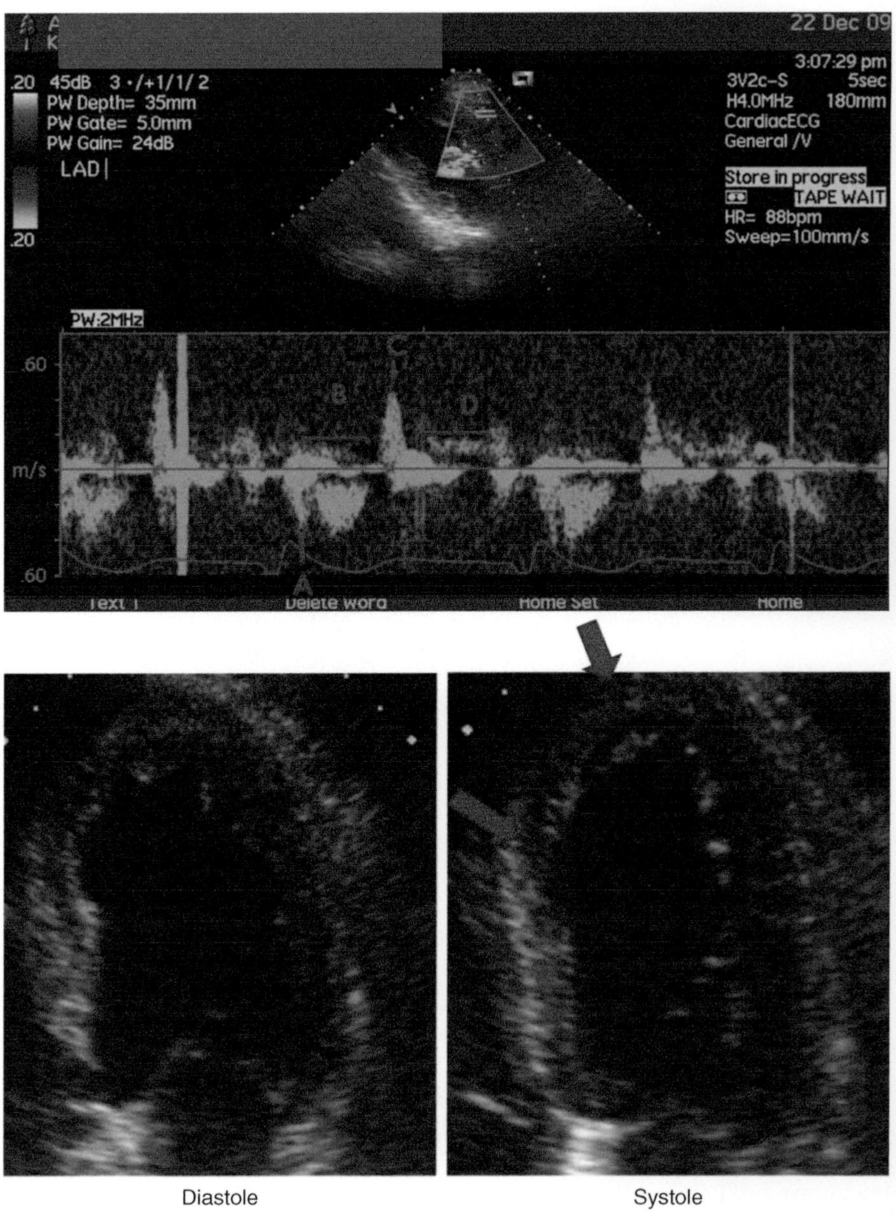

Fig. 8.4 Coronary flow and LV kinetics immediately after pPCI

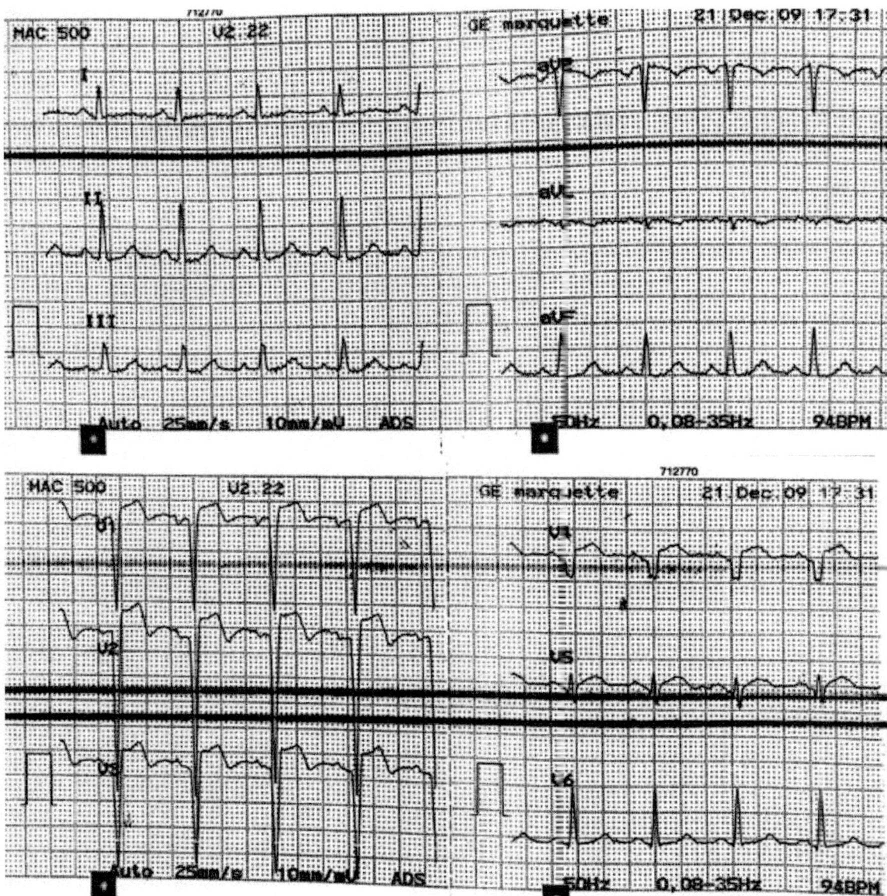

Fig. 8.5 ECG after the pPCI revealed persistence of ST segment elevation and resolution of the greatest ST segment elevation <50%

On the second day after pPCI coronary flow reserve (CFR) assessed by transthoracic Doppler echocardiography and adenosine as a stressor, was impaired (1.60), as well as LV EF (38%) with extensive akinesia encompassing LV apex, medial and apical segments of the septum and anterior wall, and apical segment of the lateral wall (Fig. 8.6). One-month after the pPCI mild LV enlargement with EF of 38% was noted by echo. By that time LAD CFR was 1.55. SPECT viability study confirmed enlarged LV (EDV 223 mL, ESV 148 mL) with impaired EF of 34%, large perfusion defect of 60% of the LV myocardium and Summed Rest Score of 42. Nonviable were LV apex, apical segments of anterior wall and septum, medial segments of septum had borderline viability, as well as basal segment of anterior wall (Fig. 8.7). By that time, patient was NYHA functional class II.

Five months after initial STEMI, patient suffered re-infarction due to in-stent thrombosis, and POBA for LAD in-stent thrombosis was done. However, 1 year

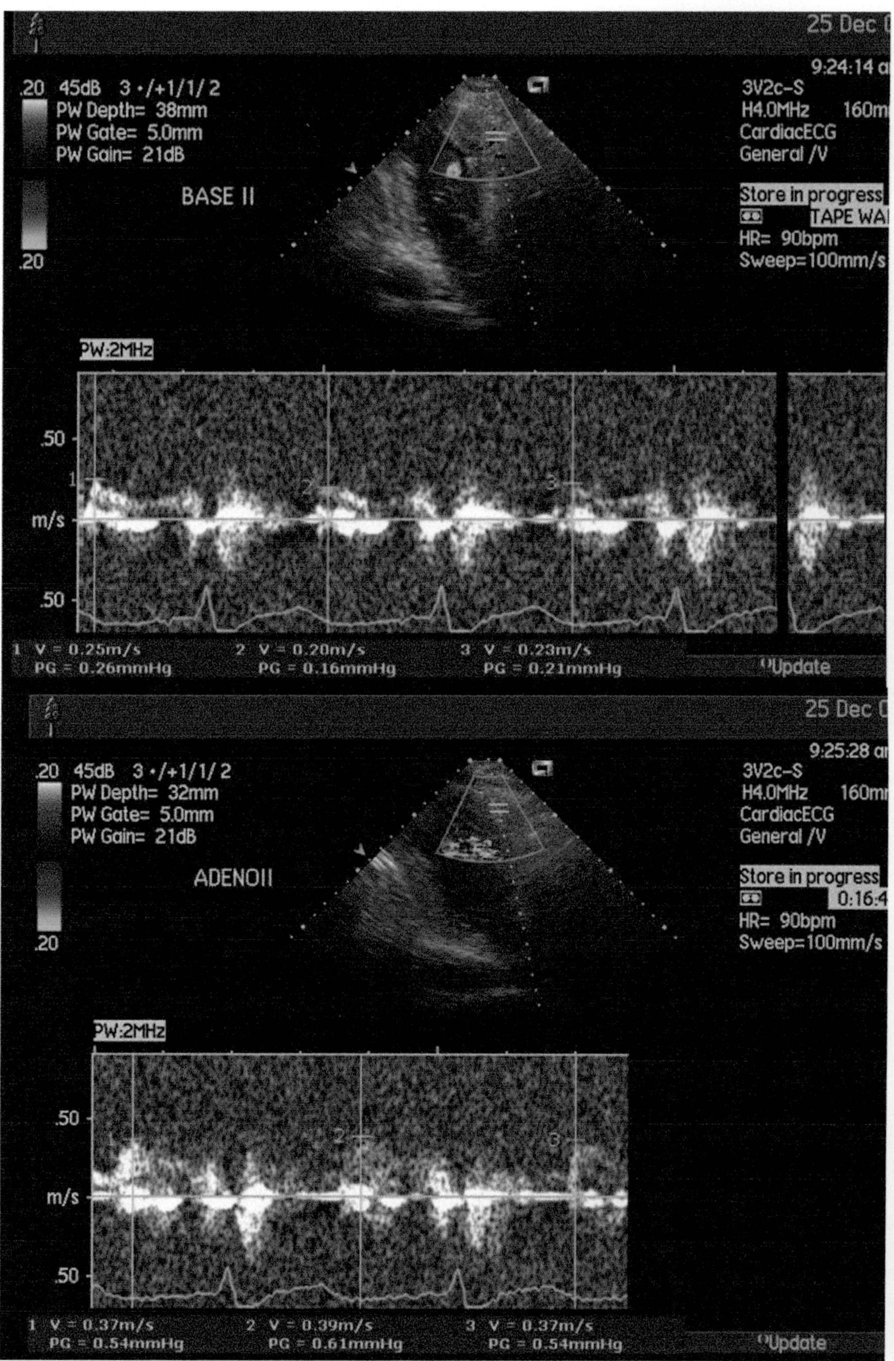

Fig. 8.6 Coronary flow reserve 2 days after pPCI

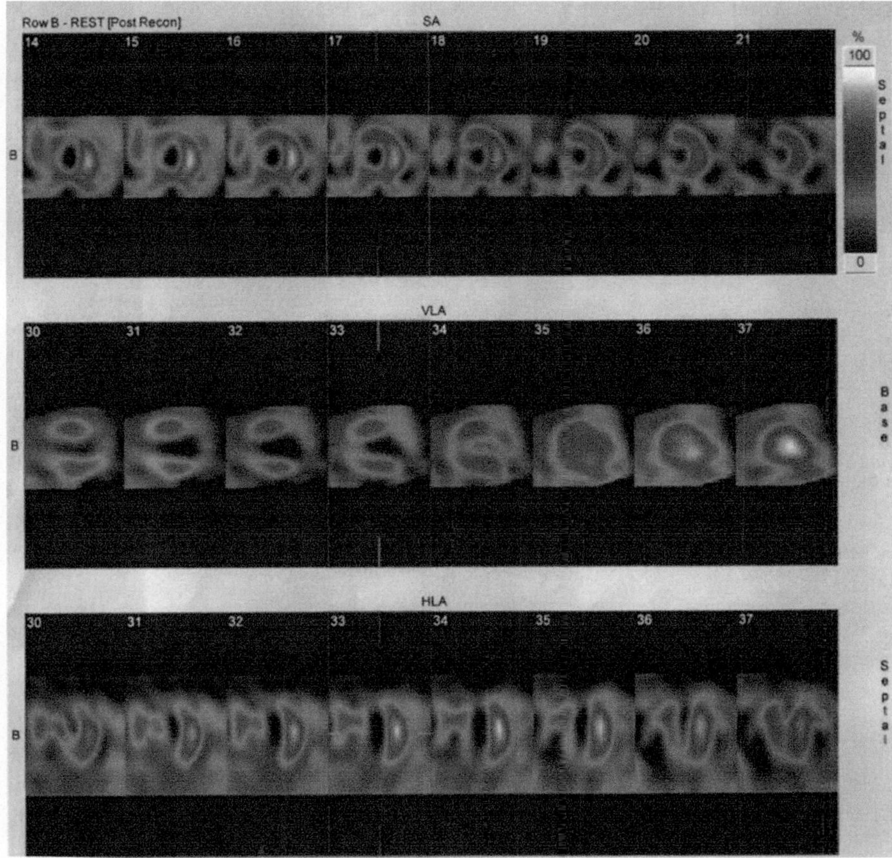

Fig. 8.7 SPECT viability study 2 months after pPCI

after initial pPCI patient developed signs and symptoms of heart failure with over decompensation. By that time echocardiography revealed significantly enlarged and spherically remodelled LV with EF of 22%, and CFR 1.4. SPECT confirmed enlarged LV (EDV 260 mL, ESV 190), with very poor systolic function (EF 27%), and extensive non-viable zone (SRS 48, perfusion defect of 80%).

Definition of No-Reflow

Myocardial infarction with ST segment elevation (STEMI) still has significant morbidity and mortality, despite achievements in contemporary therapy including primary percutaneous coronary intervention [pPCI) and modern antiplatelet regimes [1]. The principal cause of STEMI is thrombotic occlusion of the (epicardial) coronary artery, leading to the ischaemic myocardial necrosis that is proportional to the ischaemic time. Accordingly, the main therapeutic target in STEMI patients is to open infarct related artery (IRA) as soon as possible (strategy 'time is the muscle'), to obtain full reperfusion and consequently to reduce infarct size (IS). The concept of "full reperfusion" encompasses not only sufficient blood flow through epicardial coronary arteries, but also through coronary microcirculation [2]. However, despite timely and technically correct pPCI, full tissue reperfusion is not achieved in certain number of patients.

This insufficiency of distal flow through epicardial coronary artery and coronary microcirculation despite removal of epicardial occlusion, is defined as *low-, slow- or no-reflow phenomena*. It significantly impairs myocardial salvage, increases IS, promotes LV remodelling that leads to heart failure and finally translates into overall poor clinical outcomes. The problem of no-reflow may, at least partly, explain disparity between substantial reduction of door-to-balloon times for patients undergoing pPCI, that is achieved in the last few decades and virtually unchanged in-hospital mortality [3, 4].

The common pathophysiological background of *no-reflow* is functional and anatomical microvascular obstruction (MVO). MVO and final IS are the major independent predictors of long-term mortality and heart failure development in STEMI patients [5, 6].

Mechanism of Microvascular Obstruction and Dysfunction in No-Reflow

Five associated mechanisms are proposed to be involved in the pathogenesis of coronary MVO: pre-existing coronary microvascular dysfunction, ischaemia-related injury, reperfusion-related injury, distal embolization, and individual susceptibility (both genetic and due to pre-existing coronary microvascular dysfunction) [7, 8].

The important factors associated with ischemia-related injury are duration of ischemia and ischaemia extension. Ischemia-related injury manifests as severe capillary damage, endothelial protrusions, capillary lumen blebs block, endothelial gaps with extravascular erythrocytes, interstitial myocardial oedema and cell swelling [9].

The reperfusion-related injury is a result of coronary microvascular dysfunction and obstruction caused by further obliteration of vessel lumen by neutrophil-platelet aggregates, which can produce a large amount of vasoconstrictors, inflammatory mediators and reactive oxygen species [10]. It depends on the duration of ischemia and if it is more than 3 h, reperfusion injury is potentiated [11]. The reperfusion can increase infarct size due to mitochondria swelling and cell rupture as a consequence of enhanced mitochondrial membrane permeability. Ischaemia followed by reperfusion may also favour intramyocardial haemorrhage (IMH) [12]. Hypoxia can disrupt the endothelial barrier and damage the microvasculature and therefore facilitate blood cell extravasation upon reperfusion. Endothelial activation during reperfusion may also lead to consumption of coagulation factors aggravating the IMH.

Distal embolization by material from plaque and thrombotic occlusion causing STEMI, further mechanically obstruct the microcirculation. Both plaque and thrombus features are associated with the risk of distal embolization. However, above this mechanical athero-embolism, this material is biologically active representing a rich sources of vasoconstrictors and proinflamatory and procoagulant substances. Although the small size emboli during primary pPCI usually do not affect distal perfusion in microcirculation (because myocardial perfusion starts falling when microspheres obstruct >50% of coronary capillaries [13]), they may create a local reacting milieu including so call *neutrophil extracellular traps* that promote inflammation, thrombosis and vasoconstriction [13].

Genetic variability factors, as well as pre-existing coronary microvascular dysfunction in patients with traditional risk factor such as diabetes, acute hyperglycaemia, hypercholesterolaemia, modulate individual susceptibility and increase prevalence to coronary microvascular obstruction [7]. The ischaemic preconditioning (IPC), which may be present in the form of pre-infarction angina seems to protect both the myocardium and the coronary microcirculation [14].

The Incidence of No-Reflow

Since the definition of no-reflow is grounded on the impaired or absent of the flow distal to the site of (removed) epicardial obstruction, its incidence strongly depends on the technique used to estimate this flow. Incidence of MVO is variable, ranging from 10% by angiographic assessment of thrombolysis in myocardial infarction (TIMI) flow to 60% by CMR or myocardial contrast echocardiography (MCE) [15]. It is estimated, based on cumulative data from angiographic and ECG studies that ~35% of STEMI patients and ~86% of NSTEMI patients get full tissue reperfusion [7, 16].

How to Diagnose No-Reflow?

There are several invasive and non-invasive techniques used in clinical practice to detect no-reflow. Basically they can either directly measure coronary flow and myocardial perfusion or indirectly estimates consequence of inadequate myocardial reperfusion. They can be divided into invasive and non-invasive (Table 8.1).

Table 8.1 The diagnostic indices and criteria for no-reflow detection

Method	Diagnostic criteria for MVO or non-reflow
Invasive	
Angiographic parameters	
– Thrombolysis in myocardial infarction (TIMI) flow score	– Final TIMI flow <3 or final TIMI flow 3 with MBG or TIMI MPG 0–1
– Myocardial blush grade (MBG)	– MBG < 2
– Thrombolysis in myocardial infarction myocardial perfusion grade (TIMI MPG)	– TIMI MPG < 2
Intracoronary Doppler measurement	
– Pattern of epicardial coronary flow	– Systolic retrograde flow, diminished systolic anterograde flow, and rapid deceleration of diastolic flow
– Coronary flow reserve (CFR)	– CFR < 2
– Index of microvascular resistance (IMR)	– IMR> 40 U
– Doppler-derived hyperemic microvascular resistance (hMR)	– hMR $\geq$ 3.25 mmHg$*$cm^{-1}
Non-invasive	
– ST-segment resolution (STR)	– <50% or <70% 60/90 min after pPCI
– Myocardial contrast echocardiography (MCE)	– Lack of intra-myocardial contrast opacification
– Cardiac magnetic resonance (CMR)	– Lack of gadolinium enhancement during first pass and lack of late gadolinium enhancement within a necrotic region
– Hybrid positron emission tomography/cardiac computed tomography (PET/CT)	

Angiographic Detection of No-Relfow

Thrombolysis in myocardial infarction (TIMI) score grading system describes the rate of blood flow through the epicardial vessels. The values of TIMI are between no flow at all (Grade 0) to a normal flow rate (Grade 3). Microvascular obstruction is associated with angiographic TIMI flow ≤2, or TIMI=3 and myocardial blush grade = 0 or 1 [2]. However, the MVO may occur in nearly 50% of patients with TIMI flow 3 [7]. In order to improve stratification in prognosis of patients exhibiting TIMI flow 3, *TIMI frame count (TFC)* was developed. This index, defined as the number of frames required for contrast medium to reach standardized distal landmarks, correlated well with invasively assessed CFR [17].

With the intention to shift assessment of reperfusion from the epicardial to myocardial level, two angiographic methods based on the kinetics of dye penetration within the myocardium were proposed—the myocardial blush grade (MBG), and TIMI myocardial perfusion grade (TMPG) [17, 18]. *Myocardial blush grade* is a densitometric method assessing maximum intensity of contrast medium in the microcirculation and grade on a scale scored from 0–3. The TMPG assesses microvascular clearance of contrast medium on a scale of 0–3. The higher scores indicate better perfusion. Both MBG and TMPG are able to stratify the risk of patients who have TIMI flow 3 at the end of pPCI. In contemporary clinical practice it is common to define angiographic MVO, as follows: TIMI flow grade ≤3, but with MBG or TMPG 0–1 [15]. All above mentioned angiographic methods for perfusion assessment are qualitative metrics potentially with significant interobserver variability. Because of that, a more quantitative, invasive assessment of microcirculation during pPCI emerged. It includes usage of intracoronary pressure and Doppler flow wires or their combination to detect the presence of MVO [15].

Invasive Indices of Non-reflow

The most reliable assessment of coronary microvascular function is to measure directly coronary blood flow velocity using an intracoronary (IC) Doppler wire. The typical flow pattern associated with MVO is characterized by systolic retrograde flow, diminished systolic anterograde flow, and rapid deceleration of diastolic flow [19].

In the state of maximal coronary vasodilatation induced by i.c. administration of adenosine, an endothelium independent vasodilatator, increment in flow velocity, depends predominately on the functional integrity of microcirculation (in the absence of flow limiting epicardial stenosis). This ratio between hyperemic to resting flow velocity represents Coronary Flow Reserve (CFR). In case of coronary microvascular dysfunction, including MVO after pPCI, CFR is impaired. The post-PCI attenuated CFR response is associated with future cardiovascular events [20]. However, CFR is not microvascular specific and is significantly affected by resting hemodynamics.

The *index of microvascular resistance* (IMR) is calculated as the product of the distal pressure and mean transit time of a saline bolus during maximum hyperemia using a dual temperature and pressure wire. This technique is based upon thermodilution and uses a continuous infusion of a low amount of saline through a microcatheter positioned selectively in a coronary artery. Maximal hyperemia is usually induced using either a single bolus of 10–15 g of intracoronary papaverine or (more frequently) 140 g/kg/min of intravenous adenosine via a central venous catheter. IMR has been introduced as a method for evaluating the coronary microvascular circulation at the time of pPCI [21], potentially allowing the implementation of treatment to minimize MVO. IMR is more specific metric for microcirculation than CFR and is less dependent of haemodynamic parameters. Generally, an IMR <25 is accepted as a cut-off for normal microvascular function [22]. However, in STEMI, a post-stenting IMR >40 reflects severe microvascular impairment and is associated with poorer left ventricular functional recovery, higher incidence of death, myocardial infarction and readmission for heart failure [23, 24].

Despite the fact that IMR has been validated against CMR, not all studies shown a perfect concordance between increased post-procedural termodilution-derived IMR and MVO detected by CMR [25, 26]. The discordance between these two parameters was present in even 36.7% of STEMI patients, when a threshold of 40 was adopted for IMR [26]. However, in patients with MVO and higher IMR, a larger IS was observed than in those in whom MVO was associated with IMR ≤40. Those with MVO but IMR <40 experienced significant regressions of the IS at 6 months, whereas no significant change in IS was observed in patients with MVO and higher IMR [26].

The Doppler-derived hyperemic microvascular resistance (hMR) was recently introduced and compared vs conventional termodilution-derived IMR. The correlation was only modest. However, in STEMI population hMR had a clinically superior sensitivity over IMR to predict MVD determined by CMR, but not statistically significant [27].

Distal embolisation is not detectable by angiography and other methods of coronary imaging, like angioscopy and optical coherence tomography (OCT) could be useful. In this context, as suggested by a recent OCT study, the persistence of thrombus after stenting may lead to distal embolization even after stent deployment [7].

Electrocardiography

Electrocardiography is useful and long standing non-invasive, indirect method to diagnose inadequate myocardial reperfusion in STEMI patients, measuring ST segment resolution (STR) after reperfusion therapy. Different methods have been used in terms of optimal timing when to analyze STR, which lead to use as a reference (one lead with the maximal ST segment elevation or the sum of residual STR) and whether to use continuous or standard ECG [28]. Although the consensus is still lacking, it turns that the assessment of single lead STR showing maximum ST elevation at baseline is as accurate as the sum of STR measurements [17]. The only criteria indicating lack of successful reperfusion that is officially endorsed by guidelines is ST-segment regression <50% observed 60 min after pPCI [2]. It is reliable sign of either epicardial artery occlusion or microvascular obstruction [2]. Other studies, however, showed a correlation between STR <70% observed 90 min after pPCI and persistent MVO and infarct size, as assessed by CMR [28].

Myocardial Contrast Echocardiography

Myocardial contrast echocardiography (MCE) is a non-invasive imaging technique that uses intravenous contrast agents (i.e. ultrasonic enhancing agents) in the form of microbubbles that enhance ultrasound signals MCE enables assessment of the anatomic and functional integrity of cardiac microcirculation, because the path of contrast microbubbles injected into circulation is the same as the path of red blood cells, i.e. microbubbles freely flow within patent microcirculation while lack of intra-myocardial contrast opacification is due to microvascular obstruction MCE has solid temporal and spatial resolution and permits evaluation of the effectiveness of myocardial reperfusion, residual myocardial viability and infarct size after pPCI.

The first contrast study of no-reflow had been done by Ito et al. [29] applying intracoronary microbubbles immediately after restoration of anterograde flow in the infarcted artery. After that no-reflow phenomenon was successfully detected also by intravenous administration of microbubbles [30]. In the following years, several studies strongly confirmed the importance of myocardial viability detected by different modalities of MCE early after acute MI to predict functional LV recovery [31, 32]. Compared to cardiac MRI the ability of MCE to predict functional recovery of the LV reported to be similar [33].

The large multicentre study demonstrated that the extent of microvascular damage, assessed by MCE 1 day after reperfusion therapy in patients with myocardial infarction, is the most powerful independent predictor for LV remodeling compared to other indexes of post-MI reperfusion [34]. The transmurality of an infarction verified by late gadolinium enhancement on CMR, can be predicted by MCE based contrast defect intensity and reduction of resting MBF [35]. Advantage of MCE is also its suitability as a bedside tool to be the first line of investigation focus on reperfusion in post-MI patients.

Transthoracic Doppler Derived Coronary Flow Reserve

Coronary flow reserve (CFR) defined as the ratio of maximal (i.e. hyperemic) to baseline coronary blood flow velocities can be measured also noninvasively by transthoracic Doppler echocardiography (TTD). Normal values for CFR are ≥2.0, or by some authors ≥2.5.

Non-invasive CFR assessed by TTD was used to estimate coronary microcirculation of the infarct related artery after pPCI in STEMI patients in several studies. It was proved as clinically useful tool to detect no-reflow [36], to assess myocardial viability of the infarct region [37], to predict functional recovery of the infarct area [38], final infarct size [39] and left ventricular remodeling [40, 41]. Furthermore, CFR of the non IRA artery stratifies prognosis in acute coronary syndrome. These data point that coronary microvascular dysfunction is a diffuse process, not limited exclusively to infarct region, and that global atherosclerotic burden is even more important than focal epicardial disease [42]. Similar data were obtained from parallel invasive study [43].

Cardiac Magnetic Resonance

Advances in CMR have enabled comprehensive assessment including tissue characterization with imaging myocardial perfusion at rest and stress, detection of microvascular obstruction (MVO) and intramyocardial haemorrhage (IMH). CMR significantly contributes to the detection and understanding of the "no-reflow" phenomenon. Of the available modalities, CMR provides the most comprehensive assessment of MVO and IMH and numerous studies provided evidence that those CMR stigmata of no-reflow carry ominous prognosis.

On gadolinium-enhanced CMR, MVO is detected as delayed or absent wash-in of contrast agent into the infarct zone, "early" or "late" in reference to the timing of imaging relative to gadolinium administration. Early MVO is recognized as a prolonged perfusion defect on resting first-pass perfusion (FPP) imaging or as a hypointense region in the core of the infarction on T1-weighted images made 2–5 min after contrast administration [44]. Depending on the severity of MVO, the absence of wash-in of gadolinium may persist for >10 min, resulting in a region of persistent hypo enhancement within the core of the infarct on conventional late gadolinium enhancement images, referred to as "late MVO" [45]. Late gadolinium enhancement imaging used for late MVO assessment has high spatial and contrast resolution with full coverage of the LV myocardium. Currently, it is unidentified whether the rate of fill-in of the MVO area has prognostic importance and whether early or late MVO is a better predictor of LV remodeling or MACE. In overall pooled analysis, both early and late MVO are associated with lower EF [46], larger ventricular volumes [46] and infarct at baseline [47], and worse LV remodeling during follow-up [48]. Late MVO was demonstrated to have a stronger relationship with MACE and the individual outcomes of cardiac mortality, recurrent MI, and CHF/CHF hospitalization compared with early MVO [49].

IMH is a severe form of MVO and develops in the core of the infarct with a tendency to expand for several hours after PCI [50]. Ir order to assess for IMH most centers use T2-weighted short-tau inversion recovery (STIR) or T2∗-weighted gradient echo pulse sequences. IMH appears as a hypointense region within the infarct on T2-weighted sequences. Since the paramagnetic effects of hemoglobin breakdown products more strongly affect T2∗ relaxation, T2∗-weighted imaging is thought to be more sensitive for the detection of IMH. IMH detected by both T2 and T2∗ images has been correlated with the presence of hemorrhage on histopathologic analysis [51, 52]. Although intramyocardial haemorrhage is observed less frequently in patients with acute myocardial infarction than in animal models, its presence is correlated with the duration of ischaemia and infarct size, and is a predictor of adverse remodeling and outcome [53, 54] IMH also predicted MACE; however, there is a currently smaller body of literature for IMH and limited direct comparisons of IMH and MVO. Larger studies are needed.

Risk Factors to Develop No-Reflow

Delayed reperfusion, high thrombus burden on baseline angiography, and increased blood glucose level on admission can be used to stratify AMI patients into a lower or higher risk for angiographic slow/no-reflow during PCI in order to predict non-reflow [55]. Acute hyperglycemia specifically has been associated with higher incidence of coronary no-reflow, whereas glycosylated hemoglobin levels or diabetes are not, suggesting that acute hyperglycemia regardless of presence or severity of diabetes mellitus is a predictive and prognostic factor for non-reflow.

There is some evidence that the female gender is at higher risk of developing NRP [56]. Of note is that contrast agent dose shown as independent predictor of no-reflow and when the dose was >160 mL, the risk of slow/no-reflow increased significantly [57].

Recent studies have shown that some of widely used scores such as CHA2DS2-VaSc score (predict thromboembolic events in patients with atrial fibrillation rhythm) and SYNTAX score II can be used for prediction of no-reflow. CHA2DS2-VaSc and SYNTAX SCORE II consists of similar risk factors important for microvascular dysfunction [58, 59].

Clinical Importance of Non-reflow

Patients with non-reflow have poorer prognosis and higher likelihood of major adverse cardiac events (MACE). In the catheterization laboratory, the clinical presentation of no reflow during pPCI can be dramatic often with sudden hemodynamic deterioration. This can be also related to atheroembolism and slowing of blood flow in the non-culprit arteries. In the coronary care unit, the presentation is usually less dramatic. New Q waves may appear and some of those patients may be diagnosed as having infarct extensions.

The no-reflow phenomenon is linked to ventricular arrhythmias, early congestive heart failure, and even cardiac rupture [60]. Those patients also had more advanced LV remodeling, during follow-up, as detected by echocardiography. Angiographic no-reflow phenomenon strongly predicts cardiac complications independent of other well-known early predictors of long-term outcome after STMEI, such as age, Killip class and LVEF. In patients with STEMI treated by primary PCI, no-reflow phenomenon is also a strong predictor of the long term mortality, independently even from infarct size [61].

Basic Principles of Management of No-Reflow

Successful therapy of no-reflow still does not exist. Several preventive strategies were proposed, including short door to balloon time, optimization of blood pressure and blood glucose level, statin therapy, prophylactic intra-coronary administration of dilatators such as adenosine and nitroprusside and thrombus aspiration. Furthermore, few non-pharmacological therapies, including induced hypothermia were tested to improve coronary blood flow. Although some of those strategies are successful in animal studies, their effectiveness in reducing no-reflow in humans remains to be determined.

Treating no reflow may not necessarily reduce the size of myocardial infarction, because the microvascular damage is usually restrained within the area of myocardial necrosis. However, treating no reflow may enhance the delivery of blood and blood-borne elements to the necrotic area, thus speeding healing. This could reduce the presence of infarct expansion and left ventricular remodeling. Salvage of flow will ensure also drug delivery to the necrotic zone. Likewise, salvage of the small vessels may promote collateral circulation and perhaps serves as a site for neovascularization.

NO-reflow still represent a challenge in contemporary cardiology. Taking into a count importance and complexity of no re-flow as well as lack of proper and effective therapy, more studies in this field are needed.

References

1. Yeh RW, Sidney S, Chandra M, Sorel M, Selby JV, Go AS. Population trends in the incidence and outcomes of acute myocardial infarction. N Engl J Med. 2010;362:2155–65.
2. Ibanez B, James S, Agewall S, Antunes MJ, Bucciarelli-Ducci C, Bueno H, ESC Scientific Document Group, et al. 2017 ESC guidelines for the management of acute myocardial infarction in patients presenting with ST-segment elevation: the task force for the management of acute myocardial infarction in patients presenting with ST-segment elevation of the European Society of Cardiology (ESC). Eur Heart J. 2018;39(2):119–77.
3. Radovanovic D, Erne P. AMIS plus: Swiss registry of acute coronary syndrome. Heart. 2010;96:917–21.
4. Menees DS, Peterson ED, Wang Y, Curtis JP, Messenger JC, Rumsfeld JS, et al. Door-to-balloon time and mortality among patients undergoing primary PCI. N Engl J Med. 2013;369:901–9.
5. Stone GW, Selker HP, Thiele H, Patel MR, Udelson JE, Ohman EM, et al. Relationship between infarct size and outcomes following primary PCI: patient-level analysis from 10 randomized trials. J Am Coll Cardiol. 2016;67(14):1674–83.
6. Ibáñez B, Heusch G, Ovize M, Van de Werf F. Evolving therapies for myocardial ischemia/reperfusion injury. J Am Coll Cardiol. 2015;65(14):1454–71.
7. Niccoli G, Scalone G, Lerman A, Crea F. Coronary microvascular obstruction in acute myocardial infarction. Eur Heart J. 2016;37(13):1024–33.
8. Niccoli G, Kharbanda RK, Crea F, Banning AP. No-reflow: again prevention is better than treatment. Eur Heart J. 2010;31:2449–55.
9. Reffelmann T, Kloner RA. The no-reflow phenomenon: a basic mechanism of myocardial ischemia and reperfusion. Basic Res Cardiol. 2006;101:359–72.
10. Bekkers SC, Yazdani SK, Virmani R, Waltenberger J. Microvascular obstruction: underlying pathophysiology and clinical diagnosis. J Am Coll Cardiol. 2010;55:1649–60.
11. Frohlich GM, Meier P, White SK, Yellon DM, Hausenloy DJ. Myocardial reperfusion injury: looking beyond primary PCI. Eur Heart J. 2013;34:1714–22.
12. Robbers LF, Eerenberg ES, Teunissen PF, Jansen MF, Hollander MR, Horrevoets AJ, et al. Magnetic resonance imaging-defined areas of microvascular obstruction after acute myocardial infarction represent microvascular destruction and haemorrhage. Eur Heart J. 2013;34:2346–53.
13. Heusch G, Kleinbongard P, Bose D, Levkau B, Haude M, Schulz R, et al. Coronary microembolization: from bedside to bench and back to bedside. Circulation. 2009;120:1822–36.
14. Niccoli G, Burzotta F, Galiuto L, Crea F. Myocardial no-reflow in humans. J Am Coll Cardiol. 2009;54:281–92.

15. Niccoli G, Cosentino N, Spaziani C, Fracassi F, Tarantini G, Crea F. No-reflow: incidence and detection in the cath-lab. Curr Pharm Des. 2013;19:4564–75.
16. Guerra E, Hadamitzky M, Ndrepepa G, Bauer C, Ibrahim T, Ott I, et al. Microvascular obstruction in patients with non-ST-elevation myocardial infarction: a contrast-enhanced cardiac magnetic resonance study. Int J Cardiovasc Imaging. 2014;30 1087–95.
17. Gibson CM, Cannon CP, Murphy SA, Marble SJ, Barron HV, Braunwald E. Relationship of the TIMI myocardial perfusion grades, flow grades, frame count, and percutaneous coronary intervention to long-term outcomes after thrombolytic administration in acute myocardial infarction. Circulation. 2002;105:1909–13.
18. Van't Hof AW, Liem A, Suryapranata H, Hoorntje JC, de Boer MJ, Zijlstra F. Angiographic assessment of myocardial reperfusion in patients treated with primary angioplasty for acute myocardial infarction: myocardial blush grade. Zwolle Myocardial Infarction Study Group. Circulation. 1998;97:2302–6.
19. De Waha S, Patel MR, Granger CB, Ohman ME, Maehara A, Eitel I, et al. Relationship between microvascular obstruction and adverse events following primary percutaneous coronary intervention for ST-segment elevation myocardial infarction: an individual patient data pooled analysis from seven randomized trials. Eur Heart J. 2017;38:3502–10.
20. Yamamuro A, Akasaka T, Tamita K, Yamabe K, Katayama M, Takagi T, et al. Coronary flow velocity pattern immediately after percutaneous coronary intervention as a predictor of complications and in-hospital survival after acute myocardial infarction. Circulation. 2002;106:3051–6.
21. Bulluck H, Foin N, Cabrera-Fuentes HA, Yeo KK, Wong AS, Fam JM, et al. Index of microvascular resistance and microvascular obstruction in patients with acute myocardial infarction. JACC Cardiovasc Interv. 2016;9(20):2172–4.
22. Bajrangee A, Collison D, Oldroyd KG. Resistance to flow in the coronary microcirculation: we can measure it but what does it mean? EuroIntervention. 2017;13:901–3.
23. Fearon WF, Shah M, Ng M, Brinton T, Wilson A, Tremmel JA, et al. Predictive value of the index of microcirculatory resistance in patients with ST-segment elevation myocardial infarction. J Am Coll Cardiol. 2008;51:560–5.
24. Carrick D, Haig C, Ahmed N, et al. Comparative prognostic utility of indexes of microvascular function alone or in combination in patients with an acute ST-segment-elevation myocardial infarction. Circulation. 2016;134:1833–47.
25. Payne AR, Berry C, Doolin O, et al. Microvascular resistance predicts myocardial salvage and infarct characteristics in ST-elevation myocardial infarction. J Am Heart Assoc. 2012;1:e002246.
26. De Maria GL, Alkhalil M, Wolfrum M, Fahrni G, Borlotti A, Gaughran L, et al. Index of microcirculatory resistance as a tool to characterize microvascular obstruction and to predict infarct size regression in patients with STEMI undergoing primary PCI. JACC Cardiovasc Imaging. 2019;12(5):837–48.
27. Williams RP, de Waard GA, De Silva K, Lumley M, Asrress K, Arri S, et al. Doppler versus thermodilution-derived coronary microvascular resistance to predict coronary microvascular dysfunction in patients with acute myocardial infarction or stable angina pectoris. Am J Cardiol. 2018;121(1):1–8.
28. Infusino F, Niccoli G, Fracassi F, Roberto M, Falcioni E, Lanza GA, et al. The central role of conventional 12-lead ECG for the assessment of microvascular obstruction after percutaneous myocardial revascularization. J Electrocardiol. 2014;47:45–51.
29. Ito H, Tomooka T, Sakaii N, et al. Lack of myocardial perfusion. Immediately after successful thrombolysis: a predictor of poor recovery of left ventricular function in anterior myocardial infarction. Circulation. 1992;85:1699–705.
30. Lepper W, Hoffmann R, Kamp O, et al. Assessment of myocardial reperfusion by intravenous myocardial contrast echocardiography and coronary flow reserve after primary percutaneous transluminal coronary angiography in patients with acute myocardial infarction. Circulation. 2000;101:2368–74.

31. Main ML, Magalski A, Chee NK, et al. Full-motion pulse inversion power Doppler contrast echocardiography differentiates stunning from necrosis and predicts recovery of left ventricular function after acute myocardial infarction. J Am Coll Cardiol. 2001;38:1390–4.
32. Korosoglou G, Labadze N, Giannitsis E, et al. Usefulness of realtime myocardial perfusion imaging to evaluate tissue level reperfusion in patients with non ST elevation myocardial infarction. Am J Cardiol. 2005;95:1033–8.
33. Janardhanan R, Moon JC, Pennell DJ, Senior R. Myocardial contrast echocardiography accurately reflects transmurality of myocardial necrosis and predicts contractile reserve after acute myocardial infarction. Am Heart J. 2005;149:355–62.
34. Galiuto L, Garramone B, Scara A, et al. The extent of microvascular damage during myocardial contrast echocardiography is superior to other known indexes of post-infarct reperfusion in predicting left ventricular remodeling. J Am Coll Cardiol. 2008;51:552–9.
35. Choi EY, Seo HS, Park S, et al. Prediction of transmural extent of infarction with contrast echocardiographically derived index of myocardial blood flow and myocardial blood volume fraction: comparison with contrast-enhanced magnetic resonance imaging. J Am Soc Echocardiogr. 2006;19:1211–9.
36. Tesche C, De Cecco CN, Albrecht MH, et al. Coronary CT angiography-derived fractional flow reserve. Radiology. 2017;285(1):17–33.
37. Montalescot G, Sechtem U, Achenbach S, Task Force Members, et al. 2013 ESC guidelines on the management of stable coronary artery disease. Eur Heart J. 2013;34:2949–3003.
38. Wu J, Barton D, Xie F, O'Leary E, et al. Comparison of fractional flow reserve assessment with demand stress myocardial contrast echocardiography in angiographically intermediate coronary stenosis. Cir Cardiovasc Imaging. 2016;9:e004129.
39. Jayaweera AR, Wei K, Coggins M, Bin JP, Goodman C, Kaul S. Role of capillaries in determining CBF reserve: new insights using myocardial contrast echocardiography. Am J Phys. 1999;277:H2363–72.
40. Tsutsui JM, Elhendy A, Anderson JR, Xie F, McGrain AC, Porter TR. Prognostic value of dobutamine stress myocardial contrast perfusion echocardiography. Circulation. 2005;112:1444–50.
41. Gaibazzi N, Reverberi C, Lorenzoni V, Molinaro S, Porter TR. Prognostic value of high-dose dipyridamole stress myocardial contrast perfusion echocardiography. Circulation. 2012;126:1217–24.
42. Kern MJ, Bach RG, Mechem C, Caracciolo EA, et al. Variations in normal coronary vasodilatory reserve stratified by artery, gender, heart transplantation and coronary artery disease. J Am Coll Cardiol. 1996;28:1154–60.
43. Trifunovic D, Sobic-Saranovic D, Beleslin B, et al. Coronary flow of the infarct artery assessed by transthoracic Doppler after primary percutaneous coronary intervention predicts final infarct size. Int J Cardiovasc Imaging. 2014;30:1509–18.
44. Bekkers SC, Backes WH, Kim RJ, et al. Detection and characteristics of microvascular obstruction in reperfused acute myocardial infarction using an optimized protocol for contrast-enhanced cardiovascular magnetic resonance imaging. Eur Radiol. 2009;19:2904–12.
45. Mayr A, Klug G, Schocke M, et al. Late microvascular obstruction after acute myocardial infarction: relation with cardiac and inflammatory markers. Int J Cardiol. 2012;157:391–6.
46. O'Regan DP, Ariff B, Neuwirth C, Tan Y, Durighel G, Cook SA. Assessment of severe reperfusion injury with T2* cardiac MRI in patients with acute myocardial infarction. Heart. 2010;96:1885–91.
47. Bogaert J, Kalantzi M, Rademakers FE, Dymarkowski S, Janssens S. Determinants and impact of microvascular obstruction in successfully reperfused ST-segment elevation myocardial infarction. Assessment by magnetic resonance imaging. Eur Radiol. 2007;17:2572–80.
48. Mather AN, Fairbairn TA, Ball SG, Greenwood JP, Plein S. Reperfusion haemorrhage as determined by cardiovascular MRI is a predictor of adverse left ventricular remodelling and markers of late arrhythmic risk. Heart. 2011;97:453–9.
49. Wu E, Ortiz JT, Tejedor P, et al. Infarct size by contrast enhanced cardiac magnetic resonance is a stronger predictor of outcomes than left ventricular ejection fraction or end-systolic volume index: prospective cohort study. Heart. 2008;94:730–6.

50. Asanuma T, Tanabe K, Ochiai K, et al. Relationship between progressive microvascular damage and intramyocardial hemorrhage in patients with reperfused anterior myocardial infarction: myocardial contrast echocardiographic study. Circulation. 1990;96:448–53.
51. Robbers LF, Eerenberg ES, Teunissen PF, et al. Magnetic resonance imaging-defined areas of microvascular obstruction after acute myocardial infarction represent microvascular destruction and haemorrhage. Eur Heart J. 2013;34:2346–53.
52. Anderson LJ, Holden S, Davis B, et al. Cardiovascular T2-star (T2∗) magnetic resonance for the early diagnosis of myocardial iron overload. Eur Heart J. 2001;22:2171–9.
53. Kidambi A, et al. The effect of microvascular obstruction and intramyocardial hemorrhage on contractile recovery in reperfused myocardial infarction insights from cardiovascular magnetic resonance. J Cardiovasc Magn Reson. 2013;15:58.
54. Husser O, et al. Cardiovascular magnetic resonance-derived intramyocardial hemorrhage after STEMI: influence on long-term prognosis, adverse left ventricular remodeling and relationship with microvascular obstruction. Int J Cardiol. 2013;167:2047–54.
55. Dong-bao L, Qi H, Zhi L, Shan W, Wei-ying J. Predictors and long-term prognosis of angiographic slow/no-reflow phenomenon during emergency percutaneous coronary intervention for ST-elevated acute myocardial infarction. Clin Cardiol. 2010;33(12):E7–E12.
56. Celik T, Balta S, Ozturk C, et al. Predictors of no-reflow phenomenon in young patients with acute ST-segment elevation myocardial infarction undergoing primary percutaneous coronary intervention. Angiology. 2016;67(7):683–9.
57. Ding S, Shi Y, Sun X, Cao Q, Dai H, Guan J. Contrast agent dose and slow/no-reflow in percutaneous coronary interventions: a case-control study of patients with non-ST-segment elevation acute coronary syndromes. Herz. 2019;44(1):69–75.
58. Mirbolouk F, Gholipour M, Salari A, et al. CHA2DS2-VASc score predict no-reflow phenomenon in primary percutaneous coronary intervention. J Cardiovasc Thorac Res. 2018;10(1):46–52.
59. Aşkın L, Aktürk E. Association between SYNTAX II score and electrocardiographic evidence of no-reflow in patients with ST-segment elevation myocardial infarction. Turk Kardiyol Dern Ars. 2018;46(6):455–63.
60. Rezkalla SH, Robert A, Kloner RA. No-reflow phenomenon. Circulation. 2002;105:656–62.
61. Ndrepepa G, Tiroch K, Fusaro M, Keta D, Seyfarth M, Byrne RA, et al. 5-year prognostic value of no-reflow phenomenon after percutaneous coronary intervention in patients with acute myocardial infarction. J Am Coll Cardiol. 2010;55(21):2383–9.

Chapter 9
Coronary Microcirculatory Dysfunction Evaluation in Chronic Angina

Maria Dorobantu and Lucian Calmac

Introduction

Chest pain is a very common complaint, and many patients with angina-like chest pain are finally evaluated with invasive coronary angiography as it is considered the golden standard in evaluation of ischemic heart disease. In a contemporary cohort of almost 400,000 patients evaluated with elective invasive coronary angiography (ICA) for suspected obstructive epicardial coronary artery disease (excluding patients with previous documented coronary disease, ACS or other indication than coronary disease), 59% of the patients were found to have stenosis <50%, while 39% had almost normal arteries (stenosis <20%) [1]. The rate of obstructive disease (defined as >50% stenosis on left main or >70% on other vessels) was only 41.3% in patients with positive noninvasive study, so it becomes obvious that there are a lot of patients in whom even in the presence of inducible ischemia the epicardial disease does not account for ischemia/symptoms. Accordingly, these patients should be labeled and managed as Ischemia and No Obstructive Coronary Artery disease (INOCA) and in this subset of patients coronary microvascular dysfunction (CMD) and/or vasospasm are considered potential causes of ischemia [2]. We present a case illustrative for the utility of both functional vasomotor testing and microcirculatory evaluation for a precise diagnosis in a patient with ischemia and normal coronary arteries.

M. Dorobantu (✉)
Emergency Clinical Hospital Bucharest, Bucharest, Romania

University of Medicine and Pharmacy Carol Davila, Bucharest, Romania

L. Calmac
Emergency Clinical Hospital Bucharest, Bucharest, Romania

M. Dorobantu, L. Badimon (eds.), *Microcirculation*,
https://doi.org/10.1007/978-3-030-28199-1_9

Case Report

Female patient 44 years old, active, smoker (10 pack-years), BMI 23.5; she was admitted due to 2 months onset of exertion chest pain with worsening pattern. Initial evaluation was unremarkable, with normal ECG (Fig. 9.1). Initial blood tests were also unremarkable with negative troponin and myoglobin, no dyslipidemia (LDL cholesterol 130 mg/dL, triglycerides 120 mg/dL, HDL cholesterol 48 mg/dL). Transthoracic echocardiography showed normal left and right ventricular function without hypertrophy or dilatation and no valvular abnormalities. Despite low pre-test probability of angina (young female patient with typical symptoms) the patient underwent an ECG stress test which was positive for inducible ischemia (Fig. 9.2). Invasive evaluation was scheduled. Coronary angiography revealed normal coronary arteries without any parietal irregularities and TIMI 3 flow (Fig. 9.3).

Considering the "normal" aspect on angiography we decided to continue examination with evaluation of vasomotor response to acetylcholine in order to test for endothelial dependent vasomotor function. We used progressive dilutions 2–20–100 μg/5 mL saline which were slowly injected through the guiding catheter in the left coronary artery over 20 s with repeated angiography of the LAD and 12 leads ECG recording performed after each dose. There were no significant changes after the first two doses. After the 100 μg dose the patient experienced chest pain and the ECG showed significant diffuse ST segment depression with negative T waves and ST segment elevation in lead aVR suggestive for extensive ischemia. Repeated angiography (Fig. 9.4) showed moderate diffuse spasm in mid and distal LAD (maximum diameter stenosis 45%) with reduced TIMI flow (adjusted TIMI frame count 29). After 200 μg of Nitroglycerine injected through the guiding catheter the chest pain subsided as did the spastic aspect of LAD and the ECG changes, with a normal repolarization at the end.

After resolution of ECG changes we tested endothelial independent microcirculatory function using RadiAnalyzer (Abbot Vascular). A 0.014"Certus wire(Abbot Vascular) with distal sensor for both temperature and pressure was advanced through the guiding catheter in distal LAD. Three boluses of 3 mL room temperature saline were briskly injected through the guiding catheter and the procedure was repeated after induction of hyperemia using intravenous adenosine 140 μg/kgc/min (Fig. 9.5). The results demonstrated a preserved endothelial independent vasomotor function with a CFR of 2.8 and a normal resistance in the microcirculation with an IMR value of 11.

Because we succeeded to demonstrate a vasospastic microcirculatory component as responsible for our patient symptoms we recommended treatment with a calcium channel blocker (Diltiazem using a 180 mg slow release formula once daily), adding a statin (atorvastatin 80 mg in considering the endothelial dysfunction proven by the acetylcholine testing) and one antiplatelet (low dose aspirin −75 mg/day). The patient was also instructed to quit smoking, to perform physical training on regular basis and to use short acting nitrates should the chest pain recur. After initiating therapy the frequency and severity of chest pain subsided, with preserved exercise capacity.

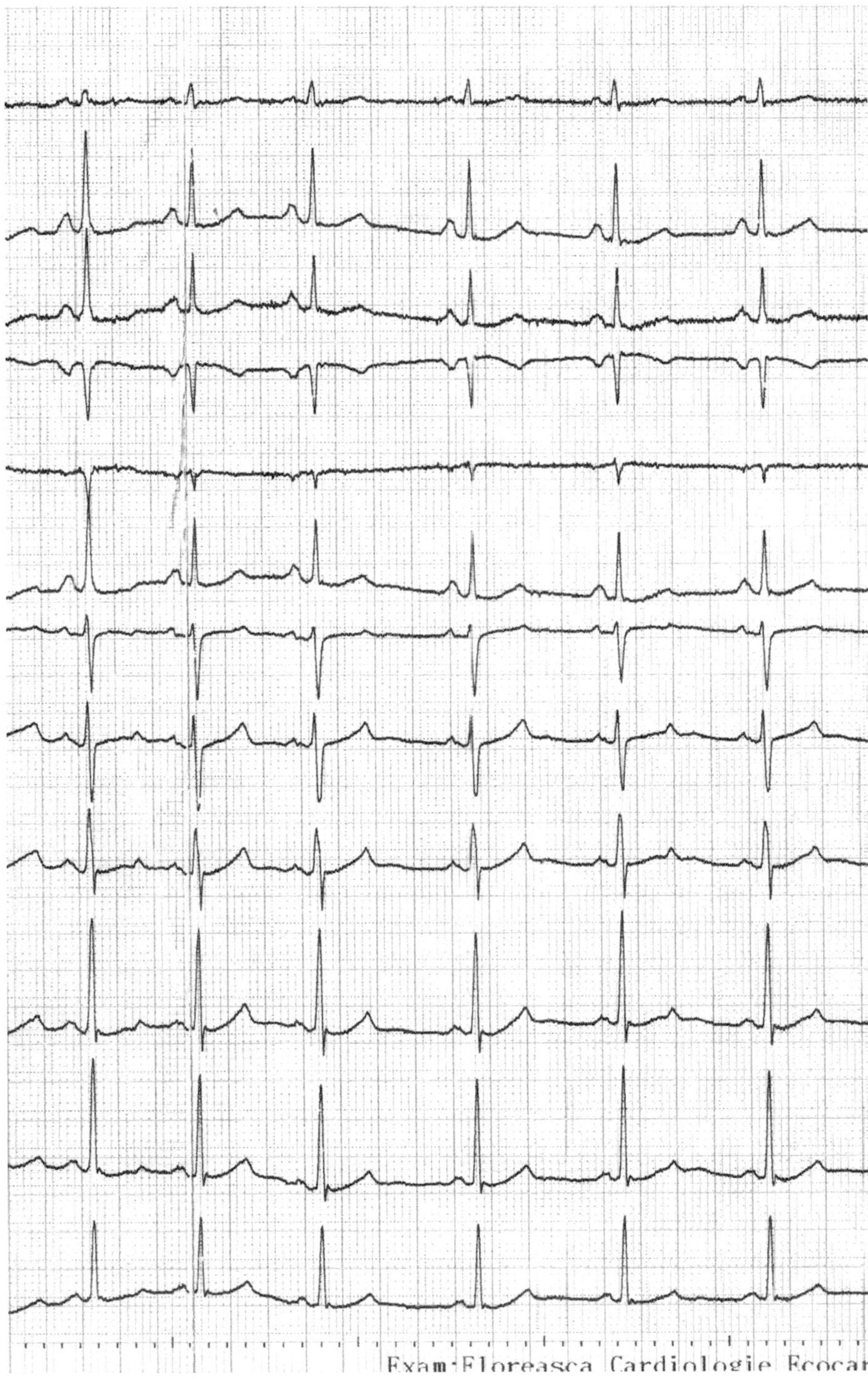

Fig. 9.1 Initial ECG—no abnormities

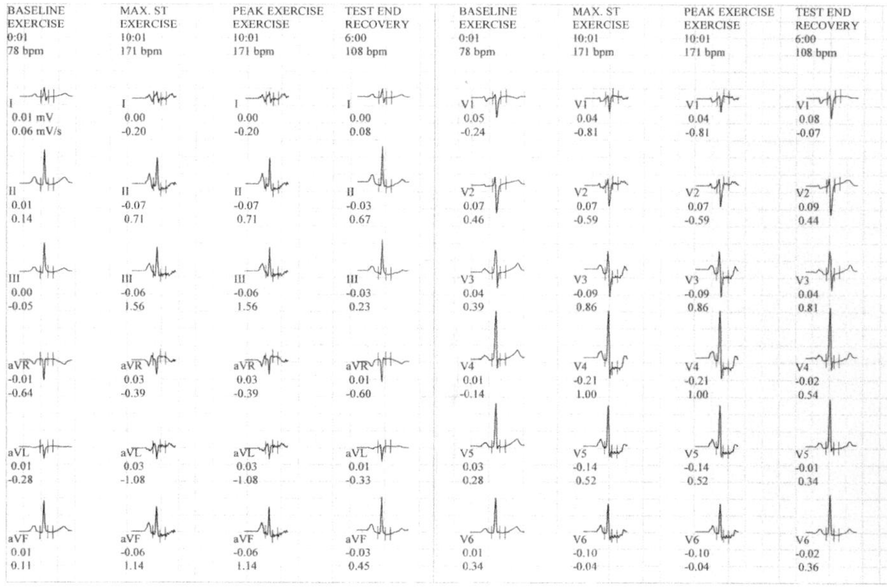

Fig. 9.2 Treadmill stress test using Bruce protocol. The test was maximal at stage 4, reaching 97% of the predicted heart rate with repolarization abnormalities (horizontal ST segment depression) mostly V3V6 which recovered after cessation of exercise, indicative for exercise induced ischemia

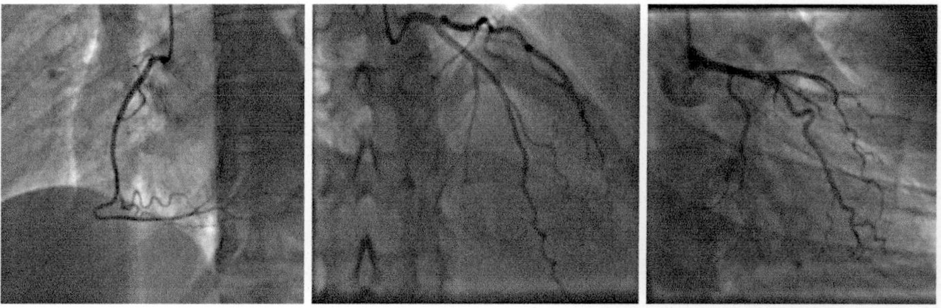

Fig. 9.3 Coronary angiography showing almost normal coronary arteries

As mentioned previously, INOCA patients are frequently encountered in clinical practice, both in men and women; however it is considered to have a higher prevalence in women [3]. It is important to mention that in these patients the risk for recurrence of symptoms in high resulting in repeated hospitalization and even repeated invasive evaluation. In WISE study the 5-year rate of repeated hospitalization for angina in women with non-obstructive coronary artery was 20%, with a 1.8 times higher rate of repeated invasive evaluation compared to those with 1 vessel disease [4] and this was associated with significant costs.

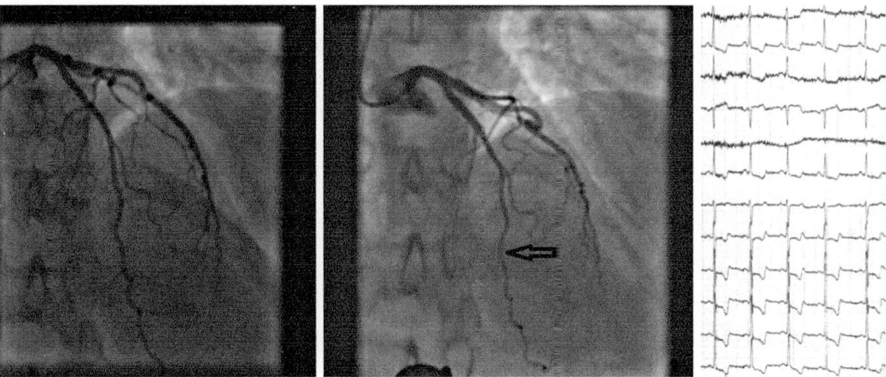

Fig. 9.4 Left: LAD angiography after nitrate. Middle: LAD angiography after 100 mcg Acetylcholine infused over 1 min. There is a diffuse spasm in the mid and distal segment of LAD of 40–45% compared to resting state with the maximum degree of spasm indicated by arrow. Right: ECG after 100 mcg Acetylcholine with diffuse ST segment depression and T wave inversion accompanied by typical angina. During Ach infusion at 100 mcg/1 min there was a slight decrease in heart rate (52/min) with normal blood pressure

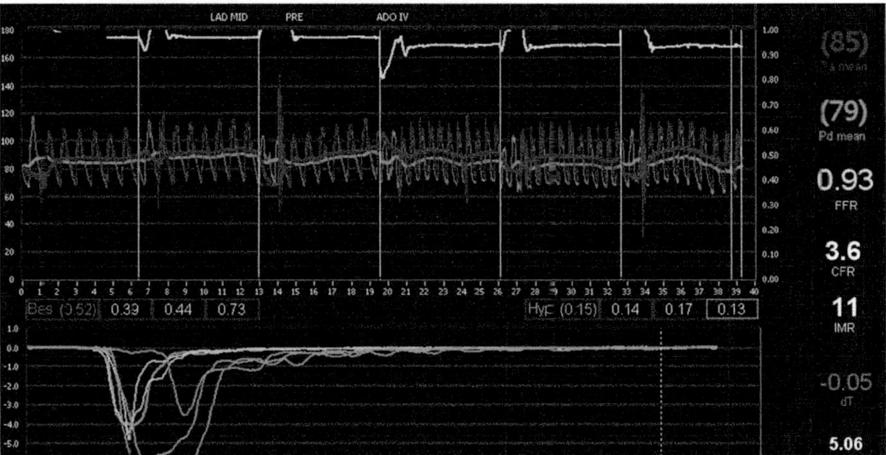

Fig. 9.5 Physiological evaluation with calculation of CFR and IMR using RadiAnalyzer and Certus Wire (Abbot Vascular). The CFR calculation was done after exclusion of one outlier value from basal evaluation (average Tmn value 0.42) with a final CFR of 2.8 and an IMR value of 11 demonstrating a normal endothelial independent response. *CFR* coronary flow reserve, *IMR* index of microcirculatory resistance, *Tmn* mean transit time

According to the 2013 ESC Guideline for stable angina, in patients with chest pain and "normal" coronary arteries the chest pain might be caused by non-cardiac causes, by coronary spasm or by anomalies in the microvascular function [5]. In our patient the chest pain was absolutely typical for angina, making an extra-cardiac etiology improbable and this was the reason for continuing investigation. Coronary epicardial spasm may be responsible for the symptoms in a minority of cases, and there are certain clinical characteristics and established criteria [6] for diagnosis of vasospastic angina.

In order to have a better and more uniform characterization of microvascular function, the COVADIS group [7] published in 2018 a report on standardization of criteria for diagnosis and evaluation of coronary microvascular dysfunction (CMD) and microvascular angina (MVA) (Table 9.1). Accordingly, *definitive* diagnosis of *MVA*, requires beside symptoms of ischemia and absence of obstructive coronary lesions, the presence of both noninvasive signs of ischemia (spontaneous or during stress testing) and microvascular dysfunction (decreased coronary flow reserve—CFR, microvascular spasm during acetylcholine testing, increased microvascular resistance or coronary slow flow). In patients without either noninvasive proof of ischemia or evidence of microvascular dysfunction the diagnosis of *suspected MVA* should be established. As we can understand from these criteria, there are several noninvasive and invasive functional testing which should be performed in order to admit or reject the diagnosis of MVA. However, aside from research purposes, functional testing the presence of MVD is rarely used in evaluation of patients with non-obstructive coronary disease.

Cardiac syndrome X is a widespread clinical entity covering cardiac chest pain in the absence of significant epicardial disease. It has some clinical features (the patients are most often women with angina-like chest pain, normal coronary arteries, and often present some evidence of ischemia, such as abnormal resting ECG or a positive stress test). However it is not well defined and is considered that includes also non-ischemic cardiac conditions like pericardial

Table 9.1 Criteria for microvascular angina [7]

Criteria
1. Symptoms of myocardial ischemia
a. Effort and/or rest angina
b. Angina equivalents (i.e. shortness of breath)
2. Absence of obstructive CAD—no stenosis with >50% diameter reduction or FFR < 0.80 (ICA or CTA)
3. Objective evidence of myocardial ischemia
a. Ischemic ECG changes during an episode of spontaneous chest pain
b. Stress testing with chest pain and/or ischemic ECG changes with or without transient/reversible abnormal myocardial perfusion and/or wall motion abnormality
4. Evidence of coronary microvascular dysfunction (CMD)
a. Reduced coronary flow reserve (cut-off values depends on methodology used ≤2.0 to 2.5)
b. Coronary microvascular spasm, defined as reproduction of symptoms, ischemic ECG changes, but no significant epicardial spasm during acetylcholine testing
c. Increased coronary microvascular resistance indices (e.g. IMR >25)
d. Coronary slow flow phenomenon (TIMI frame count >25)

IMR index of microvascular resistance, *ICA* invasive coronary angiography, *CTA* computer tomography angiography
Definitive MVA—all four criteria are fulfilled
Suspected MVA—criteria 1 and 2 + either 3 or 4

pain, abnormalities in pain perception, psychiatric conditions [8]. Accordingly, the patient fulfilling the diagnostic criteria should be labeled as MVA.

Presence of Angina

Presence of angina (especially typical angina like our patient described) despite absence of angiographic significant coronary stenosis is associated with worse prognosis even after adjusting for risk factors, as it was proven in WISE study [9]. Compared to women with risk factors only, those with angina and normal coronary arteries had a threefold increase in risk of primary endpoint (cardiovascular death, myocardial infarction, stroke or hospitalization for heart failure), while in those with non-obstructive coronary arteries (they had some coronary stenosis less than 50%) the risk was sixfold higher. Similar results were found in another cohort of almost 3500 patients (both men and women) with normal or diffuse non-obstructive coronary artery disease. In this report the presence of symptoms (angina) was associated with an increased HR for MACE even after adjusting for age, BMI, diabetes, smoking status and use of lipid-lowering and antihypertensive medication [3].

Coronary Microvascular Dysfunction (CMD)

CMD remains a challenging diagnosis as this coronary compartment cannot be imaged directly, and only functional testing may help in establishing the diagnosis. According to Camici and Crea [10] there are 4 types of CMD, with certain pathogenic mechanisms:

- type 1—in the absence of myocardial disease or obstructive coronary artery disease and this type may be related to risk factors and represent the substrate of microvascular angina
- Type 2—associated to different myocardial diseases
- Type 3—associated to obstructive epicardial disease
- Type 4—iatrogenic after percutaneous intervention or surgical revascularization

According to COVADIS criteria for CMD [7] there are 4 possibilities to prove an abnormal microcirculatory function and more data may be found in another chapter:

- Reduced coronary flow reserve (CFR) after adenosine administration; this may be done either by invasive measures at the time of diagnostic coronary angiography or noninvasively [11] using positron emission tomography [12], Doppler echocardiography and as more recently proven, magnetic resonance (either with or without contrast [13]), and cardiac CT. Invasive measures of MVD are discussed in detail in Chap. 3 and have the advantage of a better discrimination between epicardial end microcirculatory causes of reduced CFR and also the ability to study endothelial dependent variation of flow.

- Increased flow resistance—evaluated mainly with the index of microcirculatory resistance (IMR) and hyperemic microcirculatory resistance index (HMR);
- Microvascular pattern of spasm during vasomotor testing
- Decreased basal flow on angiography—also known as slow-flow phenomenon (SFP) or cardiac syndrome Y which will be discussed later

Correlation Between CMD Testing and Prognosis

Older studies indicated that chest pain with a normal CAG is associated with a good prognosis [14, 15] especially when compared to patient with significant epicardial disease. We will discuss further implications of different types MVD evaluation.

Role of Acetylcholine Vasomotor Testing (for Protocols Please Refer to Chap. 3)

In one of the largest cohort of INOCA patients (1379 patients) in Europe with Ach testing [16], one third were positive with a microvascular pattern, one quarter were positive with epicardial pattern, another third were ambiguous and less than one eights were normal. However, acetylcholine testing may be interpreted in two different ways. It might be used as a tool for coronary spasm diagnosis (especially when variant angina is suspected) or to evaluate endothelial (epicardial and microcirculatory) function in different clinical settings. When the diagnosis of coronary spasm is challenged there are certain thresholds used (>90% reduction in luminal diameter together with ECG changes and reproduction of symptoms) [6]. However, when endothelial dysfunction is tested [17] the threshold for a positive result is either a diameter reduction of >20% (for epicardial endothelial dysfunction) or a flow increase of <50% (for microcirculatory dysfunction). These are based on the fact that in coronary arteries with normal endothelial function acetylcholine infusion induces an increase in epicardial artery diameter and flow, and this finding are associated with good prognosis. Several outcome studies showed significant differences in parameters of endothelial function between patients with and without events during follow-up, especially for epicardial endothelial function, and these differences remained predictive even after adjusting for the presence of cardiovascular risk factors [18, 19]. Consequently, it is difficult to determine based on available prognostic data which is the significance of epicardial narrowing between 20% and 75% (90)% and this might be important especially in patients with inconclusive results (one third of cases in the study mentioned earlier). Moreover, the doses of acetylcholine might be a matter of debate. In previous prognostic trials testing for endothelial dysfunction [20, 21] the doses were generally 18 μg/min (1 mL/min from solution 10^{-4} M) much smaller than those used for coronary spasm testing trials [16] in (up to 200 μg in 3 min) and also from those recommended in the last consensus from Japanese Circulation Society guidelines (doses up to 100 μg injected over 20 s) [22].

Does Adenosine and Acetylcholine Testing Provide Additional Value?

In study of Reriani et al. [20] it was proven that endothelium dependent and endothelium-independent function differs. In patients considered to have EDMVD (endothelium dependent MVD) based on an increase in blood flow <50% after Ach infusion, with an average actual reduction of CBF of 11%, there was a significant increase in flow after adenosine (endothelium independent vasodilator) indicated by an average CFR of 2.78. This findings support the fact that both type of testing should be performed. The prevalence of MVD based on invasive evaluation of endothelial dependent and independent vasodilatation was found to be 67% (from 1500 non-obstructive coronary arteries patients which were evaluated) [23].

Prognostic Significance of Invasive Vasomotor Testing

An Asian study investigating 4644 patients with angina and non-obstructive coronary arteries (<50%) [17] found that although only 36% of the subjects had a definite normal response to vasoactive testing, a positive response *did not* predict hard outcomes (MACE). In this study the overall rate of MACE was low (1.6%) and did not differ according to the type of response to acetylcholine. However recurrent chest pain requiring repeated invasive evaluation was more frequent in patients with positive vasomotor test (compared to negative) in patients with fixed (non-obstructive) stenosis compared to normal arteries. In another analysis multi-vessel spastic response (with or without ECG changes or chest pain) was predictive for recurrence [24] with a HR 1.96 (CI 1.27–3.02) (vs negative result).

In a meta-analysis [25] of studies using both invasive (Ach) and noninvasive evaluation, dysfunction in the epicardial segment was associated with worse prognosis (RR 2.49 respectively 2.28 for fatal or non-fatal cardiovascular events). It was also demonstrated that vasomotor testing had additive value to classical risk factors (this study used Framingham score) in predicting cardiovascular outcomes in Caucasian patients [20].

It worth mentioning that study by Lee included Asian population while the above mentioned meta-analysis included studies performed on non-Asian population. The results of vasomotor studies should be interpreted with caution as it was observed that there are racial differences between Asian and Caucasian patients in terms of pathophysiology and prognosis [26]. Caucasian patients with positive testing were proved to have a worse prognosis (freedom of death or MI) compared to their Japanese counterparts (and this was related mostly to the presence of non-obstructive atheroma).

Vasomotor testing was studied also in patients after ACS in whom coronary angiography does not identify a culprit lesion. It was proven that vasomotor testing in this setting is safe [27, 28]. The prognostic significance appears to be more important in patients with recent myocardial infarction [28] compared to general acute coronary syndrome without a culprit lesion on angiography [29]. In study of Montone [28] there were a significantly more *death from any cause* (32.4% vs. 4.7%; P = 0.002], *cardiac death* (18.9% vs. 0; P = 0.005), and *readmission for ACS* [27.0% vs. 7.0%; P = 0.015), as well as a worse *angina status* in patients with positive testing. In the positive results group the prognosis was worse in patients with epicardial spasm pattern compared to those with a microvascular of spasm (death from any cause 45.8% vs. 7.7%; P = 0.027).

Increased Resistance in Microcirculation

The most extensive studied parameter for microcirculatory resistance is the Index of Microcirculatory Resistance (IMR). It should be mentioned it is evaluating the minimal resistance in microcirculation measured during adenosine infusion which abolishes microvascular tone in a endothelial independent fashion. For technical details please refer to Chap. 3. Generally an IMR value >25 is considered to indicate high resistance in microcirculation and this threshold is advocated in the COVADIS criteria for CMVD [7]. IMR values are also dependent on the mass of myocardium subtended to the segment of artery which is evaluated [30]. Accordingly, Lee et al. [31] identified distinct cutoff values in different coronary territories based on the 75th percentile values of IMR (using corrected values with Yong's formula [32] to account for collateral flow without measurement of wedge pressure) in a >1000 patients population with intermediate lesions. LAD had the lowest value 21.3 U, RCA had the highest value 27.1 U, while LCX had an intermediate value 23.0 U. Using these criteria Kobayashi et al. [33] found a prevalence of increased IMR in at least 1 vessel of 41% (38/93 patients) in patients with clinical suspicion of ischemic heart disease. Similar results were found in a recent publication with complex invasive and noninvasive evaluation (CRM) of patients with stable angina and indication for invasive evaluation [34], with almost half (60/125) of the vessels evaluated showing increased microvascular resistance (IMR>25), either with or without ischemic FFR.

Value of high IMR in explaining myocardial ischemia in patients with positive stress test and normal (without minor irregularities) epicardial arteries was proven by Luo et al. [35]. They identified an IMR value measured in LAD of 33.3 ± 7.6 in patients with positive stress test compared to 18.9 ± 5.6 in controls ($p < 0.001$). Moreover all IMR values in patients with ischemia were >20 and the value of IMR had a good correlation with the severity of ischemia (evaluated by Duke Treadmill Score).

Coronary Flow Reserve (CFR)

Coronary flow reserve is a measure of the capacity of increase in flood flow compared to basal conditions when both microcirculatory and epicardial resistances are as low as achievable. The stimulus used is most frequently is adenosine coupled with nitroglycerine infusion (please refer also to Chap. 3 for more details). Based on older studies is considered that the hyperemic flow is not altered by the presence of an epicardial stenosis <50% [36]. As a consequence in patients with non-obstructive coronary arteries the increase in flow is dependent only on the capacity of microcirculation to decrease resistance. It was proven that only angiographic appearance is not enough for functional characterization of epicardial disease especially in intermediate stenosis, and functional evaluation (with fractional flow reserve—FFR or instantaneous wave free ratio—iFR) is preferred. The importance of invasive functional evaluation of epicardial disease is demonstrated especially in the setting of diffuse epicardial disease where it is sometimes impossible to define a reference zone without disease which makes unreliable evaluation of angiographic degree of stenosis.

Different studies in patient with intermediate stenosis identified impaired CFR in 10–30% of the lesions with non-ischemic FFR [37–39]. Impaired CFR has been shown to predict major adverse outcomes among women evaluated for suspected ischemia [40] and also in patients with non-obstructive lesions [37]. However one potential drawback of CFR might be its dependence on resting state and it was proven that impaired CFR was associated more probably to markers of increased basal flow—increased APV at Doppler evaluation [38], or decreased transit time during thermo evaluation [37]. Considering the fact that CFR values are influenced both on extension of epicardial disease and on the basal hemodynamic conditions (and it is known that is almost impossible to maintain true resting conditions during evaluation in the cath lab), it becomes obvious that this is not the parameter of choice for evaluation of MVD [41].

CFR may also be measured noninvasively (using transthoracic Doppler, positron emission scintigraphy) and there are solid data about the prognostic value of noninvasive CFR but in this situation the relation to MVD is more difficult to be appreciated as precise information about epicardial component is missing.

Coronary Slow Flow Phenomenon–(CSFP)

This condition (known also as cardiac Syndrome Y), was first described in 1972 by Tambe et al. [42] in 6 patients evaluated invasively, 4 of them with typical angina. The diagnosis is based on angiographic demonstration of spontaneous slow flow as evidenced by slow progression of contrast dye in the coronary artery without significant coronary stenosis, coronary ectasia, in the absence of prior coronary intervention, air embolism and in the setting of a normal arterial pressure. The cut-off values used by different authors for CSFP definitions were: at least 3 cardiac cycles for the contrast media to fill entire vessel [43] or a corrected TIMI frame count >27 [44] (at 30 fps. rate, with a 1.7 correction coefficient for LAD to account for its length) [45]. This should be differentiated from secondary CSFS which may occur for example after coronary intervention due to distal debris embolization from epicardial plaque manipulation. Different reports included in this category either patients without significant coronary stenosis (<40% stenosis) or only patients without evidence of coronary atherosclerosis.

There are also transient conditions such as myocarditis in which coronary angiography may reveal slow flow in the absence of coronary stenosis [46]. Taking into consideration that this condition may mimic ACS, as generally considered for CSFP, it becomes obvious that the diagnostic workup in this situation may become more complex as final diagnosis is established after magnetic resonance imaging.

When present, the slow flow phenomenon may involve one or more coronary territories, most often LAD (up to 90 %) followed by RCA (30–45%) and left circumflex (20%) [45]. In a trial evaluating 80 patients with SCFP [47] almost three quarters were male and almost half of them were smokers. There is also an association with obesity while there are conflicting results about the association with metabolic syndrome [48]. Other clinical features of CSFP patients were described by Beltrame and col [43] in a series of 64 CSFP patients (extracted from 6000 angiographies). Seventy percent of the patients with CSFP were males, with acute presentation (rest chest pain). However, in another report [45] all the patients with CSFP had a positive non-invasive stress testing (nuclear, echo or ECG), which actually may reflect different local protocols for invasive coronary angiography prescription. In this report it is mentioned that 11 out of 15 patients had had previous invasive evaluation with documentation of CSFP pain) in 67%, myocardial infarction in another 8%, and one third were smokers. It is important to note that 84% of the patients had recurrent chest pain during follow-up and 19% were re-admitted to CCU. Based on a case control analysis in the same publication which included patients investigated for angina without slow flow as controls, male gender, acute presentation, smoking, ST/T wave abnormalities at rest were significantly more frequent present in patients with SCFP. However, stress test was positive in only 19% of CSFP patients compared to 39% in controls (difference reported as non-significant.

CSFP appears to be associated with signs of endothelial dysfunction in other vascular beds. In a previous report presence of SCFP was associated with worse flow mediated vasodilatation compared to control [49]. In that report peripheral endothelial dysfunction was improved after administration of nebivolol, together with improved exercise duration and a better control of chest pain [50].

However CSFP does not appear to be related to the other cardiovascular risk factors such as diabetes, dyslipidemia and hypertension as it was proved by Beltrame et al. [43]. In their case control study in patients with normal coronary arteries (no minor stenosis) on angiography, presence of slow flow was not associated with hypertension, dyslipidemia or a positive family history. Same results were obtained also by Hawkins et al. [44]

In a small group of patients considered to have CSFP it was proven an abnormally elevated resistance in the microcirculation (evaluated as transit time × Distal pressure) at rest but with a significant reduction during hyperemia [51] resulting in a normal CFR. An estimation of the CFR may be deduced from the ratio of TIMI frame count in the basal and hyperemic state [52]. Generally in patients with CSFP intracoronary delivery of microcirculatory active agents results in acute improvement of coronary flow (dipyridamole, adenosine, papaverine, calcium channel blockers), while nitroglycerine does not have the same effect [53, 54]. These findings support the hypothesis of a functionally increased resting microcirculatory resistance in the pathogenesis of CSFP. Moreover short-term dipyridamole oral administration results in improved coronary flow [55].

Mangieri et al. [53] proved that there were also structural abnormalities on myocardial biopsy specimens in patient with CSFP, affecting both small vessels (thickening of the vessel wall with reduced lumen) and myocites.

MVD Associated with Epicardial Disease

When we analyze the relation between MVD and epicardial disease there are several situations regarding the epicardial compartment:

- Epicardial arteries are "normal"—no parietal irregularities. There is no (identifiable) epicardial atherosclerosis.
- There is epicardial disease which is considered "non-obstructive" and in this category most of the studies used a threshold of <50% diameter stenosis. However, another possible definition might be based on functional evaluation (FFR or iFR).
- The epicardial disease is considered as "obstructive"—i.e. with stenosis >50% (or with positive functional evaluation).

MVD might be involved in the pathogenesis of ischemia also in patients with angiographic evidence of epicardial disease when a decreased CFR is found despite a non-ischemic FFR (FFR-CFR discordance) which was already presented earlier.

In a recently published report on a small cohort of 60 patients with stable angina evaluated invasively with FFR and IMR [34] abnormal IMR (>25, as an evidence of MVD) was present in 49% of the segments that were evaluated and 20% had also ischemic FFR (<0.8). In another study evaluating intermediate stenosis (40–70% diameter stenosis) Lee et al. [37] identified high IMR in 11/147 patients with ischemic FFR (7.5%) and 58/230 in patients with non-ischemic FFR (25%).

Clinical Significance

There are 2 clinical scenario for patients with ischemia and intermediate lesion:

- MVD is severe and is responsible of ischemia. Epicardial disease is just "an innocent by-stander" In this situation proceeding to revascularization may not actually alleviate ischemia and this may be responsible for post-revascularization angina [56]. In such situation proper documentation of MVD prior to revascularization, especially when documentation of ischemia is not able to indicate a specific territory (like ECG stress testing), may actually prevent unnecessary procedures with possible risks.
- MVD is borderline and the presence of epicardial lesion is further limiting the ability to increase flow during stress. However FFR is negative due to presence of MVD. Some authors suggest that in specific clinical scenario of elevated microcirculatory resistance, even negative FFR lesions revascularization may alleviate ischemia and improve symptoms [57, 58]. The predictive value of negative FFR for the ischemic potential of an epicardial lesion (evaluated with myocardial scintigraphy) was proved to be modulated by the amplitude of microcirculatory resistance (evaluated with hyperemic microcirculatory resistance index) [59].

Unfortunately we do not have enough data to establish certain cut-off values for different parameters in guiding clinical decisions regarding the need for revascularization in such special situations.

Benefits of Standardized Definition of MVA and CMD

Angina despite normal or non-obstructive coronary arteries remains a challenging diagnosis. It is frequently found in clinical practice; may be related to the local practice algorithms for indicating invasive evaluation. It is known that it has a much better prognosis compared to obstructive disease. Do we have to continue the diagnostic workup or it is enough to stop at this point to reassure the patient that his/her condition is benign and we have to control the possible risk factors?

In our patient we used acetylcholine testing to evaluate endothelium dependent vascular reactivity and also the possible involvement of vascular spasm in generation of symptoms. Another way to test endothelial dependent function would have been the cold pressor testing. We demonstrated a typical microvascular response at 100 μg with reproduction of symptoms, significant ischemic ECG changes and with moderate reduction in lumen size (less than 50%). This type of response was previously described by Ong et al. [60]. In this report different degrees of epicardial luminal reduction accompanied microvascular type of spasm: <25% in 52%, 25–50% in 36% and 50–75% in rest of the cases. Further testing for endothelium independent MVD (IMR) showed normal result.

Detection of abnormalities of coronary epicardial or microvascular compartment in patients with angina and non-obstructive unobstructed coronary arteries may reassure the patient because actually we identified a condition responsible for the symptoms which may modify the therapeutic approach (in our case calcium channel blockers were used with good control of symptoms). Other advantage for a precise diagnosis might be in evaluating other diagnostic strategies (possibly noninvasive). It is of utmost importance in this field identification of gadolinium independent magnetic resonance parameters (based on T1 map in basal conditions and during adenosine infusion) for defining microvascular dysfunction and to differentiate from epicardial involvement [13]. Standardization of diagnosis of MVA (with evidence of MVD) may help to characterize better this type of disease in terms of natural evolution, and the possibilities to influence it with different interventions. Moreover we may evaluate the efficacy of the treatment not only in terms of symptomatic recurrences, but also on certain objective measures of coronary dysfunction (extension or degree of spasm or CMVD) and even compare different therapeutic strategies which may help in developing new drugs for treatment of vasospastic conditions as it is demonstrated that currently available drugs (CCB and nitrates) are not always optimal in controlling recurrences [8, 61]. Another important issue is that during extensive testing (especially invasive) occult significant epicardial stenosis might be identified with significant therapeutic and prognostic consequences. Alternatively, in patients with negative testing (for spasm, CMVD) extra cardiac conditions should be investigated more aggressively.

In our patient due to the fact that we demonstrated presence of MVD we prescribed statin at high dose (atorvastatin 80 mg/day) as there are reports [8] on benefits of statin therapy in treating patients with MVD. We also prescribed low dose aspirin according to European guidelines recommendations [5], although the role of this therapy in the setting of MVD should be rather an interesting topic for future research. However, more attention received life style modification with smoking cessation and regular aerobic exercise training as these are considered the most important modifiers of microvascular and endothelial dysfunction [62].

References

1. Patel MR, Peterson ED, Dai D, Brennan JM, Redberg RF, Anderson HV, et al. Low diagnostic yield of elective coronary angiography. N Engl J Med. 2010;362:886–95.
2. Bairey Merz CN, Pepine CJ, Walsh MN, Fleg JL. Ischemia and no obstructive coronary artery disease (INOCA). Circulation. 2017;135(11):1075–92.
3. Jespersen L, Hvelplund A, Abildstrøm SZ, Pedersen F, Galatius S, Madsen JK, et al. Stable angina pectoris with no obstructive coronary artery disease is associated with increased risks of major adverse cardiovascular events. Eur Heart J. 2012;33(6):734–44.

4. Shaw LJ, Merz CNB, Pepine CJ, Reis SE, Bittner V, Kip KE, Health Services and Outcomes Research, et al. The economic burden of angina in women with suspected ischemic heart disease blood institute – sponsored Women's Ischemia Syndrome Evaluation. Circulation. 2006;114:894–904.
5. Montalescot G, Sechtem U, Achenbach S, Andreotti F, Arden C, Budaj A, et al. 2013 ESC guidelines on the management of stable coronary artery disease: the Task Force on the management of stable coronary artery disease of the European Society of Cardiology. Eur Heart J. 2013;34(38):2949–3003. Available from http://www.ncbi.nlm.nih.gov/pubmed/23996286.
6. Beltrame JF, Crea F, Kaski JC, Ogawa H, Ong P, Sechtem U, et al. International standardization of diagnostic criteria for vasospastic angina. Eur Heart J. 2015;38(33):2565–8.
7. Ong P, Camici PG, Beltrame JF, Crea F, Shimokawa H, Sechtem U, et al. International standardization of diagnostic criteria for microvascular angina. Int J Cardiol. 2018;250:16–20. https://doi.org/10.1016/j.ijcard.2017.08.068.
8. Marinescu MA, Löffler AI, Ouellette M, Smith L, Kramer CM, Bourque JM. Coronary microvascular dysfunction, microvascular angina, and treatment strategies. JACC Cardiovasc Imaging. 2015;8(2):210–20.
9. Gulati M, Cooper-DeHoff RM, McClure C, Johnson BD, Shaw LJ, Handberg EM, et al. Adverse cardiovascular outcomes in women with nonobstructive coronary artery disease. Arch Intern Med. 2009;169(9):843.
10. Crea F, Camici PG, Bairey Merz CN. Coronary microvascular dysfunction: an update. Eur Heart J. 2014;35(17):1101–11. Available from http://www.pubmedcentral.nih.gov/articlerender.fcgi?artid=4006091&tool=pmcentrez&rendertype=abstract.
11. Feher A, Sinusas AJ. Quantitative assessment of coronary microvascular function. Circ Cardiovasc Imaging. 2017;10(8):1–21.
12. Driessen RS, Raijmakers PG, Stuijfzand WJ, Knaapen P. Myocardial perfusion imaging with PET. Int J Cardiovasc Imaging. 2017;33(7):1021–31. https://doi.org/10.1007/s10554-017-1084-4.
13. Liu A, Wijesurendra RS, Liu JM, Greiser A, Jerosch-herold M, Forfar JC, et al. Gadolinium-free cardiac MR stress T1-mapping to distinguish epicardial from microvascular coronary disease. J Am Coll Cardiol. 2018;71(9):957–68.
14. Lichtlen P, Bargheer K, Wenzlaff P. Long-term prognosis of patients with angina- like chest pain and normal coronary angiographic findings. J Am Coll Cardiol. 1995;25:1013–8.
15. Kemp H, Kronmal R, Vlietstra R, Frye R. Seven year survival of patients with normal or near normal coronary arteriograms: a CASS registry study. J Am Coll Cardiol. 1986;7:479–83.
16. Aziz A, Hansen HS, Sechtem U, Prescott E, Ong P. Sex-related differences in vasomotor function in patients with angina and unobstructed coronary arteries. J Am Coll Cardiol. 2017;70(19):2349–58.
17. Lee EM, Choi MH, Seo HS, Kim HK, Kim NH, Choi CU, et al. Impact of vasomotion type on prognosis of coronary artery spasm induced by acetylcholine provocation test of left coronary artery. Atherosclerosis. 2017;257:195–200. https://doi.org/10.1016/j.atherosclerosis.2016.09.015.
18. Halcox JPJ, Schenke WH, Zalos G, Mincemoyer R, Prasad A, Waclawiw MA, et al. Clinical investigation and reports prognostic value of coronary vascular endothelial dysfunction. Circulation. 2002;106:653–8.
19. Von Mering GO, Arant CB, Wessel TR, Mcgorray SP, Merz CNB, Sharaf BL, et al. Abnormal coronary vasomotion as a prognostic indicator of cardiovascular events in women. Circulation. 2004;109:722–5.
20. Reriani M, Sara JD, Flammer A, Gulati R, Rihal C, Lennon R, et al. Coronary endothelial function testing provides superior discrimination compared to standard clinical risk scoring in prediction of cardiovascular events. Coron Artery Dis. 2016;27(3):213–20.
21. Halcox JPJ, Schenke WH, Zalos G, Mincemoyer R, Prasad A, Waclawiw MA, et al. Prognostic value of coronary vascular endothelial dysfunction. Circulation. 2002;106(6):653–8.
22. JCS Joint Working Group. Guidelines for diagnosis and treatment of patients with vasospastic angina (Coronary Spastic Angina) (JCS 2013). Circ J. 2014;78(11):2779–801.

23. Sara JD, Widmer RJ, Matsuzawa Y, Lennon RJ, Lerman LO, Lerman A. Prevalence of coronary microvascular dysfunction among patients with chest pain and nonobstructive coronary artery disease. JACC Cardiovasc Interv. 2015;8(11):1445–53.
24. Park S, Choi BG, Rha S, Kang TS. The multi-vessel and diffuse coronary spasm is a risk factor for persistent angina in patients received anti-angina medication. Medicine (Baltimore). 2018;97(47):e13288.
25. Brainin P, Frestad D, Prescott E. The prognostic value of coronary endothelial and microvascular dysfunction in subjects with normal or non-obstructive coronary artery disease: a systematic review and meta-analysis. Int J Cardiol. 2018;254:1–9.
26. Beltrame JF, Sasayama S, Maseri A. Racial heterogeneity in coronary artery vasomotor reactivity: differences between Japanese and Caucasian patients. J Am Coll Cardiol. 1999;33(6):1442–52. https://doi.org/10.1016/S0735-1097(99)00073-X.
27. Ong P, Athanasiadis A, Hill S, Vogelsberg H, Voehringer M, Sechtem U. Coronary artery spasm as a frequent cause of acute coronary syndrome: the CASPAR (Coronary Artery Spasm in Patients With Acute Coronary Syndrome). J Am Coll Cardiol. 2008;52(7):523–7.
28. Montone RA, Niccoli G, Fracassi F, Russo M, Gurgoglione F, Cammà G, et al. Patients with acute myocardial infarction and non-obstructive coronary arteries: safety and prognostic relevance of invasive coronary provocative tests. Eur Heart J. 2018;39(2):91–8.
29. Ong P, Athanasiadis A, Borgulya G, Voehringer M, Sechtem U. 3-year follow-up of patients with coronary artery spasm as cause of acute coronary syndrome: the CASPAR (coronary artery spasm in patients with acute coronary syndrome) study follow-up. J Am Coll Cardiol. 2011;57(2):147–52. https://doi.org/10.1016/j.jacc.2010.08.626.
30. Echavarría-Pinto M, Van De Hoef TP, Nijjer S, Gonzalo N, Nombela-Franco L, Ibañez B, et al. Influence of the amount of myocardium subtended to a coronary stenosis on the index of microcirculatory resistance. Implications for the invasive assessment of microcirculatory function in ischaemic heart disease. EuroIntervention. 2017;13(8):944–52.
31. Lee JM, Layland J, Jung JH, Lee HJ, Echavarria-Pinto M, Watkins S, et al. Integrated physiologic assessment of ischemic heart disease in real-world practice using index of microcirculatory resistance and fractional flow reserve: insights from the International Index of Microcirculatory Resistance Registry. Circ Cardiovasc Interv. 2015;8(11):e002857.
32. Yong AS, Layland J, Fearon WF, Ho M, Shah MG, Daniels D, et al. Calculation of the index of microcirculatory resistance without coronary wedge pressure measurement in the presence of epicardial stenosis. JACC Cardiovasc Interv. 2013;6(1):53–8.
33. Kobayashi Y, Lee JM, Fearon WF, Lee JH, Nishi T, Choi D-H, et al. Three-vessel assessment of coronary microvascular dysfunction in patients with clinical suspicion of ischemia. Circ Cardiovasc Interv. 2017;10(11):e005445. Available from http://circinterventions.ahajournals.org/lookup/doi/10.1161/CIRCINTERVENTIONS.117.005445.
34. Liu A, Wijesurendra RS, Liu JM, Greiser A, Jerosch-herold M, Forfar JC, et al. Gadolinium-free cardiac MR stress T1-mapping to distinguish epicardial from microvascular coronary disease. J Am Coll Cardiol. 2018;71(9):857–68.
35. Luo C, Long M, Hu X, Huang Z, Hu C, Gao X, et al. Thermodilution-derived coronary microvascular resistance and flow reserve in patients with cardiac syndrome X. Circ Cardiovasc Interv. 2014;7(1):43–8.
36. Gould KL, Lipscomb K. Effects of coronary stenoses on coronary flow reserve and resistance. Am J Cardiol. 1974;34(1):48–55.
37. Lee JM, Jung JH, Hwang D, Park J, Fan Y, Na SH, et al. Coronary flow reserve and microcirculatory resistance in patients with intermediate coronary stenosis. J Am Coll Cardiol. 2016;67(10):1158–69.
38. Van De Hoef TP, Van Lavieren MA, Damman P, Delewi R, Piek MA, Chamuleau SAJ, et al. Physiological basis and long-term clinical outcome of discordance between fractional flow reserve and coronary flow velocity reserve in coronary stenoses of intermediate severity. Circ Cardiovasc Interv. 2014;7(3):301–11.
39. Ahn J-M, Zimmermann FM, Johnson NP, Shin E-S, Koo B-K, Lee PH, et al. Fractional flow reserve and pressure-bounded coronary flow reserve to predict outcomes in coronary artery disease. Eur Heart J. 2017;38(25):1980–9. https://doi.org/10.1093/eurheartj/ehx139.

40. Pepine CJ, Anderson RD, Sharaf BL, Reis SE, Smith KM, Handberg EM, et al. Coronary microvascular reactivity to adenosine predicts adverse outcome in women evaluated for suspected ischemia: results from the NHLBI Women's Ischemia Syndrome Evaluation (WISE) study. J Am Coll Cardiol. 2010;55(25):2825–32.
41. De Bruyne B, Oldroyd KG, Pijls NHJ. Microvascular (dys)function and clinical outcome in stable coronary disease. J Am Coll Cardiol. 2016;67(10):1170–2.
42. Tambe AA, Demany MA, Zimmerman HA, Mascarenhas E. Angina pectoris and slow flow velocity of dye in coronary arteries: a new angiographic finding. Am Heart J. 1972;84:66–71.
43. Beltrame J, Ganz P. The coronary slow flow phenomenon – a new coronary microvascular disorder. Cardiology. 2002;97:197–202.
44. Hawkins BM, Stavrakis S, Rousan TA, Abu-Fadel M, Eliot S. Coronary slow flow – prevalence and clinical correlations. Circ J. 2012;76:936–42.
45. Alvarez C, Siu H. Coronary slow-flow phenomenon as an under recognized and treatable source of chest pain: case series and literature review. J Investig Med High Impact Case Rep. 2018;6:2324709618789194. Available from file:///pubmed/30038914.
46. Gori T. Coronary slow flow in a patient with myocarditis. In: Gori T, Fineschi M, editors. Atlas of FFR-guided percutaneous coronary interventions. Cham: Springer; 2016. p. 183–5.
47. Beltrame JF, Turner SP, Leslie SL, Solomon P, Freedman SB, Horowitz JD. The angiographic and clinical benefits of mibefradil in the coronary slow flow phenomenon. J Am Coll Cardiol. 2004;44(1):57–62. https://doi.org/10.1016/j.jacc.2004.03.055.
48. Yilmaz H, Demir I, Uyar Z. Clinical and coronary angiographic characteristics of patients with coronary slow flow. Acta Cardiol. 2008;63(5):579–84. https://doi.org/10.2143/AC.63.5.2033224.
49. Sezgin AT, Sigirci A, Barutcu I, Topal E, Sezgin N, Ozdemir R, Yetkin E, Tandogan I, Kosar F, Ermis N, Yologlu S, Bariskaner ECS. Vascular endothelial function in patients with slow coronary flow. Coron Artery Dis. 2003;14(2):155–61.
50. Tiryakioglu S, Tiryakioglu O, Ari H, Basel MC, Bozat T. Effects of nebivolol on endothelial function and exercise parameters in patients with slow coronary flow. Clin Med Cardiol. 2009;3:115–9.
51. Fineschi M, Bravi A, Gori T. The "slow coronary flow" phenomenon: evidence of preserved coronary flow reserve despite increased resting microvascular resistances. Int J Cardiol. 2008;127(3):358–61.
52. Manginas A, Gatzov P, Chasikidis C, Voudris V, Pavlides G, Cokkinos DV. Estimation of coronary flow reserve using the Thrombolysis In Myocardial Infarction (TIMI) frame count method. Am J Cardiol. 1999;83(11):1562–5.
53. Mangieri E, et al. Slow coronary flow: clinical and histopathological features in patients with otherwise normal epicardial coronary arteries. Cathet Cardiovasc Diagn. 1996;37:375–81.
54. Li L, Gu Y, Liu T, Bai Y, Hou L, Cheng Z, et al. A randomized, single-center double-blinded trial on the effects of diltiazem sustained-release capsules in patients with coronary slow flow phenomenon at 6-month follow-up. PLoS One. 2012;7(6):1–5.
55. Kurtoglu N, Akcay A, Dindar I. Usefulness of oral dipyridamole therapy for angiographic slow coronary artery flow. Am J Cardiol. 2001;87(6):777–9.
56. Izzo P, Macchi A, de Gennaro L, Gaglione A, Di Biase M, Brunetti ND. Recurrent angina after coronary angioplasty: mechanisms, diagnostic and therapeutic options. Eur Hear J Acute Cardiovasc Care. 2012;1(2):158–69.
57. Jabs A, Hink U, Fineschi M, Münzel T, Gori T. How should I treat a patient with typical angina, typical angiography, negative FFR? EuroIntervention. 2013;9(1):157–8.
58. Van Lavieren MA, Van De Hoef TP, Sjauw KD, Piek JJ. How should I treat a patient with refractory angina and a single stenosis with normal FFR but abnormal CFR? EuroIntervention. 2015;11(1):125–6.
59. Van De Hoef TP, Nolte F, Echavarría-Pinto M, Van Lavieren MA, Damman P, Chamuleau SAJ, et al. Impact of hyperaemic microvascular resistance on fractional flow reserve measurements in patients with stable coronary artery disease: insights from combined stenosis and microvascular resistance assessment. Heart. 2014;100(12):951–9.

60. Ong P, Athanasiadis A, Borgulya G, Mahrholdt H, Kaski JC, Sechtem U. High prevalence of a pathological response to acetylcholine testing in patients with stable angina pectoris and unobstructed coronary arteries: the ACOVA study (abnormal coronary vasomotion in patients with stable angina and unobstructed coronary arteries). J Am Coll Cardiol. 2012;59(7):655–62. Available from:. https://doi.org/10.1016/j.jacc.2011.11.015.
61. Bory M, Pierron F, Panagides D, Bonnet JL, Yvorra S, Desfossez L. Coronary artery spasm in patients with normal or near normal coronary arteries. Eur Heart J. 1996;17:1015–21.
62. Pries AR, Badimon L, Bugiardini R, Camici PG, Dorobantu M, Duncker DJ, et al. Coronary vascular regulation, remodelling, and collateralization: mechanisms and clinical implications on behalf of the working group on coronary pathophysiology and microcirculation. Eur Heart J. 2015;36(45):3134–46.

Chapter 10
Vasospastic Angina

Edina Cenko and Raffaele Bugiardini

Introduction

The hypothesis that some forms of ischemic heart disease may be caused by increased vasomotor tone of the coronary arteries is not a new, it having being proposed by William Osler over 100 years ago as the cause of angina pectoris [1]. This hypothesis was supported by evidence in 1959 with Prinzmetal' work in patients with what he first termed "variant angina" [2]. With the advent of coronary angiography, it became apparent that not all patients with clinical suspicion of myocardial ischemia had fixed obstructive stenosis in the epicardial coronary arteries. Almost 30-years later, Maseri et al. [3] concluded that the underlying pathogenetic factor of variant angina was a coronary artery spasm, which in turn was defined as, a "*local segmental spasm that produce only mild constriction in nonspastic segments of the coronary arteries*" 24 years ago, we considered whether diffused severe epicardial coronary constriction by ≥50% of lumen diameter could limit blood flow supply to the myocardium, producing myocardial ischemia and angina, in patients with normal smooth coronary arteries at angiography [4]. We proposed the term *"vasotonic angina"* as a suitable descriptor for this syndrome, commenting that as a group" *these patients show diffuse coronary epicardial vasoconstriction and the microcirculation is still the major culprit as assessed by coronary blood flow measurements in the coronary sinus. In some cases, the functional abnormalities may be exclusive to large or small arteries; in others, components of the entire coronary tree may be involved*".

The term "vasospastic angina" was officially coined by the Japanese Circulation Society in 2010 [5]. As the authors point out in their recommendations that it was,

E. Cenko · R. Bugiardini (✉)
Department of Experimental, Diagnostic and Specialty Medicine, University of Bologna, Bologna, BO, Italy
e-mail: edina.cenko2@unibo.it; raffaele.bugiardini@unibo.it

M. Dorobantu, L. Badimon (eds.), *Microcirculation*,
https://doi.org/10.1007/978-3-030-28199-1_10

perhaps, time to revise the paradigm of only one form of angina caused by coronary artery spasm and producing transient ST-segment elevation, namely variant angina. A coronary artery may be partially occluded or diffusely narrowed by spasm causing anginal attacks even with ST-segment depression.

Controversy over Clinical Guidelines

The guidelines Japanese Circulation Society established that either focal or diffuse of an epicardial coronary artery resulting in a high-grade obstruction should be collectively termed vasospastic angina [5]. However, we do not agree with this definition. Indeed, coronary spasm can be divided into 2 major categories that are distinct entities and likely should be managed differently. Focal coronary artery spasm can be treated effectively by calcium-channel blockers (CCB) and nitrates. In contrast, there have been no reports on the therapeutic management of diffuse coronary spasm. Diffuse spasm is a manifestation of endothelia dysfunction and, as so, strategies aimed at reducing cardiovascular risk factors, angiotensin-converting enzyme inhibitor therapy, supplementation with folic acid, and physical exercise may translate into an improvement in endothelial health and revert abnormal vasoconstriction.

The Mode of Presentation of Vasotonic Angina

The mode of presentation ranges from uncomplicated chest pain to severe ischemia and acute myocardial infarction (AMI). Chest pain presentation is often reported by clinicians to be more atypical. Although there is little empirical support for a different symptom profile or vocabulary, the results of a prior study suggest that differences may indeed exist in angina pain location at least in a minority of these patients [6]. The chest discomfort is often similar in quality to that of classic angina although it is usually more intense. Patients usually describe it as “constricting pain,” rather than as an “oppressive feeling,” and the pain may persist 30 min or more. Vasotonic angina may present with symptoms of both stable and unstable angina. The majority of patients seem to be between these two extremes, with a variable prevalence of the two types of symptoms. Several clues in a patient’s history may suggest the presence of vasotonic angina; these include an extremely variable threshold of physical activity that provokes angina; radiation of the discomfort to the submammary areas; and features associated with pain, such as mental arousal, or palpitation [7]. In summary, patients with vasotonic angina are often indistinguishable from those with classic angina and obstructive coronary artery disease. Although clinical presentation and outcome of chest pain may provide some insights, it is too subjective to help with individual patient diagnosis and risk stratification.

The Mode of Presentation of Variant Angina

Myocardial infarction, cardiac arrest, and sudden death can occur, although infrequently, with variant angina in the absence of obstructive coronary stenosis. Unlike vasotonic angina—which is often triggered by exertion or emotional stress—variant angina almost always occurs when a person is at rest, usually between midnight and early morning. These attacks can be very painful and can be relieved by taking sublingual nitrates. The spasms tend to come in cycles—appearing for a time, then going away. After 6–12 months of treatment, physicians may gradually reduce treatment.

Mechanisms of Focal and Diffuse Coronary Artery Spams

Abnormal coronary vasoconstriction is one manifestation of a spectrum of coronary vasoconstrictor disorders involved in ischemic heart disease ranging from classic angina in patients with predominantly fixed atheromatous lesions, to unstable angina where both fixed and dynamic lesions often occur, to variant angina and vasotonic angina where little if any fixed stenosis may exist but spasm is pathognomonic [4, 8–10]. The etiology appears non-homogenous and despite the considerable effort of research over the last four decades, there is no universally accepted understanding of the etiopathophysiology of any form of vasospastic angina. Suggested mechanisms and contributing factors of vasotonic include microvascular coronary dysfunction, altered regulation of coronary microcirculation through autonomic dysregulatory mechanisms and/or imbalance state between endothelial-derived vasodilator and vasoconstrictor factors, generalized vascular disorder, abnormal subendocardial perfusion, inflammation, hyperinsulinemia, enhanced sodium-hydrogen exchange, hormonal deficiency, abnormal pain perception and lastly inherent pathogenetic pathways. Furthermore, the notion that all forms of vasospaspic angina have “normal coronary arteries” should be reconsidered in light of some studies showing that most patients had definite coronary atherosclerosis which was concealed by positive remodeling [11].

Impairment of Parasympathetic Activity

Autonomic nervous system influences may play a role in causing focal coronary spasm or abnormal coronary vasomotor tone. Data form ECG Holter Monitoring showed a marked circadian variation in the episodes of ischemia. In one study, ischemia occurred predominantly during waking hours, none during sleep; 25% during effort; 35% during minimal physical activity; 28% during activities demanding routine mental work such as conversation, reading, or watching television; and 10%

during activities not well specified [7]. Notably, an increase in heart rate accompanied 95% of all ischemic episodes [7]. One intriguing investigation has shown that focal coronary spasm reflects inputs from the adjacent esophageal system [12]. Esophageal spasms were time-related to ischemia, from 1 to 5 min before ECG-recorded ischemia. Why? Denervation of hearts may give some insights to try to address this question. Indeed, two investigations have shown that sympathetic plexectomy at the time of coronary bypass grafting for variant angina was more effective than by-pass surgery alone [13, 14]. Perhaps, the adrenergic activity may simply modulate the threshold for symptomatic manifestation of myocardial ischemia in the presence of an underlying vasomotor dysfunction. The association of coronary spasm with other peripheral vasospastic disorders such as migraine or Raynaud's phenomenon may substantiate this hypothesis [15, 16].

Endothelial Dysfunction and Coronary Microcirculation

Endothelial dysfunction could underlie a nonspecific enhancement of the response to all vasoconstrictor stimuli [4]. Some evidence indicates that endothelial dysfunction is significantly associated with diffuse epicardial vasoconstrictor response to acetylcholine and more adverse cardiovascular events over a 2, 4, 7 and 10-year follow-up [6, 17, 18]. Assessment of endothelial function may detect early changes in endothelial vasoactive function, which is important in the development of atherosclerosis rather than identifying atherosclerosis per se [6, 19]. Indeed, endothelial abnormalities, as in hypercholesterolemia, result in abnormal dilator responses all throughout the vascular tree [20]. Loss of endothelium-dependent vasodilatation in response to acetylcholine is regarded as a sign of early stage vascular injury and atherosclerosis [6, 21–24]. An impaired ability of the endothelium to release vasoactive substances can facilitate inflammation, platelet aggregation, coronary vasoconstriction, leukocyte adhesion, and oxidative modification of low-density lipoprotein cholesterol [21]. Endothelial dysfunction has been related to oxidative stress that may result from atherosclerotic risk factors, inflammation, and genetic conditions still poorly understood [25]. All these factors may facilitate development of atherosclerosis in the vessel wall and predispose to vascular events by prothrombotic mechanisms.

Acetylcholine Testing and Endothelial Dysfunction

Techniques to detect coronary artery endothelial dysfunction are not widely used in the clinical setting. Intracoronary acetylcholine testing is considered the gold standard for detection of coronary endothelial function. Many patients diagnosed as having nonobstructive coronary artery disease exhibit a diffuse vasoconstrictor disorder of the epicardial coronary arterial tree during intracoronary acetylcholine testing. Recent work has showed that approximately 40% of patients with typical exertional chest pain had normal or near normal coronary angiograms. Of them more than two-thirds showed a vasomotor response to intracoronary acetylcholine infusion accompanied by chest pain and ischemic ECG signs [26]. Acetylcholine (Ach) testing was defined as indicative of epicardial coronary spasm in the presence of ≥75% focal or diffuse coronary artery diameter reduction. Coronary spasm occurred in approximately half of this population. If the constrictor response to acetylcholine ranged till up 75%, it was assumed that symptoms and ischemic ECG signs were due to impairment of the microvascular circulation. All vessels dilated in response to intracoronary nitroglycerin, a direct smooth muscle dilator, suggesting a disturbance of endothelial cell function in the constricting vessels. These data paralleled similar observations done by our group and others over 30 years ago during hyperventilation testing [4, 27]. There is one caveat: a constrictor response to intracoronary Ach does not necessarily indicate endothelial dysfunction. It could equally be due to the enhancement of the direct constrictor response of vascular smooth muscle [21].This can be exemplified by a shift from the normal, endothelium-dependent dilator response of human coronary artery to sympathetic stimulation to a constrictor response in association with atheroma [23]. Impairment of endothelium-dependent dilatation shifts a net dilator response to sympathetic stimulation to a net constrictor response [28].

Diagnostic Criteria for Vasospastic Angina

Vasospastic angina in the absence of obstructive CAD may not consistently cause myocardial ischemia that can be detected non-invasively [18, 29]. This can be explained by the fact that the commonly applied nuclear-based techniques for ischemia depend upon regional differences in perfusion and/or function that identified by normalizing radiotracer uptake across the myocardium [30]. This will reduce detection of diffuse microvascular coronary flow abnormalities. Prior analyses demonstrated that even in apparently normal scans, the majority of patients with vasospastic angina showed reduced thallium-201 uptake and washout in comparison to their controls [30]. Given the fact that traditional nuclear imaging techniques rely on detection of abnormalities that are compared to a normalized myocardium, diffuse vasoconstriction will appear as normal [29]. Stress cardiac magnetic resonance imaging (CMRI) is capable of defining epicardial as well as subendocardial hypoperfusion following administration of IV adenosine in women with signs and symptoms of ischemia but no obstructive CAD [31]. Adenosine may also induce global and regional left ventricular diastolic dysfunction as demonstrated by both radionuclide imaging and stress echocardiography in patients with microvascular coronary dysfunction. In prior studies, we and other have shown that ambulatory ECG monitoring have an important role in the diagnosis of patients with vasospastic angina as it can detect episode of silent ischemia. Interestingly, we have shown that during 48-h ambulatory ECG recording in patients with vasospastic angina only

9% of ischemic episodes were associated with angina [32]. Similar results were reported by another study using 24-h ambulatory ECG monitoring [33]. Ambulatory ECG monitoring may be useful also in detecting associated arrhythmias [34].

Exercise stress testing is normal in many patients with vasospastic angina. However, doing the hot phase, exercise induced coronary spasm associated with ST changes on the electrocardiogram occurs in approximately 50% of patients. Additionally, many patients with vasospastic angina have associated high-grade fixed coronary stenosis, and exercise testing can be useful in the follow-up and in selecting patients that may benefit from invasive investigation [35–37].

Coronary angiography is useful to detect the presence of fixed obstructive coronary stenosis or in the absence of coronary obstruction to pursue provocative testing. However, the expected cost of initial conventional diagnostic investigations including coronary angiography in patients with vasospastic angina approximately ranged from $3500 to 6000 [38]. Women have been found to present more often with vasospastic angina [10]. Shaw et al. reported an expected consumption of nearly $750,000 of cardiovascular health care resources related to the burden of ongoing symptoms and medications throughout the lifespan of these women [39]. Hence, a better understanding of risk relative to morbidity, mortality and cost is needed for this population.

Prognosis

The prognosis of "normal" coronary arteries in the setting of signs and symptoms of myocardial ischemia is not as benign as reported by preliminary cohort studies, and as commonly assumed by physicians. Short-term prognosis of patients with unstable angina and nonobstructive coronary artery disease includes a 2% risk of death or myocardial infarction at 30 days of follow-up [40]. Specifically, evidence of microvascular coronary dysfunction indicated by a lower coronary flow reserve determined invasively in a population of women and men or exclusively women predicts an adverse prognosis [6, 41]. Notably, among women with persistent signs and symptoms of ischemia, a relatively higher proportion of adverse events include heart failure rather than myocardial infarction suggesting possible links between microvascular coronary dysfunction and heart failure with preserved systolic function [42, 43].

Therapeutic Strategies

No randomized trials comparing therapies for the reduction of adverse cardiac events in patients with coronary artery spasm have been conducted, and available adverse outcome data are limited to cohort studies.

Calcium-channel blockers have been shown to be highly effective for reduction of coronary artery spasm episodes during daily life and are the first line treatment in patients with vasospastic angina [44, 45]. There are several potential mechanisms by which CCB may act in reducing coronary artery spasm recurrences. They prevent vasoconstriction and promote vasodilation in most patients.

Long-acting nitrates maybe useful due to their vasodilatory effect [46]. However, the occurrence of nitrate tolerance, makes them a less attractive strategy and may be used as additive to CCB in patients with persistence of symptoms.

High doses of CCB/nitrates maybe used in patients with refractory coronary artery spasm, despite optimal vasodilator therapy.

Observational evidence does not support the use of nonselective beta-blockers, in patients with vasospastic angina because they may exacerbate vasospasm with detrimental effects [47]. However, in some patients with associated fixed coronary stenosis, a reduction in the frequency of exertional angina episodes is observed [48].

Magnesium deficiency has been shown to a possible factor contributing to coronary artery spasm [49]. Magnesium supplementation may exert its benefit due to its calcium blocking effect in the vascular smooth muscle. Accordingly, in one small, study intravenous magnesium supplementation improved coronary vasodilation and symptoms in patients with vasospastic angina [50]. However, larger studies are needed before using magnesium as routine therapy for patients with vasospastic angina.

Statins improve endothelial function and may counteract oxidative stress reducing vasoconstrictor response to acetylcholine [20, 51, 52]. Another proposed mechanism is inhibition of the RhoA-associated kinase pathway [53]. Consequently, statins may prevent coronary artery spasm and symptoms in patients vasospastic angina.

Aspirin should be used with caution in patients with coronary artery spasm, as it is an inhibitor of prostacyclin production aggravating coronary vasospasm at high doses [54]. However, in patients with associated coronary atherosclerotic disease, low dose aspirin should be considered.

Percutaneous coronary intervention may be helpful in patients with associated high grade obstructive coronary lesions [55]. Results are variable in this setting and depend, in part, upon the severity of the coronary obstruction and the presence of multivessel spasm [56, 57]. Coronary stenting may be considered in selected patients with refractory coronary artery vasospasm, despite maximal optimal medical therapy, if associated with mild to moderate coronary disease [58].

In patients with a high risk of life- threatening ventricular arrhythmias and in those with aborted cardiac arrest automatic defibrillator placement is highly recommended [59].

Conclusions

Abnormality of coronary vasomotor tone can be divided into at least two major categories that are distinct entities and likely should be managed differently. Focal coronary artery spasm, characterizing variant angina, can be treated effectively by calcium-channel blockers and nitrates. Spontaneous remission may occur in these patients and in some it is possible to reduce their therapy after symptom-free periods ranging from 3 to 4 months. Diffuse coronary artery spasm, characterizing vasotonic angina, is a manifestation of endothelial dysfunction and, as so, strategies aimed at reducing cardiovascular risk factors, may translate into an improvement of symptoms and a reduction of risk of morbidity and mortality. Depending on predominant pathophysiology, individualized therapeutic approaches to patients with ischemic heart disease can be made with improved results.

Conflict of Interest The authors declare no conflict of interest, financial or otherwise.

Funding None.

References

1. Osler W. The lumleian lectures on angina pectoris. Lancet. 1910;175(4517):839–44.
2. Prinzmetal M, Kennamer R, Merliss R, Wada T, Bor N. Angina pectoris. I. A variant form of angina pectoris; preliminary report. Am J Med. 1959;27:375–88.
3. Maseri A, Severi S, Nes MD, L'Abbate A, Chierchia S, Marzilli M, Ballestra AM, Parodi O, Biagini A, Distante A. "Variant" angina: one aspect of a continuous spectrum of vasospastic myocardial ischemia. Pathogenetic mechanisms, estimated incidence and clinical and coronary arteriographic findings in 138 patients. Am J Cardiol. 1978;42(6):1019–35.
4. Bugiardini R, Pozzati A, Ottani F, Morgagni GL, Puddu P. Vasotonic angina: a spectrum of ischemic syndromes involving functional abnormalities of the epicardial and microvascular coronary circulation. J Am Coll Cardiol. 1993;22(2):417–25.
5. JCS Joint Working Group. Guidelines for diagnosis and treatment of patients with vasospastic angina (coronary spastic angina) (JCS 2008): digest version. Circ J. 2010;74(8):1745–62.
6. Bugiardini R, Manfrini O, Pizzi C, Fontana F, Morgagni G. Endothelial function predicts future development of coronary artery disease: a study of women with chest pain and normal coronary angiograms. Circulation. 2004;109(21):2518–23.
7. Bugiardini R, Borghi A, Biagetti L, Puddu P. Comparison of verapamil versus propranolol therapy in syndrome X. Am J Cardiol. 1989;63(5):286–90.
8. MacAlpin RN. Relation of coronary arterial spasm to sites of organic stenosis. Am J Cardiol. 1980;46(1):143–53.
9. Manfrini O, Pizzi C, Trerè D, Fontana F, Bugiardini R. Parasympathetic failure and risk of subsequent coronary events in unstable angina and non-ST-segment elevation myocardial infarction. Eur Heart J. 2003;24(17):1560–6.
10. Cenko E, Bugiardini R. Vasotonic angina as a cause of myocardial ischemia in women. Cardiovasc Drugs Ther. 2015;29(4):339–45.
11. Khuddus MA, Pepine CJ, Handberg EM, Bairey Merz CN, Sopko G, Bavry AA, Denardo SJ, McGorray SP, Smith KM, Sharaf BL, Nicholls SJ, Nissen SE, Anderson RD. An intravascular ultrasound analysis in women experiencing chest pain in the absence of obstructive coronary artery disease: a substudy from the National Heart, lung and blood institute-sponsored Women's ischemia syndrome evaluation (WISE). J Interv Cardiol. 2010;23(6):511–9.
12. Manfrini O, Bazzocchi G, Luati A, Borghi A, Monari P, Bugiardini R. Coronary spasm reflects inputs from adjacent esophageal system. Am J Physiol Heart Circ Physiol. 2006;290(5):H2085–91.

13. Bertrand ME, Lablanche JM, Rousseau MF, Warembourg HH, Stankowtak C, Soots G. Surgical treatment of variant angina: use of plexectomy with aortocoronary bypass. Circulation. 1980;61(5):877–82.
14. Betriu A, Pomar JL, Bourassa MG, Grondin CM. Influence of partial sympathetic denervation on the results of myocardial revascularization in variant angina. Am J Cardiol. 1983;51(5):661–7.
15. Miller D, Waters DD, Warnica W, Szlachcic J, Kreeft J, Théroux P. Is variant angina the coronary manifestation of a generalized vasospastic disorder? N Engl J Med. 1981;304(13):763–6.
16. Vanmolkot FH, Van Bortel LM, de Hoon JN. Altered arterial function in migraine of recent onset. Neurology. 2007;68(19):1563–70.
17. Halcox JP, Schenke WH, Zalos G, Mincemoyer R, Prasad A, Waclawiw MA, Nour KR, Quyyumi AA. Prognostic value of coronary vascular endothelial dysfunction. Circulation. 2002;106(6):653–8.
18. Suwaidi JA, Hamasaki S, Higano ST, Nishimura RA, Holmes DR, Lerman A. Long-term follow-up of patients with mild coronary artery disease and endothelial dysfunction. Circulation. 2000;101(9):948–54.
19. Manfrini O, Cenko E, Verna E, Salerno Uriarte JA, Bugiardini R. Endothelial dysfunction versus early atherosclerosis: a study with high resolution imaging. Int J Cardiol. 2013;168(2):1714–6.
20. Vita JA, Treasure CB, Nabel EG, McLenachan JM, Fish RD, Yeung AC, Vekshtein VI, Selwyn AP, Ganz P. Coronary vasomotor response to acetylcholine relates to risk factors for coronary artery disease. Circulation. 1990;81(2):491–7.
21. Pries AR, Badimon L, Bugiardini R, Camici PG, Dorobantu M, Duncker DJ, Escaned J, Koller A, Piek JJ, de Wit C. Coronary vascular regulation, remodelling, and collateralization: mechanisms and clinical implications on behalf of the working group on coronary pathophysiology and microcirculation. Eur Heart J. 2015;36(45):3134–46.
22. Bugiardini R, Cenko E. A short history of vasospastic angina. J Am Coll Cardiol. 2017;70(19):2359–62.
23. Zeiher AM, Drexler H, Wollschlaeger H, Saurbier B, Just H. Coronary vasomotion in response to sympathetic stimulation in humans: importance of the functional integrity of the endothelium. J Am Coll Cardiol. 1989;14(5):1181–90.
24. Bugiardini R, Badimon L, Collins P, Erbel R, Fox K, Hamm C, Pinto F, Rosengren A, Stefanadis C, Wallentin L, Van de Werf F. Angina, "normal" coronary angiography, and vascular dysfunction: risk assessment strategies. PLoS Med. 2007;4(2):e12.
25. Badimon L, Bugiardini R, Cenko E, Cubedo J, Dorobantu M, Duncker DJ, Estruch R, Milicic D, Tousoulis D, Vasiljevic Z, Vilahur G, De Wit C, Koller A. Position paper of the European Society of Cardiology-working group of coronary pathophysiology andmicrocirculation: obesity and heart disease. Eur Heart J. 2017;38(25):1951–8.
26. Ong P, Athanasiadis A, Borgulya G, Mahrholdt H, Kaski JC, Sechtem U. High prevalence of a pathological response to acetylcholine testing in patients with stable angina pectoris and unobstructed coronary arteries. The ACOVA study (abnormal COronary VAsomotion in patients with stable angina and unobstructed coronary arteries). J Am Coll Cardiol. 2012;59(7):655–62.
27. Crea F, Davies G, Chierchia S, Romeo F, Bugiardini R, Kaski JC, Freedman B, Maseri A. Different susceptibility to myocardial ischemia provoked by hyperventilation and cold pressor test in exertional and variant angina pectoris. Am J Cardiol. 1985;56(1):18–22.
28. Vrints CJ, Bult H, Hitter E, Herman AG, Snoeck JP. Impaired endothelium-dependent cholinergic coronary vasodilation in patients with angina and normal coronary arteriograms. J Am Coll Cardiol. 1992;19(1):21–31.
29. Bugiardini R, Bairey Merz CN. Angina with "normal" coronary arteries: a changing philosophy. JAMA. 2005;293(4):477–84.
30. Rosano GM, Peters NS, Kaski JC, Mavrogeni SI, Collins P, Underwood RS, Poole-Wilson PA. Abnormal uptake and washout of thallium-201 in patients with syndrome X and normal-appearing scans. Am J Cardiol. 1995;75(5):400–2.

31. Panting JR, Gatehouse PD, Yang GZ, Grothues F, Firmin DN, Collins P, Pennell DJ. Abnormal subendocardial perfusion in cardiac syndrome X detected by cardiovascular magnetic resonance imaging. N Engl J Med. 2002;346(25):1948–53.
32. Bugiardini R, Borghi A, Sassone B, Pozzati A, Puddu P. Prognostic significance of silent myocardial ischemia in variant angina pectoris. Am J Cardiol. 1991;68(17):1581–6.
33. Araki H, Koiwaya Y, Nakagaki O, Nakamura M. Diurnal distribution of ST-segment elevation and related arrhythmias in patients with variant angina: a study by ambulatory ECG monitoring. Circulation. 1983;67(5):995–1000.
34. Pozzati A, Pancaldi LG, Di Pasquale G, Pinelli G, Bugiardini R. Transient sympathovagal imbalance triggers "ischemic" sudden death in patients undergoing electrocardiographic Holter monitoring. J Am Coll Cardiol. 1996;27(4):847–52.
35. Waters DD, Szlachcic J, Bourassa MG, Scholl JM, Théroux P. Exercise testing in patients with variant angina: results, correlation with clinical and angiographic features and prognostic significance. Circulation. 1982;65(2):265–74.
36. de Servi S, Falcone C, Gavazzi A, Mussini A, Bramucci E, Curti MT, Vecchio C, Specchia G, Bobba P. The exercise test in variant angina: results in 114 patients. Circulation. 1981;64(4):684–8.
37. Minoda K, Yasue H, Kugiyama K, Okumura K, Motomura K, Shimomura O, Takahashi M. Comparison of the distribution of myocardial blood flow between exercise-induced and hyperventilation-induced attacks of coronary spasm: a study with thallium-201 myocardial scintigraphy. Am Heart J. 1994;127(6):1474–80.
38. Bairey Merz CN, Shaw LJ, Reis SE, Bittner V, Kelsey SF, Olson M, Johnson BD, Pepine CJ, Mankad S, Sharaf BL, Rogers WJ, Pohost GM, Lerman A, Quyyumi AA, Sopko G, Investigators W. Insights from the NHLBI-sponsored Women's ischemia syndrome evaluation (WISE) study: part II: gender differences in presentation, diagnosis, and outcome with regard to gender-based pathophysiology of atherosclerosis and macrovascular and microvascular coronary disease. J Am Coll Cardiol. 2006;47(3 Suppl):S21–9.
39. Shaw LJ, Merz CN, Pepine CJ, Reis SE, Bittner V, Kip KE, Kelsey SF, Olson M, Johnson BD, Mankad S, Sharaf BL, Rogers WJ, Pohost GM, Sopko G. Investigators WsISEW. The economic burden of angina in women with suspected ischemic heart disease: results from the National Institutes of Health--National Heart, Lung, and Blood Institute--sponsored Women's ischemia syndrome evaluation. Circulation. 2006;114(9):894–904.
40. Bugiardini R, Manfrini O, De Ferrari GM. Unanswered questions for management of acute coronary syndrome: risk stratification of patients with minimal disease or normal findings on coronary angiography. Arch Intern Med. 2006;166(13):1391–5.
41. Vaccarino V, Badimon L, Corti R, de Wit C, Dorobantu M, Manfrini O, Koller A, Pries A, Cenko E, Bugiardini R. Presentation, management, and outcomes of ischaemic heart disease in women. Nat Rev Cardiol. 2013;10(9):508–18.
42. Britten MB, Zeiher AM, Schächinger V. Microvascular dysfunction in angiographically normal or mildly diseased coronary arteries predicts adverse cardiovascular long-term outcome. Coron Artery Dis. 2004;15(5):259–64.
43. Vaccarino V, Badimon L, Corti R, de Wit C, Dorobantu M, Hall A, Koller A, Marzilli M, Pries A, Bugiardini R. Ischaemic heart disease in women: are there sex differences in pathophysiology and risk factors? Position paper from the working group on coronary pathophysiology and microcirculation of the European society of cardiology. Cardiovasc Res. 2011;90(1):9–17.
44. Braun LT. Calcium channel blockers for the treatment of coronary artery spasm: rationale, effects, and nursing responsibilities. Heart Lung. 1983;12(3):226–32.
45. Yasue H, Takizawa A, Nagao M, Nishida S, Horie M, Kubota J, Omote S, Takaoka K, Okumura K. Long-term prognosis for patients with variant angina and influential factors. Circulation. 1988;78(1):1–9.
46. Lombardi M, Morales MA, Michelassi C, Moscarelli E, Distante A, L'Abbate A. Efficacy of isosorbide-5-mononitrate versus nifedipine in preventing spontaneous and ergonovine-induced myocardial ischaemia. A double-blind, placebo-controlled study. Eur Heart J. 1993;14(6):845–51.

47. Robertson RM, Wood AJ, Vaughn WK, Robertson D. Exacerbation of vasotonic angina pectoris by propranolol. Circulation. 1982;65(2):281–5.
48. Cannon CPBE. Unstable angina and non-ST elevation myocardial infarction. 8th ed. Philadelphia: Saunders Elsevier; 2008.
49. Satake K, Lee JD, Shimizu H, Ueda T, Nakamura T. Relation between severity of magnesium deficiency and frequency of anginal attacks in men with variant angina. J Am Coll Cardiol. 1996;28(4):897–902.
50. Teragawa H, Kato M, Yamagata T, Matsuura H, Kajiyama G. The preventive effect of magnesium on coronary spasm in patients with vasospastic angina. Chest. 2000;118(6):1690–5.
51. Pizzi C, Manfrini O, Fontana F, Bugiardini R. Angiotensin-converting enzyme inhibitors and 3-hydroxy-3-methylglutaryl coenzyme a reductase in cardiac syndrome X: role of superoxide dismutase activity. Circulation. 2004;109(1):53–8.
52. Manfrini O, Pizzi C, Morgagni G, Fontana F, Bugiardini R. Effect of pravastatin on myocardial perfusion after percutaneous transluminal coronary angioplasty. Am J Cardiol. 2004;93(11):1391–3, A6.
53. Yasue H, Mizuno Y, Harada E, Itoh T, Nakagawa H, Nakayama M, Ogawa H, Tayama S, Honda T, Hokimoto S, Ohshima S, Hokamura Y, Kugiyama K, Horie M, Yoshimura M, Harada M, Uemura S, Saito Y. Investigators SSaCAST. Effects of a 3-hydroxy-3-methylglutaryl coenzyme a reductase inhibitor, fluvastatin, on coronary spasm after withdrawal of calcium-channel blockers. J Am Coll Cardiol. 2008;51(18):1742–8.
54. Miwa K, Kambara H, Kawai C. Effect of aspirin in large doses on attacks of variant angina. Am Heart J. 1983;105(2):351–5.
55. Sueda S, Suzuki J, Watanabe K, Mineoi K, Kondou T, Yano K, Ochi T, Ochi N, Kawada H, Hayashi Y, Uraoka A. Comparative results of coronary intervention in patients with variant angina versus those with non-variant angina. Jpn Heart J. 2001;42(6):657–67.
56. Tanabe Y, Itoh E, Suzuki K, Ito M, Hosaka Y, Nakagawa I, Kumakura M. Limited role of coronary angioplasty and stenting in coronary spastic angina with organic stenosis. J Am Coll Cardiol. 2002;39(7):1120–6.
57. Corcos T, David PR, Bourassa MG, Val PG, Robert J, Mata LA, Waters DD. Percutaneous transluminal coronary angioplasty for the treatment of variant angina. J Am Coll Cardiol. 1985;5(5):1046–54.
58. Gaspardone A, Tomai F, Versaci F, Ghini AS, Polisca P, Crea F, Chiariello L, Gioffrè PA. Coronary artery stent placement in patients with variant angina refractory to medical treatment. Am J Cardiol. 1999;84(1):96–8, A8.
59. Matsue Y, Suzuki M, Nishizaki M, Hojo R, Hashimoto Y, Sakurada H. Clinical implications of an implantable cardioverter-defibrillator in patients with vasospastic angina and lethal ventricular arrhythmia. J Am Coll Cardiol. 2012;60(10):908–13.

Chapter 11
Brain Microcirculation and Silent Cerebral Damage

Cristina Sierra and Antonio Coca

Introduction

Regardless of age, hypertension is undoubtedly the cardiovascular risk factor (CVRF) most closely related to cerebrovascular pathology [1]. In fact, hypertension is the most important risk factor for stroke, both ischemic and hemorrhagic, as well as other cerebral vascular diseases including lacunar infarction, cerebral white matter lesions (WML), microbleeds, cognitive impairment and vascular dementia [1, 2]. Hypertension seems to predispose to early cognitive deterioration, which evolves to dementia and stroke after a time period that may vary from a few years to several decades. During this time, in which the majority of hypertensives remain asymptomatic, elevated blood pressure (BP) predisposes to the development of subtle alterations, based on arteriolar narrowing or microvascular changes that lead to chronic small vessel ischemia, focal or diffuse (lacunar or WML), as well as deposits of hemosiderin in the perivascular spaces, mainly of the deep perforating arteries (microbleeds). These lesions are detected mainly by means of brain magnetic resonance imaging (MRI) and, for the most part, in asymptomatic patients.

These silent cerebrovascular lesions are associated with several CVRF (hypertension, dyslipidemia, diabetes mellitus, smoking), although hypertension is undoubtedly the most important [3]. It is widely accepted that cerebral small vessel disease (lacunar, WML, cerebral microbleeds) is part of the silent cerebrovascular injury in by high blood pressure in hypertensive patients [1, 4, 5]. Despite the undoubted epidemiological relationship, the etiopathogenic mechanisms through which hypertension leads to cerebral pathology are diverse, complex and not completely clarified.

C. Sierra (✉) · A. Coca
Hypertension and Vascular Risk Unit, Department of Internal Medicine, Hospital Clinic, IDIBAPS, University of Barcelona, Barcelona, Spain
e-mail: CSIERRA@clinic.cat; csierra@clinic.ub.es

M. Dorobantu, L. Badimon (eds.), *Microcirculation*,
https://doi.org/10.1007/978-3-030-28199-1_11

Cerebral Blood Flow and Blood Pressure

The brain is an organ with high metabolic activity and, despite representing only 2% of body weight, consumes 20–30% of blood oxygen, for which it receives approximately 15–20% of cardiac output. The oxygen consumption in the different parts of the nervous system depends on the density of the neurons and the state of their functional activation. As a result of these high demands, the central nervous system is especially vulnerable to alterations in cerebral circulation. Under normal conditions cerebral blood flow (CBF) is approximately 50–60 ml/100 g/min [6, 7]. CBF is determined by the following formula:

$$\text{CBF} = \text{Cerebral perfusion pressure} / \text{Cerebral vascular resistance}$$

Cerebral perfusion pressure (CPP) represents the difference between the pressure in the artery when entering the cerebral circulation and the venous pressure of return. Under normal conditions, the return venous pressure is minimal and, therefore, CPP is similar to systemic BP. Thus, when CPP is normal, the changes in CBF are due to changes in cerebral vascular resistance (CVR). Several mechanisms regulate CBF, the most important being autoregulation, mediated by changes in CVR and through which the cerebral blood vessels dilate in response to a fall in BP and contract when BP increases (Fig. 11.1). This ensures that the CBF remains constant

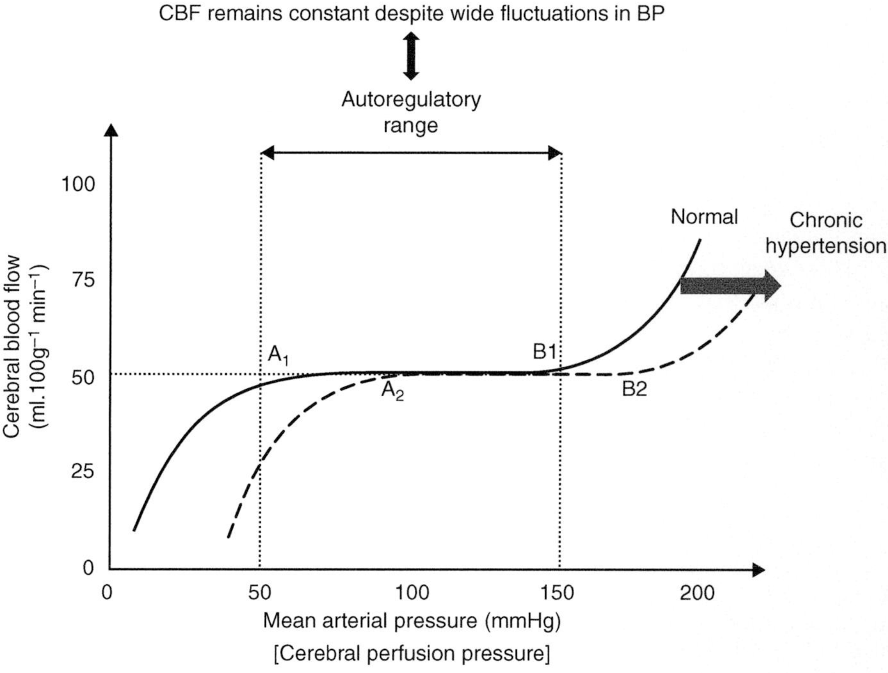

Fig. 11.1 Diagram of the limits of autoregulation of cerebral blood flow according to variations in blood pressure. The displacement of the lower limit of pressure to the right, from the A1 to A2 values, in hypertensive patients, means that, in this pressure range, the cerebral blood flow corresponding to each pressure value is lower than that of normotensive subjects

despite wide fluctuations in BP, which can range between 50 and 160 mmHg (lower and upper limit, respectively). Therefore, the autoregulation of cerebral circulation is the set of mechanisms that protect the brain from ischemia in situations of low cerebral perfusion and prevent the risk of cerebral edema in the face of elevations in BP. The mechanisms involved in brain autoregulation include endothelial, neurogenic, metabolic and myogenic factors. The sympathetic nervous system also plays a role in CBF regulation (its activation displaces the upper limit of autoregulation towards higher blood pressures) and in the renin-angiotensin system (its activation shifts the auto-regulation curve to the right). In experimental models, angiotensin-converting enzyme (ACE) inhibitors increase the interval of the autoregulating plateau, displacing both its upper and lower limits, at the expense of dilation and contraction of the large arteries, but not of the cerebral microcirculation [8]. Thus, some studies have shown that, during cerebral ischemia, renin-angiotensin system blockade reduces BP without modifying CBF [9]. Another factor that conditions CBF is plasma viscosity, which depends on the hematocrit, the situation of cellular aggregation and protein concentrations, especially fibrinogen.

Cerebral Autoregulation and Hypertension

In hypertensive subjects, the absolute value of CBF is the same as in normotensives because the curve of cerebral autoregulation is displaced to the right with respect to both the lower and upper limits. Thus, although higher BP values are tolerated, tolerance to hypotension decreases, which may result in tissue hypoxia by decreasing cerebral perfusion pressure. However, despite the physiological phenomenon of cerebral autoregulation, the sustained increase in BP levels characteristic of established hypertension, involves sustained vasoconstriction in the arterioles and small cerebral arteries that induces structural changes in the vessels and favors the appearance of various types of brain injuries. These changes are characterized by hypertrophy of the vascular wall and decreases in the internal and external diameter of the vessels, a phenomenon known as "vascular remodeling" [6].

Studies of cerebral hemodynamics performed in hypertensive patients have shown that young individuals with hypertension have a higher cerebral blood flow velocity than patients with "chronic" hypertension and a history of stroke [10]. Likewise, a reduction in cerebral blood flow velocity and an increase in distal vascular resistance have also been objectified in patients with hypertension of long evolution (>5 years), in comparison with patients with short-term hypertension (<5 years) [11]. In addition, middle-aged hypertensive patients with silent cerebral WML show an increase in cerebrovascular tone compared with hypertensive patients without these lesions [12].

Hypertension and Arteriosclerosis

Hypertension is a risk factor for arteriosclerosis, and the incidence of arteriosclerosis in the arteries of hypertensive patients is higher than that observed in normotensive patients of the same age and sex. In fact, arteriosclerosis occurs much more frequently in the vascular areas that support greater pressure, and is more intense and progressive when other vascular risk factors are associated, such as diabetes, dyslipidemia or smoking. Table 11.1 show several physiopathological mechanisms which have been implicated in the genesis of hypertensive cerebral arterial disease. The hypertension-induced alterations related to early brain involvement may be classified as functional or structural (Table 11.2). Functional alterations, such as a decrease in the cerebral hemodynamic reserve or mild cognitive impairment, may be caused, in turn, by structural lesions associated with the cerebral atherosclerotic process caused by hypertension.

However, the chronopathology of these alterations and their interrelationships are not clear. The physiopathological mechanisms that trigger them include:

- An increase in intraluminal pressure that would cause an alteration in endothelial function and the smooth muscle of the arterial wall. This would increase the permeability of the blood-brain barrier and cause focal or multifocal cerebral edema;
- Endothelial lesions: which would also cause the local formation of thrombi and ischemic lesions;
- Fibrinoid necrosis: which would cause lacunar infarcts through stenosis or focal occlusions;

Table 11.1 Pathophysiology of cerebrovascular changes associated with high blood pressure (Adapted from Sierra et al. [2])

Mechanical stress (endothelial lesion)—Endothelial dysfunction (loss of vasodilatory capacity)
↑ Vascular permeability
Opened ionic channels
Hypertrophy of smooth muscle vascular vessels (reduced lumen)
Contraction of smooth muscle vascular vessels (increased vascular resistance)
Synthesis of collagen fiber (vascular stiffness)
Transudation of plasmatic products to the arterial wall

Table 11.2 Early cerebrovascular damage associated with hypertension

Functional abnormalities
– Reduced cerebral blood flow
– Increased cerebrovascular resistance
– Reduced cerebral vasomotor reactivity
– Incipient cognitive impairment
Structural abnormalities
– Arterial remodeling
– Lacunar infarcts: small deep infarcts caused by penetrating arteriolar occlusive disease
– White matter lesions: periventricular and subcortical white matter lesions caused by subcortical hypertensive small vessel disease
– Cerebral microbleeds

- Degenerative changes in the endothelium and vascular vessel muscle that predispose to cerebral hemorrhages;
- Adaptive structural changes in the resistance vessels. Despite the positive effect of reducing vessel pressure, increased distal vascular resistance may compromise the collateral circulation and increase the risk of ischemic episodes related to hypotension phenomena, or those located distal to a stenosis;
- Hypertension mediated stenotic lesions or embolisms of the large extra-cranial vessels, the aortic arch and the heart;
- Lesions in the perforating arteries, small caliber vessels that arise directly from the trunks of the main cerebral arteries, which are more sensitive to BP. In these cases there are different types of lesions: lipohyalinosis, Charcot-Bouchard micro-aneurysms and/or microatheromas.

Studies have indicated that hypertension and arteriosclerosis may have a common pathogenic pathway—alteration of the endothelium [13]. In hypertension, this alteration could be due to a defect in the endothelial production of nitric oxide or to excess degradation. In any case, this would result in deficient vasodilator capacity mediated by the endothelium which, in turn, would enhance the endothelial dysfunction present in the early stages of atheromatosis. In arteriosclerosis, the first step in the formation of atheromatous plaque is a functional alteration of the endothelium, characterized by an increase in the production of vasoconstrictive substances and growth promoters (endothelin, vasoconstrictor prostaglandins) with respect to vasodilators (nitric oxide, and prostacyclin, a hyperpolarizing factor derived from the endothelium), with no morphological changes being apparent. This endothelial dysfunction is mainly caused by the shearing effect of the bloodstream and is located in the vascular areas with greater blood flow turbulence, mainly at arterial bifurcations. Hypertension contributes to a greater shearing effect. Subsequent to this endothelial dysfunction and, probably, as a consequence of it, there is greater adhesion and platelet aggregation, monocyte infiltration and intracellular and extracellular accumulation of lipids in the injured vascular wall; these processes cause a proliferation of vascular smooth muscle cells and cellular necrosis with calcium deposits, which finally results in the formation of atheromatous plaque.

The physiopathological consequences of atheromatosis in the cerebral arteries which, like the coronary arteries are medium-sized muscular arteries, are decreased vascular adaptability, with the consequent loss of vasodilator capacity against oxygen needs, resulting in a reduction in the cerebral vascular reserve. Studies of cerebral hemodynamics in hypertensives have shown that hypertensive patients have decreased cerebrovascular reactivity (or vasodilatory capacity) compared with normotensive individuals, but of less intensity compared with hypertensive patients with a previous cerebral lacunar infarction [14].

The rupture of an atheroma plaque produces the phenomenon of thrombosis, reorganization of the thrombus and enlargement of the atheroma plaque with the consequent reduction or occlusion of the vascular lumen, which results, depending on the vascular territory affected, in various clinical syndromes. These lesions are responsible for ischemic strokes, including both those of atherothrombotic etiology and non-cardiac embolisms, which are caused by the detachment of atheromatous plaque. In addition, in large arteries affected by arteriosclerosis, dilatations and ectopic elongations, whose rupture causes a hemorrhagic stroke, may also occur.

Cerebrovascular Aging

The changes associated with the aging process itself also lead to greater susceptibility of the vessels to the harmful effects of CVRF and CV diseases [15]. Table 11.3 summarizes the changes related to vascular aging and the changes associated with brain aging itself. The alterations related to brain aging contribute to small vessel disease, ischemic and hemorrhagic stroke and cognitive deterioration.

The cerebral microvasculature that forms the blood-brain barrier (BBB) changes during the aging process. Studies have shown that there is an increase in the permeability of BBB with aging, which may be one of the possible etiopathogenic mechanisms of both the onset and progression of cerebral microvascular disease [16]. The area of the capillary surface decreases while the diameter, volume and total length increase [17]. This degeneration associated with the structural and functional aging of the cerebral vasculature results in alterations in local perfusion. This cerebral hypoperfusion would not necessarily cause ischemia as severe as that observed in a stroke, but would lead to hypovolemia and the subsequent alteration of the microcirculation and damage to the cerebral endothelium [18].

In summary, the alterations associated with the aging of the cerebral vasculature would reduce the cerebrovascular reserve and increase the susceptibility of the brain to ischemic and hemorrhagic lesions.

Hypertension and Cerebral White Matter Lesions

The etiopathogenesis of WML is not yet completely clarified. The most widely accepted hypothesis in the pathogenesis of these lesions is that they are mediated by a vascular mechanism, given the high prevalence of cerebral WML in patients with

Table 11.3 Mechanisms of vascular aging, and age-related brain changes that cause vulnerability in the elderly and increase the risk of cerebrovascular disease (Adapted from Sierra et al. [2])

Vascular aging	Age-related brain changes
• Low-grade inflammation	• ↑ Brain-blood barrier permeability
• Oxidative stress and endothelial dysfunction	• Tortuosity of white matter arterioles
• Increased arterial stiffness	• ↓Brain weight, expanded ventricles, ↑ choroid plexus weight
• Upregulation of renin-angiotensin system	• Small vessel disease
• Impaired endothelial progenitor cell function	• Cerebral amyloid angiopathy

CVRF. Post-mortem studies have shown that the presence of WML is associated with degenerative changes in arterioles [19], suggesting that arteriosclerosis of the penetrating cerebral vessels is the main factor in the pathogenesis of WML. Cross-sectional studies have associated indirect measures of atherosclerosis, such as carotid intima media thickness [20] or the elasticity index [21, 22] with WML. In this arteriosclerosis continuum, markers of endothelial dysfunction (intercellular adhesion molecules -ICAM-) [23], as well as inflammation (C reactive protein) [24], have also been linked to WML. Although mostly associated with ischemic phenomena related to arteriosclerosis, the hemodynamic component favoring hypoxia (with a decrease in perfusion pressure) caused by the loss of cerebral autoregulation observed in hypertension may also be related to WML.

Studies with both transversal and longitudinal designs have established the relationship between BP levels and WML, as well as the influence of antihypertensive treatment and optimal BP control [2, 25–30]. In the review by Pantoni et al. [31], which included more than 160 publications related to the presence of WML, hypertension, together with age, were the risk factors most closely associated with WML.

Finally, the circadian BP profile has also been associated with the existence of WML in studies performed in elderly hypertensives, which found that patients who present a nocturnal reduction in SBP of ≥20% of daytime systolic pressure ("extreme dippers") have greater silent cerebrovascular injury (lacunar infarcts and WML) than the remaining hypertensive patients [32]. In contrast, hypertensive patients without nocturnal BP descent ("non dippers") also have a greater incidence of cerebral vascular injury than those with a decrease of between 10% and 20% ("dippers") [33].

References

1. Meschia JF, Bushnell CD, Boden-Albala B, Braun LY, Bravata DM, Chaturvedi S, et al. Guidelines for the primary prevention of stroke. A statement for healthcare professionals from the American Heart Association/American Stroke Association. Stroke. 2014;45:3754–832.
2. Sierra C, Coca A, Schiffrin EL. Vascular mechanisms in the pathogenesis of stroke. Curr Hypertens Rep. 2011;13:200–7.
3. Pantoni L. Cerebral small vessel disease: from pathogenesis and clinical characteristics to therapeutic challenges. Lancet Neurol. 2010;9:689–701.
4. Williams B, Mancia G, Spiering W, Agabiti Rosei E, Azizi M, Burnier M, et al. 2018 ESC/ESH Guidelines for the management of arterial hypertension: The Task Force for the management of arterial hypertension of the European Society of Cardiology and the European Society of Hypertension: The Task Force for the management of arterial hypertension of the European Society of Cardiology and the European Society of Hypertension. J Hypertens. 2018;36:1953–2041.
5. Sierra C, Coca A. Brain damage. In: Mancia G, Grassi G, Redon J, editors. Manual of hypertension of the European Society of Hypertension. 2nd ed. Boca Raton: CRC Press Taylor & Francis Group; 2014. p. 177–89. (Print ISBN: 978-1-84184-997-6).
6. Strandgaard S, Paulson OB. Cerebral blood flow and its pathophysiology in hypertension. Am J Hypertens. 1989;2:486–92.
7. Veglio F, Paglieri C, Rabbia F, Bisbocci D, Bergui M, Cerrato P. Hypertension and cerebrovascular damage. Atherosclerosis. 2009;205:331–41.

8. Powers WJ, Grubb RL Jr, Darriet D, Raichle ME. Cerebral blood flow and cerebral metabolic rate of oxygen requirements for cerebral function and viability in humans. J Cereb Blood Flow Metab. 1985;5:600–8.
9. Postiglione A, Bobkiewicz T, Vinholdt-Pedersen E, Lassen NA, Paulson OB, Barry DI. Cerebrovascular effects of angiotensin converting-enzyme inhibition involve large artery dilation in rats. Stroke. 1991;22:1363–8.
10. Sugimori H, Ibayashi S, Irie K, Ooboshi H, Nagao T, Fujii K, Sadoshima S, Fujishima M. Cerebral hemodynamics in hypertensive patients compared with normotensive volunteers. A transcranial Doppler study. Stroke. 1994;25:1384–9.
11. Cho SJ, Sohn YH, Kim JS. Blood flow velocity changes in the middle cerebral artery as an index of the chronicity of hypertension. J Neurol Sci. 1997;150:77–80.
12. Sierra C, de la Sierra A, Chamorro A, Larrousse M, Domenech M, Coca A. Cerebral hemodynamics and silent cerebral white matter lesions in middle-aged essential hypertensive patients. Blood Press. 2004;13:304–9.
13. Bondjers G, Glukhova M, Hansson GK, Postnov YV, Reidy MA, Schwartz SM. Hypertension and atherosclerosis. Cause and effect, or two effects with one unknown cause? Circulation. 1991;84:VI-2–VI-16.
14. Maeda H, Matsumoto M, Handa N, Hougaku H, Ogawa S, Itoh T, Tsukamoto Y, Kamada T. Reactivity of cerebral blood flow velocity to carbon dioxide in hypertensive patients: a transcranial Doppler method. J Hypertens. 1994;12:191–7.
15. Chrissobolis S, Faraci FM. The role of oxidative stress and NADPH oxidase in cerebrovascular disease. Trends Mol Med. 2008;14:495–501.
16. Farrall AJ, Wardlaw JM. Blood-brain barrier: ageing and microvascular disease –systematic review and meta-analysis. Neurobiol Aging. 2009;30:337–52.
17. Chen RL, Balami JS, Esiri MM, et al. Ischemic stroke in the elderly: an overview of evidence. Nat Rev Neurol. 2010;6:256–65.
18. Stoquart-ElSankari S, Baledent O, Gondry-Jouet C, et al. Aging effects on cerebral blood and cerebrospinal fluid flows. J Cereb Blood Flow Metab. 2007;27:1563–72.
19. Van Swieten JC, van den Hout JH, van Ketel BA, Hijdra A, Wokke JH, van Gijn J. Periventricular lesions in the white matter on magnetic resonance imaging in the elderly: a morphometric correlation with arteriolosclerosis and dilated perivascular spaces. Brain. 1991;114:761–74.
20. Henskens L, Kroon A, van Oostenbrugge RJ, Gronenschild E, Fuss-Lejeune M, Hofman P, et al. Increased aortic pulse wave velocity is associated with silent cerebral small-vesssel disease in hypertensive patients. Hypertension. 2008;52:1120–6.
21. Manolio TA, Burke GL, O'Leary DH, Evans G, Beauchamp N, Knepper L, for the CHS Collaborative Research Group, et al. Relationships of cerebral MRI findings to ultrasonographic carotid atherosclerosis in older adults. The Cardiovascular Health Study. Arterioscler Thromb Vasc Biol. 1999;19:356–65.
22. Duprez DA, De Buyzere ML, Van den Noortgate N, Simoens J, Achten E, Clement DL, et al. Relationship between periventricular or deep white matter lesions and arterial elasticity indices in very old people. Age Ageing. 2001;30:325–30.
23. Markus HS, Hunt B, Palmer K, Enzinger C, Schmidt H, Schmidt R. Markers of endothelial and hemostatic activation and progression of cerebral white matter hyperintensities: longitudinal results of the Austrian Stroke Prevention Study. Stroke. 2005;36:1410–4.
24. Van Dijk EJ, Prins ND, Vermeer SE, Vrooman HA, Hofman A, Koudstaal PJ, et al. C-reactive protein and cerebral small-vessel disease: the Rotterdam Scan Study. Circulation. 2005;112:900–5.
25. Liao D, Cooper L, Cai J, Toole JF, Bryan NR, Hutchinson RG, et al. Presence and severity of cerebral white matter lesions and hypertension, its treatment, and its control. The ARIC Study. Stroke. 1996;27:2262–70.
26. Sierra C, de la Sierra A, Mercader J, Gómez-Angelats E, Urbano-Márquez A, Coca A. Silent cerebral white matter lesions in middle-aged essential hypertensive patients. J Hypertens. 2002;20:519–24.

27. Longstreth WT, Manolio TA, Arnold A, Burke GL, Bryan N, Jungreis CA, for the Cardiovascular Health Study Collaborative Research Group, et al. Clinical correlates of white matter findings on cranial magnetic resonance imaging of 3301 elderly people. The Cardiovascular Health Study. Stroke. 1996;27:1274–82.
28. Breteler MM, van Swieten JC, Bots ML, Grobbee DE, Claus JJ, van den Hout JH, et al. Cerebral white matter lesions, vascular risk factors, and cognitive function in a population-based study: the Rotterdam Study. Neurology. 1994;44:1246–52.
29. Schmidt R, Fazekas F, Kapeller P, Schmidt H, Hartung HP. MRI white matter hyperintensities. Three-year follow-up of the Austrian Stroke Prevention Study. Neurology. 1999;53:132–9.
30. Dufouil C, de Kersaint-Gilly A, Besancon V, Levy C, Auffray E, Brunnereau L, et al. Longitudinal study on blood pressure and white matter hyperintensities. The EVA MRI cohort. Neurology. 2001;56:921–6.
31. Pantoni L, García JH. The significance of cerebral white matter abnormalities 100 years after Binswanger's report. A review. Stroke. 1995;26:1293–301.
32. Shimada K, Kawamoto A, Matsubayashi K, Ozawa T. Silent cerebrovascular disease in the elderly. Correlation with ambulatory pressure. Hypertension. 1990;16:692–9.
33. Kario K, Matsuo T, Kobayashi H, Imiya M, Matsuo M, Shimada K. Nocturnal fall of blood pressure and silent cerebrovascular damage in elderly hypertensive patients. Advanced silent cerebrovascular damage in extreme dippers. Hypertension. 1996;27:130–5.

Chapter 12
Coronary Microcirculation and Left Ventricular Hypertrophy

Sebastian Onciul, Oana Popa, and Lucian Dorobantu

Clinical Case

A 45-year-old male, without any known medical history presents with progressive dyspnea and episodes of chest pain both at rest and during exercise. On clinical examination, there were signs of both pulmonary and systemic congestion with basal pulmonary rales on auscultation and bilateral leg oedema; the patient was tachycardic with a rate of 114 bpm and his blood pressure was 90/40 mmHg. The ECG showed low voltage in the limb leads, normal duration of QRS complex and infero-lateral ST depression (Fig. 12.1). The echocardiography showed a dilated and hypertrophied left ventricle (LV) with severely impaired systolic function, with an ejection fraction of 25%. The two-dimensional speckle tracking assessment showed a severely impaired LV longitudinal strain of the basal and mid- ventricular segments, with a typical pattern of apical sparing. There was restrictive mitral filling pattern and both atria were enlarged with a thickened inter-atrial septum (Fig. 12.2). The right ventricle (RV) longitudinal function was also impaired and there were criteria for severe pulmonary hypertension. A small pericardial effusion was surrounding the heart. The invasive coronary angiogram showed normal epicardial coronary arteries.

Sebastian Onciul and Oana Popa contributed equally with all other contributors.

S. Onciul (✉)
Carol Davila University of Medicine and Pharmacy, Bucharest, Romania

Cardiology Department, Clinical Emergency Hospital, Bucharest, Romania

O. Popa
Agrippa Ionescu Hospital, Bucharest, Romania

L. Dorobantu
Monza Hospital, Bucharest, Romania

M. Dorobantu, L. Badimon (eds.), *Microcirculation*,
https://doi.org/10.1007/978-3-030-28199-1_12

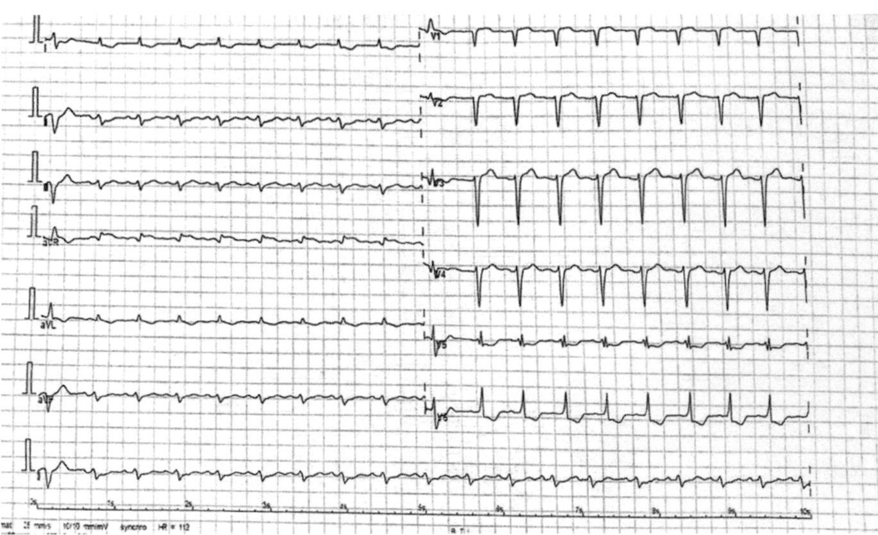

Fig. 12.1 ECG showing sinus tachycardia, normal PR interval, low voltage in limb leads, Q wave in V1 and V2, slow R wave progression in the anterior leads. There are no voltage criteria for left ventricular hypertrophy, however the infero-lateral ST downslopping depression is suggestive of LV strain

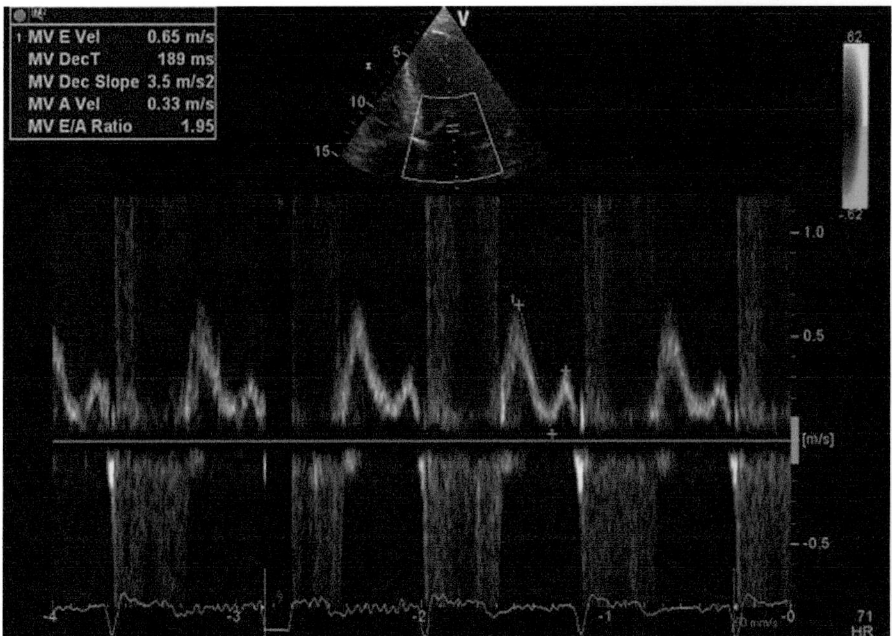

Fig. 12.2 Pulsed-wave Doppler echocardiography showing a restrictive mitral filling pattern

Given the LVH and dilatation but with low voltage in limb leads on ECG, a diagnosis of cardiac amyloidosis (CA) was suspected and a CMR exam was performed.

The CMR Examination

The CMR cine acquisitions showed an asymmetrical septal hypertrophy (basal interventricular septum measured 15 mm, all other walls were 9 mm thick) (Fig. 12.3). The LV was severely dilated (142 ml/m^2)with a severely impaired systolic function (LVEF 26%) due to global hypokinesia with severe impairment of the longitudinal contraction. The RV was also dilated (129 ml/m^2) and dysfunctional (RV EF 41%). There was also severe bi-atrial dilatation and thickening of the left atrial walls (9 mm thick) with impaired atrial pump function. A small circumferential pericardial effusion was also noted.

Early Gadolinium enhancement (EGE) images showed a circumferential, thin area of subendocardial hypo-enhancement surrounded by normally enhancing myocardium (Fig. 12.4a). No intracavitary thrombus was seen.

The Late Gadolinium Enhancement (LGE) images were difficult to acquire due to suboptimal nulling of the myocardial signal despite using different inversion times. There was diffuse myocardial hyper enhancement, which was transmural in some areas (intraventricular septum and basal lateral wall) (Fig. 12.5).

T2 weighted imaging displayed homogenous signal intensity without any focal hyperintense areas, suggesting the absence of focal myocardial oedema. However, the T2 mapping showed diffusely high values (54 ms) suggesting diffuse, global myocardial oedema.

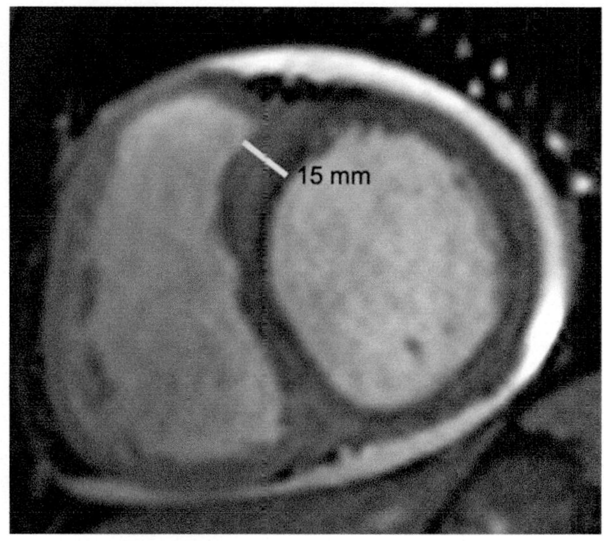

Fig. 12.3 Diastolic phase of a balanced steady-state free precession (bSSFP) cine sequence. The basal antero-septum is 15 mm thick, while the other walls are not hypertrophied. Small, circumferential pericardial effusion is also noted

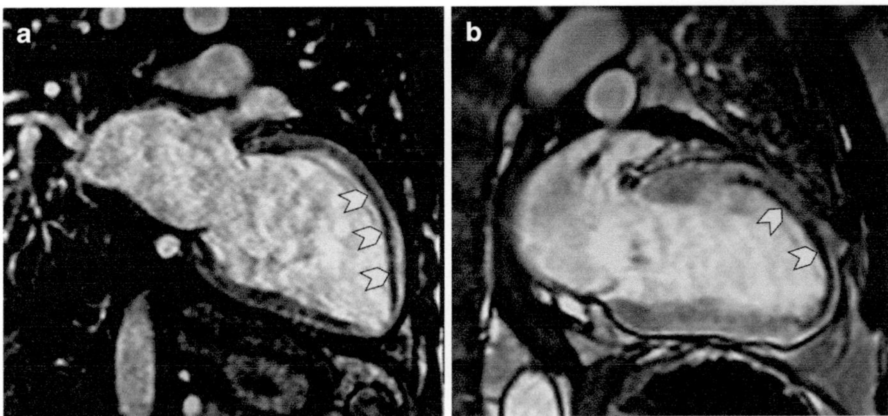

Fig. 12.4 Comparison between early Gadolinium enhancement (EGE) 2 chamber longitudinal axis images of the patient with AL amyloidosis (**a**) and a patient with acute anterior myocardial infarction (**b**). In both images a dark subendocardial area (yellow arrowheads) can be seen surrounded by bright myocardium. In the first 3 min after contrast administration, the normal myocardium becomes bright. However, areas of microvascular obstruction appear dark, as contrast cannot penetrate immediately in the respective areas

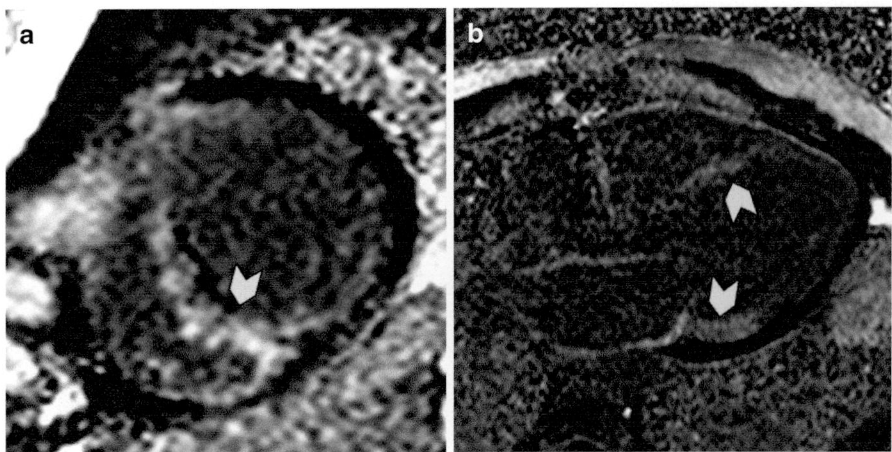

Fig. 12.5 Late Gadolinium Enhancement (LGE) images aquired in short axis (**a**) and longitudinal 4 chamber (**b**) views, respectively. Difficult nulling of myocardium, with areas of transmural hyperenhancement (yellow arrow heads) without respecting a coronary artery distribution

T1 mapping demonstrated extremely high native T1 values (1200 ms), as well as severe expansion of the interstitium: extracellular volume fraction (ECV) 51% (normal values 22–29%).

The constellation of these CMR findings were highly suggestive of CA, and thus a complete hematological work-up was performed in order to establish the precise etiology of cardiac amyloid deposition. AL type systemic amyloidosis was demonstrated, and specific chemotherapy was subsequently initiated.

Discussion

We present a case of LVH in which the diagnostic work-up identified the amyloid deposition as the substrate of wall thickening. Alterations of coronary microcirculation have been described in the context of cardiac amyloidosis on endomyocardial biopsy and post-mortem studies. However, in vivo demonstration of MVO in the setting of cardiac amyloid deposition has not been reported before. In our case, the images acquired after Gadolinium-based contrast administration were highly suggestive of MVO.

Structural and Functional Alterations of Coronary Microcirculation

Coronary microcirculatory abnormalities are present along the whole spectrum of LVH etiologies, either in the form of abnormal coronary flow reserve (CFR), or more infrequently as MVO.

Non-invasive quantification of myocardial blood flow (MBF) at rest and during maximal coronary dilatation is able to confirm the microvascular dysfunction (MVD). Both Rubidium-82 positron-emission tomography (PET) imaging and CMR are able to demonstrate impaired myocardial blood flow during vasodilator stress with adenosine. The ratio between MBF under basal conditions and in conditions of maximal coronary vasodilatation represents the coronary flow reserve (CFR) [1].

However, the most severe form of MVD is MVO which can be demonstrated histologically but also by non-invasive imaging. In this regard, MVO has been well characterized by CMR in the setting of acute myocardial infarction (MI) [2].

Coronary Microvascular Dysfunction Across the Spectrum of LVH Etiologies

Left ventricular hypertrophy is encountered in a variety of clinical settings. LVH may appear secondary to increased afterload conditions such asarterial hypertension or aortic stenosis. However, LVH may also be the expression of primary cardiomyopathic processes such as HCM or infiltrative diseases. In all these conditions the extracellular compartment of the myocardium may be disorganized with alterations of the interstitial matrix architecture. The intramyocardial capillaries lumen is narrowed secondary to both increased capillary wall thickness, but also due to extrinsic compression by an expanded extracellular matrix.

Consequently, alterations of the coronary microcirculation consist in either abnormal CFR, or the most extreme alteration of the microcirculation, namely MVO.

Coronary Microvascular Dysfunction in Hypertrophic Cardiomyopathy

The structural alterations of coronary microcirculation in HCM are well documented.

Maron proposedthattheprimarystructural substrate for microvasculardysfunction in HCMisthethickening of the intima and/or medial layers of thearterial wallsresulting in narrowing of theintramuralcoronaryarterioleslumen [1] (Fig. 12.6). The increased myocardial oxygen demand due to increased LV mass as well as the LV outflow obstruction can lead to periods of ischaemia which may result in areas of replacement fibrosis.

Patients with HCM have normal MBF at rest, but exhibit a blunted response during vasodilatatory stress, i.e. the MBF does not increase during the infusion of adenosine or dypiridamole [1, 3, 4].

Petersen et al. demonstrated using CMR imaging that patients with HCM have decreased CFR, and patients with higher degree of hypertrophy have more severe microcirculatory dysfunction [4]. Furthermore, the reductions in MBF were associated with increasing wall thickness and the amount of segmental LGE.

However, MVD is present not only in the hypertrophied segments, but also in the non-hypertrophied walls suggesting that MVD is part of a diffuse impairment of microcirculation in HCM [1, 3]. As such, the occurrence of MVD in the non-hypertrophied segments may be an early marker of the HCM phenotype [5].

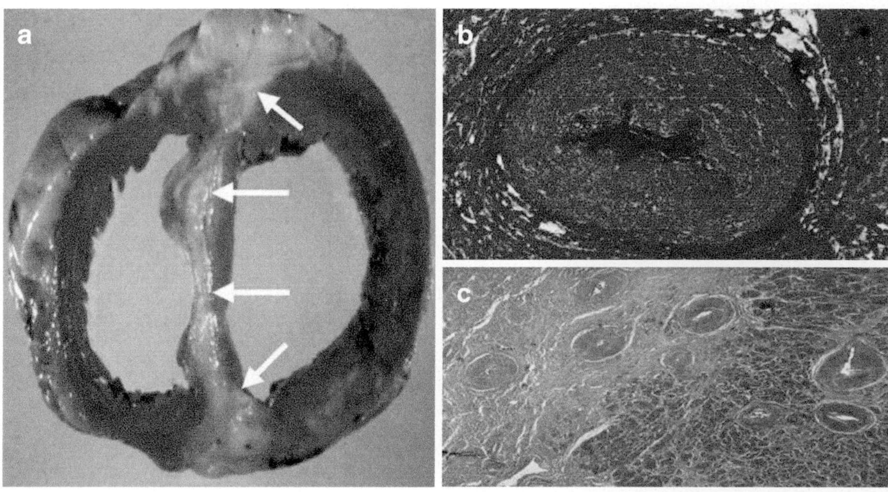

Fig. 12.6 Small-Vessel Disease and the Morphologic Basis for Myocardial Ischemia in HCM. (**a**) Native heart of a patient with end-stage HCM who underwent transplantation. Large areas of gross macroscopic scarring are evident throughout the LV myocardium (white arrows). (**b**) Intramural coronary artery in cross-section showing thickened intimal and medial layers of the vessel wall associated with small luminal area. (**c**) Area of myocardium with numerous abnormal intramural coronary arteries within a region of scarring, adjacent to an area of normal myocardium. Original magnification ×55. With permission from M. S. Maron et al., "The Case for Myocardial Ischemia in Hypertrophic Cardiomyopathy," J. Am. Coll. Cardiol., vol. 54, no. 9, pp. 866–875, 2009

Anderson-Fabry Disease

Patients with Anderson-Fabry (AFD) disease frequently present with angina, positive non-invasive testing for ischaemia but no epicardial coronary obstructive disease [6, 7]. PET imaging has demonstrated that male patients with Anderson Fabry disease have an impaired CFR [7].

In these patients, myocardial ischaemia may result from capillary rarefaction in the context of a thickened myocardium, but this is not the sole mechanism. Coronary microvascular dysfunction may occur in AFD patients independently of the LV wall thickness, including females without LVH [8]. This observation suggest that intrinsic alterations of capillary wall may contribute to CMD. Indeed, histological studies have shown that the lumen of the intramural arteries is narrowed because of hypertrophy and proliferation of smooth muscle and endothelial cells, both engulfed by glycosphingolipids [6].

As CMD may appear early in the course of AFD, this may have important consequences for the optimal timing of enzyme replacement therapy in the pre-hypertrophic stages of the disease [8].

Endomyocardial biopsies before and after treatment with recombinant human α-galactosidase A have shown that replacement therapy resulted in successful clearance of globotriaosylceramide accumulation on cardiac biopsies [9]. However, the coronary microvascular function does not seem to recover after enzyme replacement therapy [7].

Amyloidosis

Angina is a common presentation of patients with cardiac amyloidosis (CA). They usually have positive exercise or pharmacological stress tests, in the absence of epicardial coronary artery disease. These patients are initially diagnosed as having cardiac syndrome X, but they do not respond to anti-anginal medication that is usually prescribed for this condition [10, 11].

Reduced vasodilator coronary flow reserve was demonstrated in CA patients using vasodilator stress N-13 ammonia PET: peak stress myocardial blood flow (MBF) was significantly lower in cardiac amyloidosis patients compared to healthy volunteers and to patients with hypertension related LVH (0.91 vs 1.94 vs 2.1 ml/g/min, $p < 0.0001$) [12].

According to Dorbala et al., CMD in amyloidosis has three major mechanisms:

- structural (amyloid deposition in the vessel wall causing wall thickening and luminal stenosis)
- extravascular (extrinsic compression of the microvasculature from perivascular and interstitial amyloid deposits and decreased diastolic perfusion)
- functional (autonomic and endothelial dysfunction) [13].

Apart from this, post-mortem histologic examination of hearts of patients with AL amyloidosis identified severe obstructive alterations of the intramural coronary arteries with amyloid leading to significant luminal narrowing or occlusion [11]. Fresh myocardial necrosis was found in the myocardial areas with small-vessel obstruction [11].

Thus, cardiac amyloidosis is one of the LVH conditions which may associate coronary MVO and the non-invasive diagnosis of MVO may be of interest for therapeutic and prognostic purposes in patients with CA. CMR imaging is unique among the cardiac imaging modalities as it has the capacity to provide detailed information about the structure of the myocardium including the identification of areas of MVO.

Diagnosis of Microvascular Obstruction by Cardiovascular Magnetic Resonance

During a standard contrast enhanced CMR protocol, MVO can be identified at 3 different steps:

- the first-pass perfusion
- the early Gadolinium enhancement (EGE) and
- the late Gadolinium enhancement (LGE) [14].

On these images, MVO appears as a dark core in the middle of bright areas of contrast enhancement. The dark appearance is explained by the non-penetrance of Gadolinium-based contrast inside de MVO territory. EGE images are usually acquired in the first 3 min after contrast administration, while LGE images are acquired 10–15 min after contrast administration. All along this time, contrast may penetrate the periphery of the MVO area, resulting in a smaller MVO area appearance on LGE than on EGE images [2].

MVO has been well documented in the setting of reperfused acute MI (example in Fig. 12.4b) as an expression of no-reflow phenomenon. In these patients, MVO detection by CMR is a poor prognostic indicator and marker of subsequent adverse LV remodeling [2].

The Potential of CMR to Diagnose MVO in Cardiac Amyloidosis

To our knowledge, diagnosis of MVO by CMR has not been reported in the setting of cardiac diseases other than acute reperfused MI. However, endomyocardial biopsy and post-mortem studies have clearly described severe MVO in the setting of CA [11, 10].

The EGE and LGE images in our patient show a circumferential area of subendocardial hypo-enhancement, which may represent reduced subendocardial flow, possibly due to MVO (Fig. 12.4). The persistence of the dark core even 15 min after contrast infusion suggest the failure of Gadolinium to penetrate the area of reduced blood flow. Our assumption that the dark core on EGE/LGE images is the expression of MVO, is based on the similar aspect of MVO in acute reperfused MI (Fig. 12.4b). However, an endomyocardial biopsy has not been performed in this patient, and therefore our belief is shadowed by uncertainty for the moment.

Conclusions

Coronary MVD occurs across the entire spectrum of LVH etiologies mainly as impaired CFR. This can result in angina in the absence of epicardial coronary obstructive disease and may be quantified non-invasively by measuring the myocardial blood flow during vasodilator stress. However, cardiac amyloidosis represents a particular condition, structurally characterized not only by decreased CFR but also by obvious MVO. CMR may be a patent method to non-invasively diagnose MVO in the setting of cardiac amyloidosis with important clinical significance.

References

1. Maron MS, et al. The case for myocardial ischemia in hypertrophic cardiomyopathy. J Am Coll Cardiol. 2009;54(9):866–75.
2. Wu KC. CMR of microvascular obstruction and hemorrhage in myocardial infarction. J Cardiovasc Magn Reson. 2012;14(1):68.
3. Camici P, et al. Coronary vasodilation is impaired in both hypertrophied and nonhypertrophied myocardium of patients with hypertrophic cardiomyopathy: a study with nitrogen-13 ammonia and positron emission tomography. J Am Coll Cardiol. 1991;17(4):879–86.
4. Petersen SE, et al. Evidence for microvascular dysfunction in hypertrophic cardiomyopathy. Circulation. May 2007;115(18):2418–25.
5. Camaioni C, et al. 004 perfusion mapping in hypertrophic cardiomyopathy: microvascular dysfunction occurs regardless of hypertrophy. Heart. 2017;103(Suppl 1):A4.
6. Chimenti C, et al. Angina in fabry disease reflects coronary small vessel disease. Circ Heart Fail. 2008;1(3):161–9.
7. Elliott PM, et al. Coronary microvascular dysfunction in male patients with Anderson-Fabry disease and the effect of treatment with alpha galactosidase A. Heart. 2006;92(3):357–60.
8. Tomberli B, et al. Coronary microvascular dysfunction is an early feature of cardiac involvement in patients with Anderson-Fabry disease. Eur J Heart Fail. 2013;15(12):1363–73.
9. Thurberg BL, Fallon JT, Mitchell R, Aretz T, Gordon RE, O'Callaghan MW. Cardiac microvascular pathology in Fabry disease: evaluation of endomyocardial biopsies before and after enzyme replacement therapy. Circulation. 2009;119(19):2561–7.
10. Yagishita A, et al. Cardiac amyloidosis presumptively diagnosed as cardiac syndrome X. Circ J. 2009;73(7):1349–51.

11. Ogawa H, et al. Cardiac amyloidosis presenting as microvascular angina--a case report. Angiology. 2001;52(4):273–8.
12. Dorbala S, et al. Coronary microvascular function in cardiac amyloidosis. J Nucl Med. 2012;53(Suppl 1):297.
13. Dorbala S, et al. Coronary microvascular dysfunction is related to abnormalities in myocardial structure and function in cardiac amyloidosis. JACC Heart Fail. 2014;2(4):358–67.
14. Mather AN, et al. Appearance of microvascular obstruction on high resolution first-pass perfusion, early and late gadolinium enhancement CMR in patients with acute myocardial infarction. J Cardiovasc Magn Reson. 2009;11(1):33.

Chapter 13
Microcirculatory Dysfunction in Acute Heart Failure

Ovidiu Chioncel and Alexandre Mebazaa

Introduction

Acute heart failure (AHF) is characterized by an acute or sub-acute deterioration in cardiac function resulting from numerous possible underlying heart diseases and precipitating factors [1].

The diversity in etiologies, precipitants, and comorbidities suggests that multiple pathophysiologic targets contribute to HF progression, and substantial heterogeneity in the response to therapy might be expected.

Despite significant advances in diagnosis and therapy over the past 20 years [1, 2], HF patients still have a poor prognosis. European registries [2–4] showed that 1-yearoutcome rates remain unacceptably high, and confirm that hospitalization for AHF represents a change in the natural history of the disease process.

This finding can be explained by the incomplete understanding of pathophysiology of the disease and by the fact that in-hospital therapeutic approaches to these patients have remained practically unchanged during the last few decades [5].

Furthermore, AHF represents a broad spectrum of disease states, varying from hypertensive heart failure to CS [4], and consequently, there is a diversity of pathophysiological mechanisms and therapeutic approaches.

Cardiogenic shock (CS) is the most severe manifestation of acute heart failure (AHF) [1], with in-hospital mortality between 30 and 60% [2–4].

O. Chioncel (✉)
Emergency Institute for Cardiovascular Diseases "Prof. C.C. Iliescu", Bucharest, Romania

University of Medicine Carol Davila, Bucharest, Romania

A. Mebazaa
Université de Paris, Hôpitaux Universitaires Saint Louis Lariboisière, APHP, U 942 Inserm-MASCOT, F-CRIN INI-CRCT, Paris, France
e-mail: alexandre.mebazaa@aphp.fr

M. Dorobantu, L. Badimon (eds.), *Microcirculation*,
https://doi.org/10.1007/978-3-030-28199-1_13

Vital organ hypoperfusionis, the hallmark of CS, and compensatory mechanisms by vasoconstriction lead to intermittent improvement in coronary and peripheral perfusion at the cost of increased afterload [6, 7].

Compensatory vasoconstriction is reversed by inflammatory mediators, which determine nitric oxide (NO) dependent pathological vasodilation [6, 7]. The occurrence of the systemic inflammatory response syndrome (SIRS) contributes to the further worsening of hypoperfusion and development of multi-organ dysfunction syndrome (MODS) through excessive vasodilation, the key element being the impairment of microcirculation [6, 7].

In addition, bleeding, transfusion and even hemolysis induced by some MCS further contribute to the inflammatory response [7, 8].

Development of SIRS and MODS are considered to be major contributors to the high in-hospital mortality beyond hemodynamic abnormalities [6–8].

However, there is a limited understanding of the pathophysiology of CS and AHF, and current therapies focus rather on central macro-hemodynamic abnormalities (e.g. preload, afterload) as opposed to targeting specific organ pathways.

Several conceptual frameworks have been proposed to explore the underlying pathogenesis of AHF, and recently emerging evidence has suggested a potential impact of microcirculatory dysfunction. Although, the clinical consequences of macro-circulatory abnormalities, congestion or hypoperfusion, can lead to organ injury and, ultimately, the failure of target organs (i.e. heart, lungs, kidneys, liver, intestine, brain), which are associated with increased mortality, the intermediary link between central hemodynamics and organ failure is represented by microcirculatory dysfunction.

Clinicians have no ability to assess the microcirculation and the balance of metabolic supply and demand at the bedside. Hence, more readily available macrocirculatory measures, such as cardiac output, mean arterial pressure, centralvenous pressure, serum lactate, and mixed venous oxygen saturation, are used as surrogates, making the assumption that microcirculatory perfusion is strictly coupled to the macro-circulation. Even though a minimal cardiac output and arterial pressure is mandatory to sustain the microcirculation, this level is not yet well defined and has a high organ and individual variability. Above this level, microcirculation and systemic circulation are relatively dissociated, so that microcirculatory alterations can be observed even when systemic hemodynamics are within satisfactory goals, and furthermore, the response of the microcirculation to therapeutic interventions is often dissociated from systemic effects [9–11].

Data from SHOCK registry [12], demonstrated that 45% of non-survivors of CS die with a normal cardiac index (i.e. >2.2 l/min/m^2), indicating that optimization of macro-hemodynamic parameters alone may fail to improve outcomes.

In addition, patients with AHF, may present with distinct clinical phenotypes, varying from hypertensive heart failure to CS [4], and whether the severity of microcirculatory alterations and the response to therapy differs among these clinical conditions needs to be investigated.

Pathophysiology of Microcirculatory Dysfunction in AHF

The cardiovascular system, including macro-circulation and microcirculation, are closely controlled to warrant that oxygen delivery is matched to the metabolic demands of the whole organism. Systemic perfusion pressure is a key element of the macro circulation but is strongly influenced by vascular tone within the micro-circulation. Individual organs adjust their microcirculatory perfusion to regulate the local supply of oxygen in order to meet their metabolic needs [13].

Because oxygen has to diffuse from capillaries to tissue cells, every organ has a rich network of microvessels [13], and density of this network depend on the metabolic requirement of each specific tissue [13].

The microcirculation consists of a network of blood vessels less than 100 μm in diameter (arterioles, capillaries and venules) [9, 14]

Arterioles are tiny branches of arteries that lead to capillaries and form the major resistive component of the microcirculation. The smooth muscle cells from arteriolar wall are under the control of the sympathetic nervous system. Vascular endothelial cells can respond to mechanical stimuli (alterations in local shear stress), biochemical stimuli (pH, lactate, tissue concentration of O_2 and CO_2), neurohormonal mediators [9, 14].

These central and local control mechanisms regulate constriction and dilatation of the arterioles depending on the perfusion pressure and metabolic requirements of the tissue cells. Under abnormal conditions, such as CS or AHF, the balance between vascular resistance to preserve arterial pressure (by constriction of the resistance vessels) and peripheral tissue flow may be lost, causing insufficient blood flow to sustain metabolism in specific organs (Fig. 13.1). For instance, the temporary compromise as a response to a sudden decline in blood pressure (e.g., in shock states) is an increase in arterial resistance and reduced bloodflow to the less vital organs such as the skin and the splanchnic system.

Capillaries consist of a single layer of epithelium and a basement membrane. The main function of capillaries is to allow exchange of molecules between blood and tissues [9, 13, 14].

Capillary blood flow (a product of driving pressure, arteriolar tone, and hemorheology) and capillary patency are the main determinants of capillary perfusion [14, 15].

Blood flow in one single capillary is not a good indicator of oxygen delivery to the tissue under evaluation due to the temporal and spatial heterogeneity of capillary blood flow [14–16].

Capillary patency is reflected by functional capillary density (FCD), defined as the number of functional capillaries in a given area where functional is defined as capillaries filled with flowing red blood cells [14–16].

FCD is tightly coupled to cellular metabolic requirements such that increased requirements result in decreased terminal arteriolar tone, increased FCD, and increased substrate supply. Decreasing in FCD reduce the surface area for capillary exchange, increase diffusion distance, and increase the degree of arterio-venous shunting of blood through tissues [14–16] (Fig. 13.2).

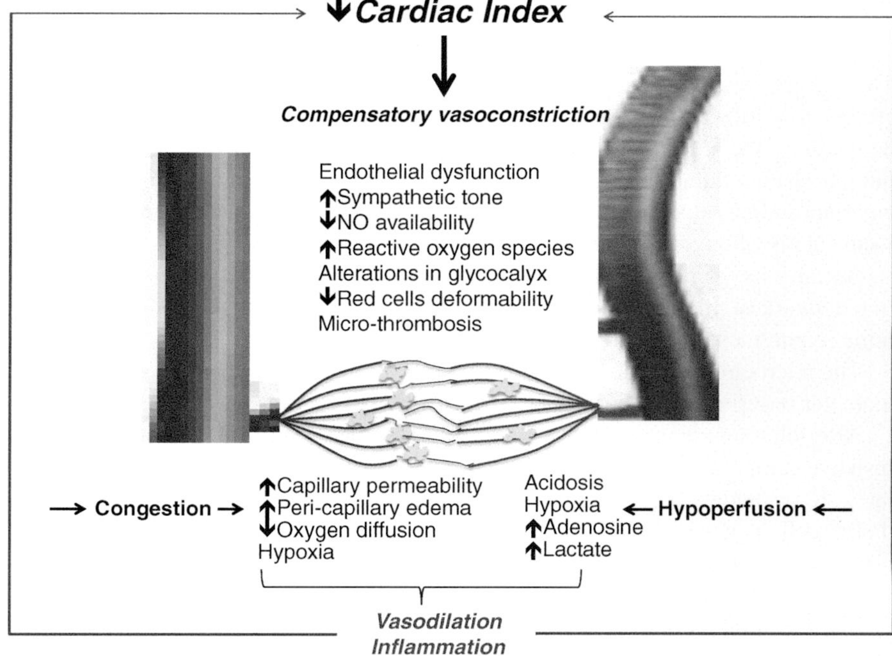

Fig. 13.1 Pathophysiology of microcirculatory dysfunction in AF

In normal conditions, the microcirculation is responsible for fine-tuning of perfusion to meet local oxygen requirements. This is achieved by recruiting and de-recruiting capillaries, shutting down or limiting flow in capillaries which perfuse areas with low oxygen requirements and increasing flow in areas with high oxygen requirements [16] (Fig. 13.2).

The venular part of the microcirculation serves as a large low-pressure reservoir and it may contain as much as 75% of total blood volume [17]. Active and passive changes of venous vascular tone alter the quantity of venous blood, which thereby change cardiac preload and cardiac output and guarantee maintenance of the circulating blood pool [17].

Microcirculatory perfusion is subject to myogenic, metabolic, and neurohumoral mechanisms that control loco-regional bloodflow [13–16].

Myogenic auto-regulation is the intrinsic ability of a blood vessel to constrict or dilate in response to a change in intraluminal pressure and is tempered by shear stress-induced release of nitric oxide (NO) [15, 16].

Myogenic responses, mediated by changes in vascular smooth muscle contractility, serve to regulate capillary pressure and FCD across a wide range of systemic perfusion pressures. These responses provide a basal level of tone but also interact with other vascular control mechanisms to influence regional perfusion [15, 16].

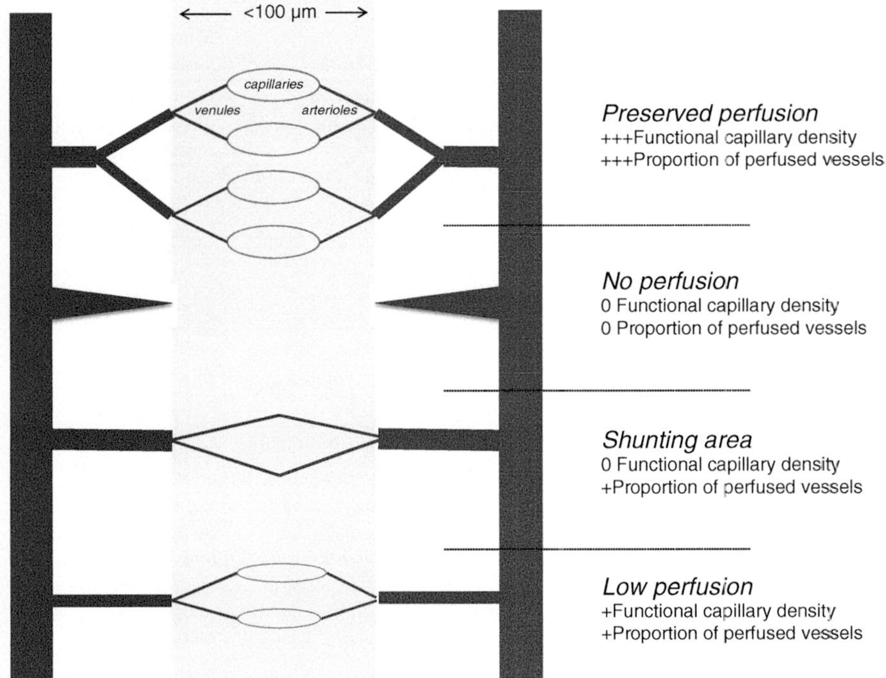

Fig. 13.2 Heterogeneity of microcirculation and tisular perfusion in AHF

The metabolic theory of auto-regulation describes the matching of local capillary blood flow to the metabolic needs of the underlying tissue [18].

Hypoxia results in rapid, endotheliummediatedvasodilation via release of vasodilating prostaglandins and NO. The release of metabolites, such as adenosine, lactate, H^+, and K^+, from the underlying tissues induces amore delayed vasodilator response [15, 16, 18].

Also, the degree of arteriolar vasodilation is dependent on the distribution of adrenergic receptors particular to a given organ [19].

Based on these regulatory mechanisms, endothelium could modulate the number of well-perfused capillary, i.e., the functional capillary density, in order to supply tissue metabolic requirements [13–16, 20].

Numerous experimental and clinical studies have reported that microvascular blood flow is altered in patients with AHF and CS (Table 13.1), and tissue perfusion can remain altered even after achievement of within-target cardiac output and arterial pressure. Multiple organ failure is common in these patients, often despite correction of mean arterial pressure and cardiac output (Fig. 13.3). Low-flow conditions are associated with a substantial decrease in FCD as a result of shutting down some capillaries while others remain perfused with reduced flow [10, 14–16].

The severity of the decrease in FCD is directly related to a poor outcome [10, 21, 22].

Table 13.1 Studies enrolling AHF patients and documenting microcirculatory dysfunction

	Clinical settings	N	Lot control	Technique	Microcirculatory variable
Kirschenbaum et al. [23]	CS post MI	8	6 ICU patients and 6 septic shock patients	Venous air plethysmography	Decreased forearm blood flow during reactive hyperemia
De Backer et al. [10]	AHF and CS	40	15 patients	OPS, sublingual	Low PPSV
Jung et al. [21]	CS	7	17 ICU patients without shock	OPS, sublingual	Low microflow
Den Uil et al. [54]	ADHF	24	20 healthy volunteers	SDF, sublingual	Low PCD
Lauten et al. [11]	ADHF	27	No	SDF, sublingual	Low MFI
Lam et al. [71]	CS post MI with Impella support	6	3 healthy volunteers	SDF, sublingual	Low MFI, PVD

ADHF acute decompensated heart failure, *CS* cardiogenic shock, *ICU* intensive care unit, *MFI* microcirculatory flow index, *MI* myocardial infarction, *PCD* perfused capillary density, *PPV* proportion of perfused vessels, *PVD* perfused vessel density, *SDF* Side-stream Dark-Field, *TCD* total capillary density

Hypoperfusion of microcirculation may be an etiologic factor in the pathogenesis of multiple organ failure and may contribute to mortality in a considerable proportion of patients with CS [10, 21, 22].

The severity and the duration of microcirculatory alterations are related to the occurrence of organ dysfunction and risk of death [9].

Different mechanisms have been implicated in the development of these alterations including, impaired endothelial vasoreactivity, alterations in red blood cell rheology, alteration in endothelial glycocalyx, platelet aggregation, and microthrombosis (Fig. 13.1). Further on, alteration in microvascular endothelium is associated with activation of coagulation and inflammation, reactive oxygen species generation, and permeability alterations [20, 21].

In one of the first studies [10], despite of the fact that the perfusion of large vessels was preserved in all groups, the proportion of perfused small (<20 μm) vessels was lower in patients with severe AHF and CS than in control patients, and acetylcholine totally reversed microcirculatory dysfunction.

Furthermore, the response to reactive hyperemia is attenuated in CS, and this may reflect increased vasoconstriction and an impaired capacity for vasodilation [23].

This may be explained by augmented sensitivity to an already increased sympathetic output. There may also be a systemic reduction in NO production as a result of reduced activity of the endothelial isoform of NO synthase, as is seen in chronic left ventricular failure [24].

Rheological factors, such as decreased erythrocyte deformability may also be important in limiting systemic microvascular flow [23].

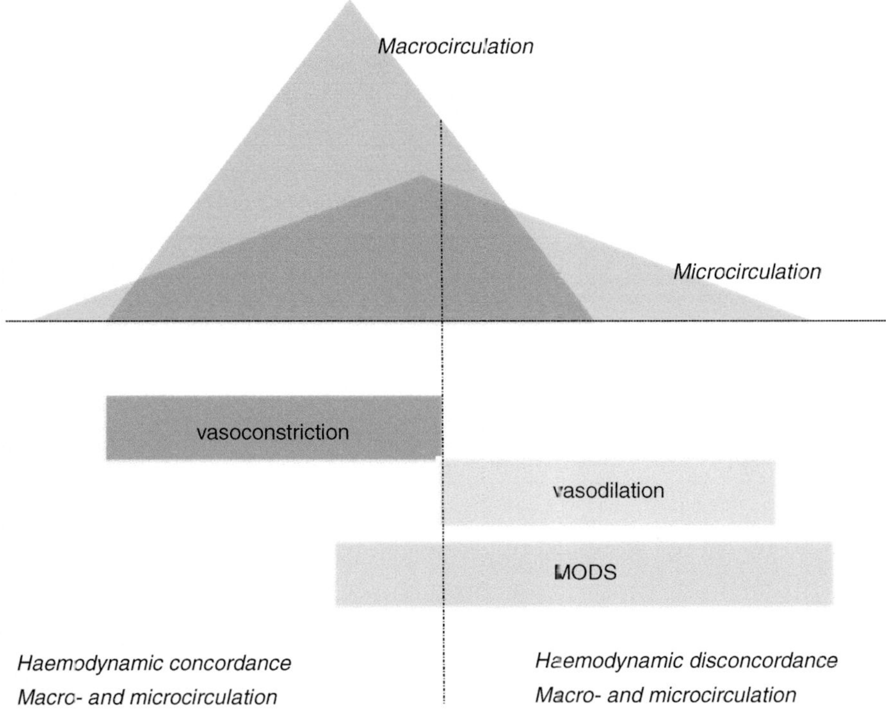

Fig. 13.3 Time course of microcirculatory dysfunction

As the degree of sympathetic activation and vasoconstriction are proportional to severity of HF, decreased microvascular tissue perfusion is likely to occur even in patients with no global hemodynamic compromise or laboratory signs of hypoperfusion. Microcirculatory dysfunction, consisting of a decrease in sublingual vessel density and in the proportion of perfused capillaries, was observed in patients with ADHF even in the absence of clinical or laboratory signs of hypoperfusion [11].

These findings indicate microcirculatory impairment as a pathophysiological mechanism involved in the development of organ failure, which is frequently observed in AHF and associated with a significant morbidity and mortality (Table 13.2).

Using global hemodynamic markers as target to therapy in AHF may not be sufficient to avoid subsequent organ failure [9, 10, 25].

This may at least in part be explained by the fact that organ perfusion is mostly determined by microvascular perfusion, which can be affected independently of global and/or regional perfusion (Fig. 13.3). However, distinct to the sepsis, in CS microvascular alterations are not completely independent from changes in macrocirculation [9, 14–16], and at least in the early phase, a clear relationship between cardiac output and microcirculatory status can be seen.

Table 13.2 Parameters of microcirculatory dysfunction and their prognosis role in AHF studies

	Clinical settings	Control group	N	Technique	Serial measurements	Prognostic variable	Outcome
De Backer [10]	AHF and CS	Yes	40	OPS	No	PPSV	In-hospital mortality
Den Uil [22]	CS	No	68	SDF	Yes	PCD	30-day mortality
Jung [69]	CS post MI with IABP	Yes	41	SDF	Yes	PCD,PVD,TCD	30-day mortality
Kara [73]	CS with VA ECMO	No	24	IDF	Yes	PVD	ICU-mortality
Yeh [74]	CS with VA ECMO	No	48	IDF	Yes	PVD, PPV	28-day mortality

ICU intensive care unit, *IDF* Incident Dark Field Imaging, *PCD* perfused capillary density, *PPV* proportion of perfused vessels, *PVD* perfused vessel density, *OPS* Orthogonal Polarization Spectral imaging, *SDF* side-stream dark field imaging, *TCD* total capillary density

Thus, the use of some measurements of microcirculation function in conjunction with global hemodynamic data (such as cardiac index, lactate level, SaO_2, SVO_2), in order to appropriately guide therapy, would be more clinical relevant than only relying on macro-hemodynamics [25].

Techniques Used to Monitor Microcirculation

Microcirculation assessment was possible only in experimental condition until very recently. Due to the improvement of technology, clinicians are able to evaluate both anatomy and metabolism of microcirculation at the bedside [9, 10, 15, 16, 20].

The microcirculation in humans can be evaluated directly by videomicroscopy or indirectly by vascular occlusion tests. Of note, direct videomicroscopic techniques evaluates the actual state of the microcirculation, whereas the vascular occlusion test evaluates microvascular reserve. In clinical experiences, AHF and CS have been associated with a decrease in perfused capillary density and an increase in the heterogeneity of microcirculatory perfusion, with non-perfused capillaries in close vicinity to perfused capillaries (Table 13.1).

Microvideoscopic techniques, such as orthogonal polarization spectral (OPS) and side stream dark field (SDF) imaging, directly evaluate microvascular networks covered by a thin epithelium. The most investigated site in humans is the sublingual mucosa. In the sublingual area, which has a common embryologic origin with splanchnic microcirculation, capillaries and venules of variable size can be visualized. These techniques use a light source directed on a tissue and the light is reflected by deeper layers providing transillumination of the superficial layers of the tissue. In both techniques, the wavelength of the emitting light, 548 nm (wavelength which is both deoxy and oxyhemoglobin light absorption), is absorbed by the hemoglobin contained in the red blood cells (both deoxy and oxyhemoglobin), independently of its oxygenation state, so that these can be seen as black/gray bodies [14–16].

The Orthogonal Polarization Spectral (OPS) imaging technique is a relatively non-invasive method developed for the assessment of the human microcirculation, ideal to study capillaries under thin mucosa layer such as those of tongue, conjunctiva, and serosa. In OPS, the examined tissue is illuminated with polarized light and the reflected light is depolarized, due to multiple hits on cells in the deep layers of the tissue.

Sidestream Dark-Field (SDF) is a further development of OPS technique and it allows a better resolution and clarity [26]. Hand-held SDF imaging produces high-resolution video of the microcirculation and can be used non-invasively on the sublingual mucosa or invasively on a wide variety of tissues. The indices of microcirculatory perfusion generated with this technique provide an estimate of capillary density, magnitude of blood flow, and heterogeneity of perfusion [14, 26].

The following parameters have been suggested: assessment of perfusion quality for small, medium, and large vessels (Microvascular flow index-MFI), a measure of vessel density (total or perfused vessel density TVD and PVD), two indices of vascular perfusion (proportion of perfused vessels-PPV and microcirculatory flow index-MFI), and a flow heterogeneity index [14–16, 26, 27].

Recently, introduction of Incident Dark Field Imaging (IDF) imaging allows for a faster and more stable and precise measurement to be made [28].

This new device with improved optics detects 30% more sublingual vessels than the SDF, and has a faster measurement acquisition time, requiring only 3–5 s to assess the quality of the microcirculation [28].

Laser Doppler and near-infrared spectroscopy (NIRS) measurements detect the dynamic response of the microcirculation to a stress test [15, 16].

Laser Doppler is based on the Doppler shift of the emitted laser light when it travels through tissue and is reflected off the moving objects, such as the moving erythrocytes.

Laser Doppler devices allow a vasoreactivity test, based on the fact that after transient ischemia obtained by arterial occlusion with a cuff placed around the arm, the speed of flow recovery will mostly be determined by the capacity of the microvasculature to recruit arterioles and capillaries [14–16]. An adequaterestoration of blood supply requires a microcirculation that is functional enough to recruit vascular beds in response to metabolic need after mild ischemia.

NIRS is a non-invasive method assessing hemoglobin oxygen saturation measured in a volume of illuminated tissue with a near infrared wavelength [15, 16, 26, 27].

Near-infrared spectroscopy (NIRS) is a technique that utilizes near-infrared light (wavelengths between 700 and 900 nm) which easily penetrate biological tissues and allows a quantification of the oxygenation of chromophores such as haemoglobin and myoglobin, as well as of the redox state of the intracellular cytochromes (Aa3).

The fractions of oxy- and deoxyhemoglobin are used to calculate tissue O_2 saturation (StO_2), and total light absorption is used to compute total tissue hemoglobin (HbT) and the absolute tissue hemoglobinindex (THI) [14–16].

The analysis of changes in StO_2 during a brief episode of forearm ischemia enables quantification of the rate of falling-off of microcirculatory oxygen saturation, representing the metabolic status of the underlying tissue [29]. The rate of return of normal microcirculatory saturation is hypothesized to represent microcirculatory reserve [15, 16, 29].

Tissue CO_2 represents the balance between CO_2 production and flow to the tissue [24, 25, 40]. The PCO_2 gap (the difference between tissue and arterial concentration of CO_2) reflects more the adequacy of flow than the presence of tissue hypoxia. TissuePCO_2 can be measured by probes in contact with the tissue, or tonometry [15, 16, 26]. This measurement can detect zones of impaired regional perfusion and/or tissue hypoxia even when total perfusion is preserved but heterogeneous.

A gastric PCO_2 gap above 20 mmHg discriminated survivors from non-survivors in critically-ill patients [30]. However, this technique, although attractive, has some technical problems related to duodeno-gastric reflux and feeding can interfere with PCO_2 measurements [30].

Clinical Consequences of Microcirculatory Dysfunction in AHF

Organ injury or/and failure and impairment are commonly observed in patients with AHF, and the abnormalities in hemodynamic status related to both congestion and hypoperfusion are the essential pathophysiological mechanism of impaired organ function [25].

Microcirculatory dysfunction is the main facilitator of organ failure in both hemodynamic conditions (Fig. 13.4). In fact, degrees of microvascular abnormalities have been correlated with organ dysfunction and mortality in AHF and CS [10, 22].

Additionally, microcirculatory alterations can be already detected in the very early stage of disease, and may persist regardless of macro-hemodynamic status [11].

To note, some studies have reported that microvascular variables predicted more accurately organ dysfunction and mortality than traditional hemodynamic parameters [22].

Heart

Although in AHF, heart and brain perfusion are relatively preserved due to redistribution of cardiac output via compensatory vasoconstriction in other territories, microcirculatory dysfunction is a systemic condition resulting in multi-organ injury/failure [9, 25].

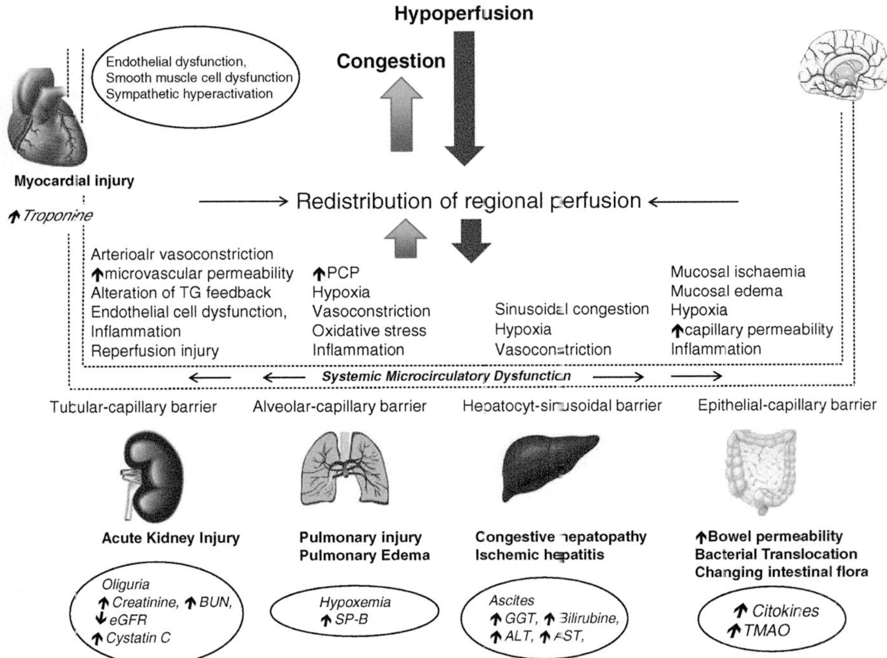

Fig. 13.4 The role of microcirculatory dysfunction in end-organ injury/failure

Even if troponin testing is the biomarker gold standard for the diagnosis of acute myocardial infarction (MI), elevation of troponin may occur in situations other than acute coronary ischemia [31], and elevated serum troponin is common during AHF decompensation [32], and even more, troponin elevation persists long term after discharge [33].

During HF decompensation, prolonged episodes of reduced myocardial perfusion may result in coronary microvascular dysfunction [25].

The mechanisms responsible for microvascular dysfunction include endothelial dysfunction, smooth muscle cell dysfunction, and the dysregulation of sympathetic innervation [31].

Kidney

Kidney injury and renal dysfunction are common in AHF settings being reported in 25–30% of patients [34].

Kidney injury can be detected and quantified using a combination of urine output (oliguria) and blood biomarkers of renal function (e.g. cystatin C, serum creatinine, blood urea nitrogen, GFR, albuminuria) [34].

In AHF, vasoconstriction of afferent artery as result of the redistribution of cardiac output is followed by vasoconstriction of efferent artery, in order to preserve glomerular filtration rate [34].

Because peri-tubular capillaries are derived from the efferent glomerular arterioles, any disturbance of glomerular blood flow will impair peri-tubular perfusion.

Intra-renal microcirculatory dysfunction can be the result of both congestion and hypoperfusion, but the unique microvascular architecture of the kidney, having both series and parallel components, preserves the renal flow if microvascular vasoconstriction or obstruction occurs in certain areas [35].

To note, systemic congestion was a stronger predictor of worsening renal function than cardiac output or mean arterial pressure, suggesting that worsening renal function cannot be predominantly attributed to reduced cardiac output [36].

Elevated central venous pressure may produce microcirculatory dysfunction and worsen renal function through several different mechanisms, including increasing capillary permeability, pressure-induced reduction in renal blood flow via tubule-glomerular feedback activation and renal hypoxia [37].

However, the mechanisms that contribute to peri-tubular capillary dysfunction in AHF are multifactorial, including increased microvascular permeability, endothelialcell dysfunction, inflammation, imbalance between vasodilating and vasoconstricting factors, and reperfusion injury [34, 36, 37].

Gout

The circulatory adaptations that occur in patients with AHF may favour microcirculatory injuries leading to a disruption in the intestinal barrier and change in intestinal bacterial composition, thereby amplifying inflammation [38–40].

Gut barrier function is maintained by well-balanced intestinal flora, an intact mucosa and a normal functioning immune system. If these mechanisms are disrupted, viable bacteria or their degradation products like endotoxin (i.e. lipopolysaccharide-LPS), or bacterial toxic metabolites like trimethylamine N-oxide (TMAO) may cross the gut mucosa and spread to systemic circulation and distant organs [38, 39].

In the intestinal villi, arterioles and venules form a countercurrent microcirculatory system. Therefore, arteriolar oxygen shunts to venules before reaching the villus tip, resulting in the lowest oxygen concentration occurring at the villus tip. In patients with HF, there are microcirculatory disturbances in the gut due to reduced perfusion, increased congestion, and sympathetically mediated vasoconstriction [38].

These hemodynamic alterations lead to exaggerated hypoxia, especially at the villus tip. Both, bowel mucosal ischaemia and mucosal edema cause epithelial cell dysfunction and disruption in intestinal barrier function in turn can lead to increased gut permeability, loss of the barrier function of the intestine, increased bacterial translocation which allows lipopolysaccharide or endotoxin produced by gram-negative gut bacteria to enter the circulatory system [38, 39].

These effects trigger systemic inflammation, cytokine generation [38, 39] and elevated circulating levels of TMAO [40], which further contributes to increasing intestinal capillaries permeability.

In addition, due to the gut microcirculatory dysfunction, mucosa intestinal hypoxia, hypercapnia and changes in local pH, all known to be potent activators of bacterial virulence in microbiota [40], the composition of intestinal microbiota in AHF may shift rapidly amplifying inflammatory cascades [40].

Liver

The basic structural unit of the hepatic microcirculation is the hepatic lobule, in which a terminal hepatic venule (~25 μm) is located at the center, and several portal venules (50 μm) at the periphery, with the hepatic sinusoids (5–8 μm) running from the terminal portal venules to the terminal hepatic venule, forming a hexagonal vascular structure [41]. Sinusoids are small endothelium-lined capillaries in the liver that have open pores, which greatly increase the permeability of the liver [41].

Congestive hepatopathy is the most common cause of liver dysfunction in HF, more common than reduced cardiac output. In HF, elevated central venous pressure is transmitted to the sinusoidal bed without any significant attenuation owing to a lack of hepaticvenous valves [42]. Sinusoidal congestion, resulting in peri-sinusoidal edema, which decreases oxygen diffusion to the hepatocytes [42].

In the setting of venous congestion, cholestasis is observed with elevation of alkaline phosphatase, bilirubin and γ-glutamyltransferase (GGT) [41–42].

Sinusoidal congestion can also cause exudation of protein-rich fluid into the space of Disse. Excess fluid in the space of Disse is usually drained into hepatic lymphatics, but when the lymph formation exceeds the capacity of the lymphatics, high-protein fluid may fooze from the surface of the liver and drain into the peritoneal cavity.

Hypoxic liver injury, or hypoxic hepatitis refers to diffuse hepatic injury from a sudden drop in cardiac output and may be more likely in the presence of hepatic congestion [43].

From a laboratory perspective, ischemic hepatitis is characterized by rapid increases in serum aminotransferases (ALT, AST) and lactatedehydrogenase (LDH). The aminotransferases peak $\approx$1 to 3 days after the hemodynamic insult and return to normal within 7–10 days in the absence of any further hemodynamic insult [43].

Increasing transaminases was a strong risk factor for mortality for the full spectrum of severity of AHF patients [44].

Brain

In contrast to marked reduction in cardiac output and arterial pressures together with reduction sublingual microcirculatory flow, cerebral cortical microcirculation was fully preserved during CS [45].

These findings further document a dissociation between the systemic and cerebral circulations, and potentially explain earlier clinical and experimental observations that the brain is selectively protected during severe states of cardiogenic shock in the absence of cardiac arrest [45].

Hypoxaemia is the primary cause of cerebral dysfunction in AHF, which can manifest as cognitive dysfunction, and delirium [25].

Lungs

Pulmonary congestion is defined as accumulation of fluid in the lungs, as result of high pulmonary capillary hydrostatic pressures which disturb Starling's equilibrium while the alveolar-capillary barrier remains intact [46].

Several experimental models have shown that pressure-induced trauma leads to ultrastructural changes of the blood-gas barrier involving disruption of the pulmonary capillary endothelial layer as well as the alveolar epithelial layer, with acute increase in permeability of microcirculation [46–48].

The result is a progressive transition from a low permeability form to a high permeability form of PE. Lung epithelium–specific proteins, such as surfactant protein-B (SP-B), can leak across the alveolar-capillary barrier into the circulation and may serve as markers of barrier damage in cardiogenic and non-cardiogenic PE [47].

However, even in cardiogenic PE, there is a combination of high hydrostatic pulmonary capillary pressure and high permeability of the alveolar-capillary barrier, resulting in impaired gas exchange and arterial hypoxemia [48].

An inflammation-triggered increase in permeability of the pulmonary microcirculation may play a role in patients who develop PE despite relatively low hydrostatic pressures [48, 49].

Hydrostatic lung injury in the setting of AHF causes acute alveolar inflammation, which maybe a direct response to mechanical stress of the pulmonary microcirculation [48].

Capillary pulmonary endothelium can transduce the mechanical signal into a biological response by inducing several intracellular signaling pathways, which may result in increased inflammatory cytokine production, macrophage activation, acute inflammation, activation of reactive oxygen species and barrier dysfunction [45, 48].

Repetitive or severe decompensations, when elevation of pulmonary capillary pressure is sustained and persistent, may result in "pulmonary remodeling" and alveolar-capillary barrier responds by an exaggerate thickening protecting the lungs to the development of recurrent PE, but causing a significant decrease in alveolar diffusion capacity and gas transfer, pulmonary vasoconstriction and, finally, pulmonary hypertension [48, 49].

Therapies

One important characteristics of microcirculation in AHF, distinct to sepsis, is that microvascular dysfunction in AHF is not completely independent from changes in macro-circulation. Consequently, at least in theory, any attempts to correct hemodynamics should ameliorate microcirculatory dysfunction. However, in CS states, this relationship is disrupted such that microcirculatory organ perfusion may be abnormal despite restitution of seemingly adequate macro-circulatory parameters [9–11].

Of interest, two groups have reported that standard medical treatment alone is successful in restoring microcirculatory flow in decompensated AHF, but not in CS patients [11, 50].

Also, time course of microcirculatory alterations during AHF decompensation is longer than abnormalities in macro-hemodynamics, and tissue perfusion can remain altered even after achievement of within-target cardiac output and arterial pressure. In the later stages of the disease, microcirculatory dysfunction attains a "point of no return", when it is partially or completely decoupled to macro-hemodynamics, and furthermore, the attempts to correct central hemodynamics may aggravate microcirculatory disorders and supplementary trigger the development of multi-organ failure. Evidence is robust that cellular metabolism reduces in multi-organ failure such that supply of oxygen at physiological levels may be, useless or even potentially harmful, as inferred from models of ischaemia– reperfusion injury [51].

Despite of a robust pathophysiological background and significant prognosis association, very few studies have targeted microcirculatory dysfunction in AHF.

To note, there is only one randomized clinical trial investigating the non-selective NO synthase inhibitor tilarginine (L-NG-monomethylarginine) that failed to improve outcomes [52].

Although in AHF, different treatment strategies, including pharmacological interventions and mechanical circulatory support (MCS) devices, may theoretically improve microcirculatory dysfunction, the evidence data are provided by small sample size observational studies on base of "single centre experience".

In one study enrolling 27 patients with ADHF, optimization of standard pharmacological treatment to decrease neurohumoral activation (beta blockers, angiotensin-converting enzyme inhibitors/angiotensin-II-receptor blockers, Spironolactone) significantly improves sublingual microvascular perfusion evaluated by SDF imaging [11].

Interestingly, improvement in microcirculation was associated to decreasing plasma levels of neurohormonal mediators endotheline (ET) and norepinephrine (NE). To note, at the time of discharge, the MFI did not reach the maximum value, which is considered to represent microcirculation in healthy subjects without cardiovascular disease. This may be due to incomplete recovery at this time point, which is also reflected by the elevated plasma BNP levels observed at discharge. This is an important finding, linking residual hemodynamic congestion reflected by high value of BNP [53], to persistent microcirculatory dysfunction.

Similar results were provided by other study, where IV and oral therapies given in ED, promptly improved microcirculation in a cohort of 36 patients with ADHF [50].

Two other studies specifically investigated the effect of NTG in patients with AHF without hypotension or signs of hypoperfusion, and demonstrated that the NO donor NTG can increase the number of patent capillaries in patients admitted for AHF [54, 55].

First study investigated whether low-dose nitroglycerin (NTG) improves microcirculatory perfusion in 20 patients admitted for AHF [54]. Sublingual microcirculation has been evaluated by SDF imaging at baseline, 15 min after initiation of NTG, and after NTG had been stopped for 20 min.

After the administration of low-dose, intravenous NTG at a fixed dose of 33 mg/min, a significant increase in perfused capillary density (PCD) was reported in 14 patients, and the improvement in microcirculation was reversed after the discontinuation of NTG [54].

The patients who did not respond had a smaller decrease in central venous pressure (CVP) after NTG, suggesting vascular resistance to NTG or less venodilation than responders due to an insufficient dose of NTG.

To explore the maximum response of the microcirculation to NTG, a dose-response study investigated association between titration of NTG doses and changes of microcirculation in 17 patients with severe AHF [55]. The investigators reported a gradual and consistent increase of tissue perfusion by titration of NTG [55].

NTG dose-dependently improves tissue perfusion, as demonstrated by a gradual decrease in temperature gradient and a progressive increase in perfused capillary density in patients with AHF. Improvement in microcirculation (delta PCD) occurred earlier, at a lower dose of NTG, than did changes in global hemodynamics (CVP). In addition, these changes occurred independently of changes in cardiac index. These findings underline the great value of monitoring microcirculation in critically ill patients. Demonstrating the feasibility of serial monitoring of the microcirculation. Whether monitoring of tissue microcirculation optimizes current treatment strategies in patients with severe HF, and whether such a strategy will favorably affect outcome, warrants further investigation.

Inotropic therapy is often considered in patients with CS to improve the hemodynamic status, but short-term and long-term safety concerns have been reported regarding their use [56], and notably, the utility of inotropic therapy in restoring end-organ perfusion in patients with CS is based primarily on clinical experience rather than clinical trial data [57].

Also, global hemodynamic parameters, such as mean arterial blood pressure do not reflect differential patterns of regional organ blood flow or compromised tissue perfusion associated with shock states [9].

First clinical experiences with the effect of inotropic agents on microcirculation were reported in septic shock patients [57]. Dobutamine may recruit a poorly perfused microcirculation independent of its haemodynamic effects [57], but this outcome has not been reproduced in a randomized control trial [58].

In a study enrolling 30 patients with CS, microcirculation was improved by enoximone, but not by dobutamine or norepinephrine [59]. Dobutamine decreased central-to-peripheral temperature gradient but no increased the number of sublingual patent capillaries [59].

A positive signal came from the inodilatatory agent, levosimendan, recruiting the microcirculation in CS [60].

Although vasopressors might be able to stabilize the mean arterial pressure, their use has been associated to a direct cytotoxic effect, and negative consequences for tissue viability [59].

In AHF, the effects of norepinephrine on tissue perfusion are largely unknown. In one study, norepinephrine significantly decreased sublingual PCD, whereas cardiac index remained constant and SvO_2 increased [59].

These findings also suggest development of microcirculatory shunting induced by norepinephrine in patients with CS.

Mechanical circulatory support (MCS) devices can be used to maintain organ perfusion in patients with CS and decompensated chronic HF [6–8].

However, correction of global hemodynamic parameters by MCS do not always cause a parallel improvement in microcirculatory perfusion and oxygenation of the organ systems, a condition referred to as a loss of hemodynamic coherence between macro- and microcirculation [8–12].

The improvement of macro-hemodynamics following MCS implant may be only a measure of technical success of MCS, and without limiting the progression of MODS within the first few days, these hemodynamic improvements may be futile and may not translate into improved survival [6, 7, 61].

Most of the studies suggest that preventing or limiting progression of microcirculatory dysfunction by MCS devices is a key factor responsible for improvement of outcome in patients with CS, and preservation of microcirculation with adequate tissue perfusion rather than maintenance of more normal arterial pressure is a crucial determinant of outcome [22].

The achievement of hemodynamic coherence between the micro- and the macrocirculation must be considered as a success of MCS since these devices target mainly the support of the systemic circulation and organ perfusion [62].

Current literature in monitoring tissue perfusion in patients with MCSs is very heterogenic due to the variety of monitoring techniques, type of MCS, time frame of monitoring and type of the study. However, majority of the studies concerning the microcirculation were performed with SDF imaging.

Intra Aortic Baloon Pump (IABP)

To date, the most rigorously studied device is the IABP, which failed to demonstrate benefit in the IABP-SHOCK II (Intra-Aortic Balloon Pump in Cardiogenic Shock II) trial [63, 64]. Also, other recent meta-analysis [65] have also suggested limited utility of IABP therapy in CS. The 2017 ESC STEMI guidelines [66] gave IIIB recommendation for the routine use of the IABP in CS, and consider IABP only in patients with mechanical complications post AMI (class IIa, level C).

In two small studies [67, 68], circulatory support with IABP increases microcirculatory flow in the smallest vessels of the sublingual mucosa.

In another study, although parameters of the microcirculation might be helpful to identify high-risk patients, there is no effect of IABP treatment on microvascular perfusion in patients with CS [69].

Distinct to the previous studies, monitoring microcirculation during and after withdrawal of IABP, SDF imaging showed an increase of microcirculatory flow of small vessels after withdrawal of IABP therapy [70]. This study seems to suggest that longer support using IABP may impair microvascular perfusion.

To conclude, understanding of improved microvascular perfusion in response to IABP-support is still based on limited and conflicting data, even though the same technique for microcirculatory measurements were used.

Impella

Microcirculation assessed by SDF improved in CS STEMI patients treated with the Impella 2.5 to levels observed in healthy persons and remained suboptimal after 72 h inpatients without support [71].

Restoration of the microcirculation, monitored by sublingual SDF imaging, was already observed after 24 h of circulatory support in hemodynamically compromised patients, simultaneous to the correction of systemic hemodynamics through the Impella LP2.5 [71].

Moreover, not only an increase in the microcirculatory flow did occur, but also this effect remained up to 72 h of support. This was the first study describing a positive relationship between macro-circulation and improvement in sublingual microcirculation, paralleling the left ventricular function improvement after STEMI [71].

V-A ECMO

VA-ECMO is increasingly being used following CS to support the cardiovascular system temporarily as a bridge to recovery, transplantation or bridge to durable LVAD [72]. This flow support, results in a significant increase in blood pressure and strongly improves end-organs perfusion [72].

Monitoring microcirculatory parameters (PVD) in 24 CS patients treated with VA-ECMO, has showed a significant difference in the microcirculatory parameters at all time points between the survivors and non-survivors [73].

Furthermore, PVD of the sublingual microcirculation at initiation of VA-ECMO can be used to predict ICU mortalityin patients with cardiogenic shock (Table 13.2).

In other study, microcirculatory dysfunction was more severe in 28-day non-survivors than in survivors with VA-ECMO support, and this study revealed that the PVD in the following 12 h after initiation of ECMO could be used to predict the survival [74]. To note, sublingual PVD at 12 h post ECMO initiation, was significantly lower in non-survivors compared with survivors, even if mean arterial pressure, inotropic score, and lactate level at 12 h did not differ significantly between the two groups [74].

Although there is a massive return of circulation via VA-ECMO, the exposure of a patient's blood to the non-endothelialised surface of the ECMO circuit, results in the widespread activation of the innate immune system and reperfusion damage, that may result in inflammation, microcirculatory dysfunction and organ injury [75].

This may explain even though indexes of microcirculatory dysfunction did improve as result of VA-ECMO, these did not return toward the values observed in healthy subjects [72, 73].

Timing of weaning following "normalization" of the cardiovascular system from any MCS device, in particular VA-ECMO, is an important goal in the management of MCS. Too early or too late weaning can cause treatment failure and various complications. Conventionally hemodynamic and echocardiographic parameters are used to wean from ECMO, but few studies have evaluated outcome predictors following ECMO [76].

In a recent study, successful weaning was associated with sustained improvement of sublingual microcirculatory function during ECMO flow reduction [77].

Sustained values of single-spot measurements of perfused vessel density during 50% flow reduction of ECMO were found to be more specific and more sensitive indicators of successful weaning from VA-ECMO as compared to echocardiographic parameters [77], suggesting that weaning from VA-ECMO could be performed by imaging of the microcirculation.

LVAD

In one of the first studies, showed that pulsatile unloading of the heart by LVAD resulted in increased microvascular density [78].

Microvascular function was assessed in the forearm during reactive hyperemia using laser Doppler perfusion imaging and pulsed wave Doppler [78].

Improvements in microvascular perfusion was reported also after implantation of a continuous flow LVAD [79].

However, destruction of blood cells may contribute to residual endothelial dysfunction potentially by increasing NO scavenging capacity. In addition, the lower pulsatility and associated changes in shear stress, due to the continuous-flow mechanical support may explain reduced microcirculatory functional reserve, despite of the central hemodynamic improvements afforded by a continuous flow LVAD [80].

Further studies investigating whether treatment strategies that improve sublingual microcirculation are effective in improving survival of CS patients are needed.

Future Research

Direct monitoring of the microcirculation by using currently available techniques, in conjunction with global hemodynamic data can be expected to help in the understanding of the pathophysiological role of microcirculatory dysfunction during AHF decompensation. Furthermore, the integration of microcirculatory data in risk stratification model can help to identify "at risk" patients, even in the absence of macro-hemodynamic abnormalities. However, further clinical research will be needed to evaluate if including microcirculatory dysfunction in the risk stratification of patients with AHF could improve clinical outcome and resources allocation.

The vast majority of scientific evidences regarding the role of microcirculatory alterations in pathophysiology of AHF patients, are provided by single centre experiences with a small sample, using a non-randomized design. In addition, patients with acute heart failure may present with distinct clinical condition, varying from hypertensive heart failure to cardiogenic shock, and whether the severity of microcirculatory alterations and the response to therapy differs among these clinical conditions need to be further investigated. To investigate this more comprehensively, more robust, preferably randomized controlled trials of well defined patient categories will be needed. Also, the relationship between microcirculatory dysfunction and mortality, should be prospectively validated in larger studies.

Understanding the time-course of microcirculatory abnormalities during CS may assist to guide the therapies, and could possibly help in identifying the optimal moment for MCS implant, timing of MCS weaning or bridging these patients towards a durable LVAD's or cardiac transplantation.

Clinical Case

A 68 year-old male presented in ED for prolonged chest pain and shortness of breath. Onset of pain was 4 h before admission with crescendo intensity.

Vital signs collected in ED showed: SBP = 80 mmHg, HR = 100/min, Respiratory rate = 28/min, T = 36.8 °C and peripheral O^2 saturation of 92%. Clinical examination focused on cardiovascular system revealed systolic murmur of mitral regurgitation 4/6 and S3 sound, pulmonary rales on both pulmonary fields, cold extremities and altered mental status.

No relevant medical history has been found for the patient, except a previous diagnosis of hypercholesterolemia and a recent Echocardiography documenting a moderate mitral regurgitation (MR).

ECG showed sinus rhythm (96/min) elevation of J point and ST elevation in V1–V5, with maximum of 8 mm in V2 (Fig. 13.5a) findings suggesting of anterior wall ST elevation myocardial infarction. Panel of biomarkers, available in 15 min since presentation, shows NT-pro-BNP = 3400 pg/ml, Hs-Troponin I = 885 ng/l and venous lactate of 5.2 mmol/l. Focus Echocardiography revealed LV global akinesia

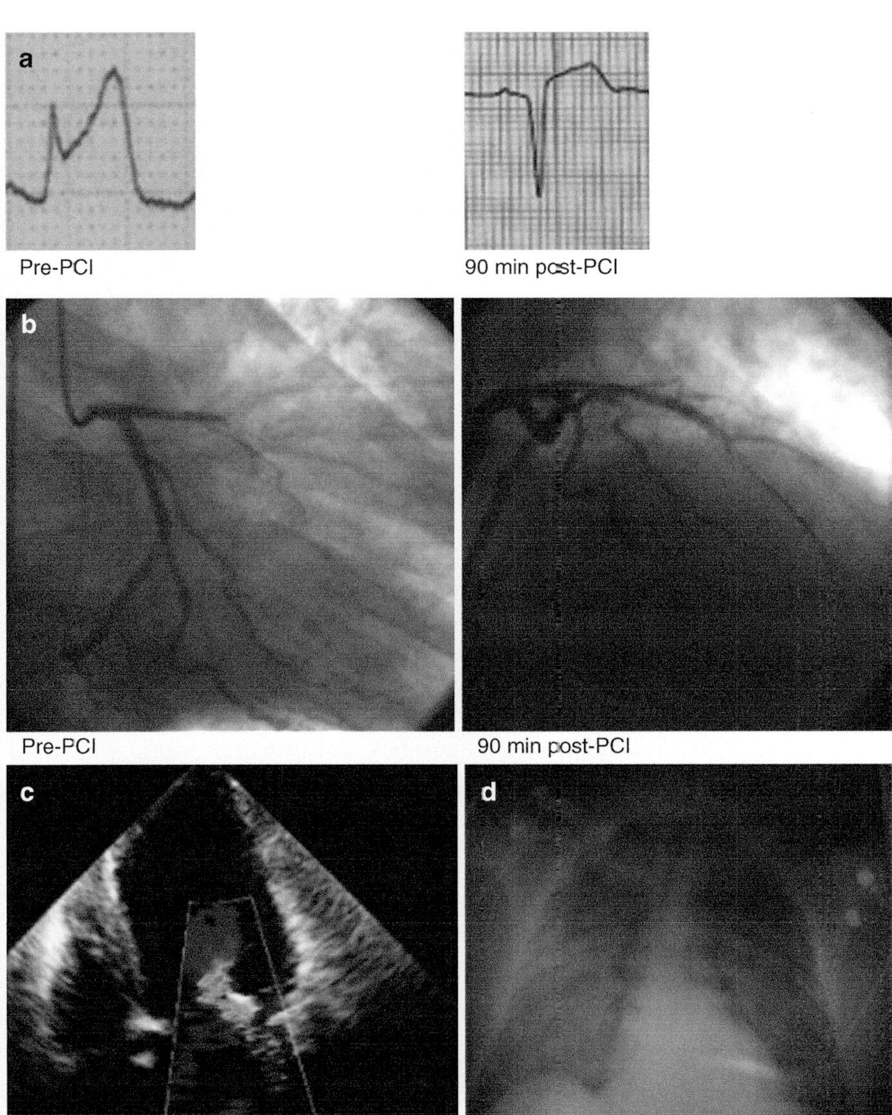

Fig. 13.5 (**a**) ST elevation in V3 lead before and after 90 min post PCI; (**b**) Coronary angiography before and after stenting (arrow shows the site of LAD occlusion); (**c**) Echocardiography showing dilated LV, apical akinesia, severe mitral regurgitation. (**d**) Chest X-ray showing moderate cardiomegaly, redistribution with upper vessel enlargement, perihilar haze, and bilateral pulmonary infiltrates

with severe MR, preserved RV function and did not detect other alternative causes of myocardial ischemia.

At this moment the diagnosis was anterior STEMI Killip IV class, and a loading dose of 180 mg Ticagrelor and 325 mg Aspirin were given to the patient.

We decided to activate the Heart Team for Cardiogenic Shock (CS) and to transfer the patient to Cath Lab. Due to hypoxia (SaO_2 = 92% under 4 L Oxygen flow) and high respiratory rate (30/min), and in the context of low SBP (75–80 mmHg), we considered first of all mechanical ventilation via IOT concomitant with administration of Dobutamine 5 mcg/kg/min. Furthermore, because of persistent low SBP, Heart Team decision was to implant a short-term mechanical circulatory support before coronary intervention, and only available option in that moment was Intra-Aortic Balloon Pump (IABP). Coronary angiography revealed occlusion of the first segment of LAD and interventionist performed direct stenting on culprit lesion with TIMI 3 flow (Fig. 13.5b). After angioplasty, the patient is transferred in Intensive care Unit (ICU) with IABP support 1:1 and mechanical ventilation. ECG performed at 90 min post angioplasty revealed resolution with more than 50% of ST elevation in V2 (Fig. 13.5a). BP was 85/45 mmHg and urinary output (via bladder catheter) was 30 ml/h. In ICU, information provided by Echocardiography confirmed severe MR, with LVEF 25% and good RV function (Fig. 13.5c). Blood lactate was 5.8 mmol/l and the result of other blood sample collected in ED showed Hemoglobin = 12.9 g/dl, WBC = 12,400/mm^3, CK-MB = 76 serum creatinine = 1.9 mg/dl, ALT = 45UI/L, AST = 58UI/L, GGT = 71UI/L. A Swann-Ganz catheter was inserted and this option was determined by the need to adequately monitor hemodynamic parameters in a STEMI with IABP and persistent hypoperfusion secondary to CS. Invasive hemodynamic data showed Cardiac Index (CI) = 1.7 l/min/m^2, Pulmonary Capillary Wedge Pressure (PCWP) = 24 mmHg, Systemic Vascular Resistances (SVR = 21 Wood units) and Central Venous Pressure (CVP) = 14 mmHg (Fig. 13.6). IV vaso-active treatment included Dobutamine 7 mcg/kg/min and Furosemide 4 mg/h and it was continued for the next 18 h.

Chest X-ray detected moderate cardiomegaly, redistribution with upper vessel enlargement, perihilar haze, and bilateral pulmonary infiltrates (Fig. 13.5d).

In the day 2 in ICU, hemodynamic data showed increased of CI, but a substantial decrease in SVR (10 Wood units). This finding, in conjunction with worsening of multi-organ injury and radiological findings were supportive for the occurrence of Systemic Inflammatory Syndrome (SIRS) and dictated initiation of IV vasoconstrictor Norepinephrine at doses of 0.3 and then 0.5 mcg/kg/min. In the day 3, SBP was constantly higher than 95 mmHg with urinary output of 100 ml/h, CI increased at 2.4 l/min/m^2 and PCWP ranged between 15 and 17 mmHg (Fig. 13.6). Furthermore, blood lactate decreased at 2.2 mmol/l. TTE reported decreasing severity of MR. Dobutamine dose decreased at 5 mcg/kg/min. However, despite of the improving of the hemodynamics and of the global metabolic deficit, multi-organ injury remains persistent. During day 4, SBP and urinary output increased comparative with previous days and SVR increased toward normal value (1–14 Wood units) (Fig. 13.6). Blood lactate was 1.7 mmol/l. Norepinephrine dose was decreased and then stopped while

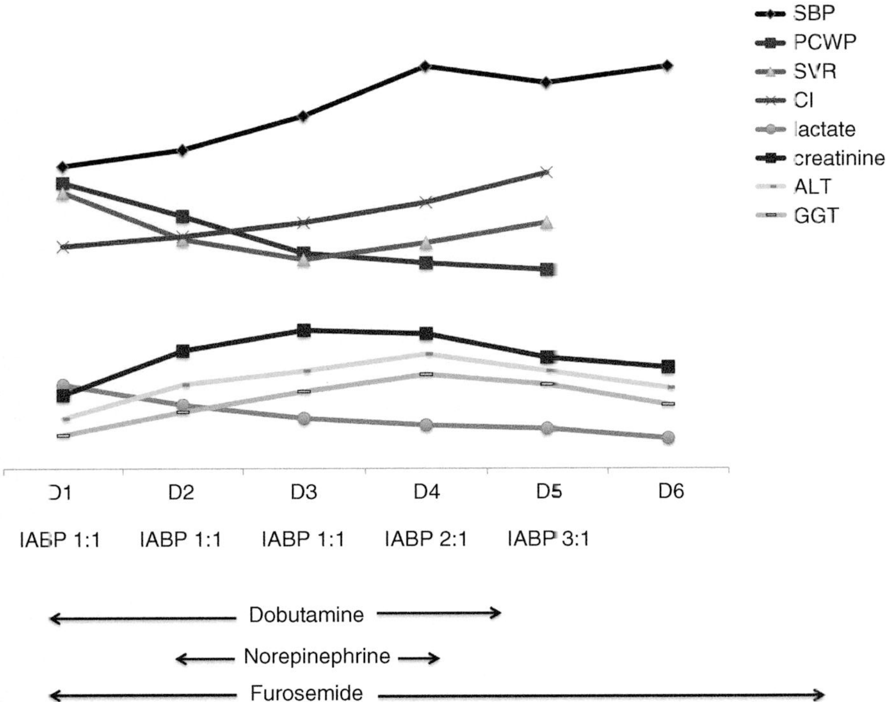

Fig. 13.6 Time course of the hemodynamic abnormalities and markers of organ dysfunction during the first 6 days of hospitalization. *ALT* alanine amin-transferaza, *CI* cardiac index, *GGT* gama glutamil transpeptidaza, *IABP* Intra-Aortic Baloon Pump, *PCWP* pulmonary capillary wedge pressure, *SVR* systemic vascular resistance

Dobutamine dose has remained unchanged. Even if multi-organ injury continued to evolve, IABP assistance was switched from 1:1 to 2:1, without significant variations in SBP and without decrease of sub-aortic velocity time integral (VTI) at Echo. In the day 5, clinical examination reported no evident clinical signs of hypoperfusion and only mild congestion (basal pulmonary rales). All hemodynamic parameters have entered in normal range and to note, markers of organ dysfunction improved. IABP was switched at 3:1 during the next 6 h and then stopped. Dobutamine dose decreased at 2 mcg/kg/min. In the day six patient was transferred in Cardiology Unit. In Cardiology, the patient has been monitored clinically, ECG and biologic. Echocardiography demonstrated a substantial improvement in global contractility with EF = 35–37% and MR remained moderate. The markers of organ injury further decreased during hospitalization, but without attaining the normal values. The therapies with ACE-inhibitors and beta-blocker was initiated as soon as the patient became stable.

The patient was discharged in day 13 without signs of residual congestion and with a very good mobility. The patient and family have been instructed for effort and dietetic regimen, and a follow up visit at 2 weeks post discharge has been planned.

Comments

The clinical case is very illustrative for the in-hospital course of post MI-CS associated with SIRS and multi-organ injury (kidney, liver and lung). Multi-organ injury is the consequence of the various degree of microvascular abnormalities, and actually microcirculatory dysfunction is the main facilitator of organ injury/failure in CS.

In this case, the time course of microcirculatory alterations during hospitalization was longer than abnormalities in macro-hemodynamics, and tissue perfusion remained altered even after achievement of within-target cardiac index and SBP. In D3, D4 and D5 was a disconnection between improving in hemodynamic measurements and markers of organ injury.

Notably, although in this case revascularization has been associated to re-establishing of coronary microcirculatory perfusion, suggested by TIMI 3 flow and a >50% resolution of ST elevation, recovery of LV function is a long term process, unable to prevent early occurrence of multi-organ injury. In addition, the microcirculatory dysfunction initiated by systemic hypoperfusion to other organs may evolve independent of central hemodynamics.

Mechanical circulatory support (MCS) device has been used to reverse hemodynamic abnormalities and to maintain organ perfusion. Despite of the recent evidences showing limited outcome benefit, IABP remained the most utilized MCS. IABP has shown to improve coronary blood flow by augmenting coronary diastolic blood pressure and increasing cardiac index by reducing left ventricular afterload. These effects have been proved very useful in a patient with large anterior MI, where a substantial area of stunning may be responsible of persistent LV dysfunction despite of prompt revascularization, and furthermore in conditions of severe MR, potentially improved by decreasing afterload.

However, correction of global hemodynamic parameters by IABP did not cause a parallel improvement in microcirculatory perfusion and oxygenation of the organ systems, a condition referred to as a loss of hemodynamic coherence between macro- and microcirculation.

Beyond of technical success, reflected by improvement of macro-hemodynamics, preventing or limiting progression of microcirculatory dysfunction by MCS devices is a key factor responsible for improvement of outcome in patients with CS, and preservation of microcirculation with adequate tissue perfusion rather than maintenance of more normal arterial pressure is the crucial determinant of outcome.

References

1. Ponikowski P, Voors AA, Anker SD, et al. 2016 ESC Guidelines for the diagnosis and treatment of acute and chronic heart failure: The Task Force for the diagnosis and treatment of acute and chronic heart failure of the European Society of Cardiology (ESC). Developed with the special contribution of the Heart Failure Association (HFA) of the ESC. Eur Heart J. 2016;37(27):2129–200.

2. Maggioni AP, Dahlstrom U, Filippatos G, et al. EURObservational Research Programme: the Heart Failure Pilot Survey (ESC-HF Pilot). Eur J Heart Fail. 2010;12(10):1076–84.
3. Chioncel O, Vinereanu D, Datcu M, et al. The Romanian Acute Heart Failure Syndromes (RO-AHFS) registry. Am Heart J. 2011;162(1):142–53 e1.
4. Chioncel O, Mebazaa A, Harjola VP, et al. Clinical phenotypes and outcome of patients hospitalized for acute heart failure: the ESC Heart Failure Long-Term Registry. Eur J Heart Fail. 2017;19(10):1242–54.
5. Hamo CE, Butler J, Gheorghiade M, Chioncel O. The bumpy road to drug development for acute heart failure. Eur Heart J Suppl. 2016;18(suppl G):G19–32.
6. Chioncel O, Collins SP, Ambrosy AP, Pang PS, Radu IR, Antohi EA, Masip J, Butler J and Iliescu VA. Therapeutic Advances in the Management of Cardiogenic Shock. Am J Ther. 2019;26(2):e234–47.
7. Thiele H, Ohman EM, Desch S, et al. Management of cardiogenic shock. Eur Heart J. 2015;36(20):1223–30.
8. van Diepen S, Katz JN, Albert NM, et al. Contemporary management of cardiogenic shock: a scientific statement from the American Heart Association. Circulation. 2017;136(16): e232–e68.
9. den Uil CA, Klijn E, Lagrand WK, Brugts JJ, Ince C, Spronk PE, Simons ML. The microcirculation in health and critical disease. Prog Cardiovasc Dis. 2008;51(2):161–70.
10. De Backer D, Creteur J, Dubois MJ, Sakr Y, Vincent JL. Microvascular alterations in patients with acute severe heart failure and cardiogenic shock. Am Heart J. 2004;147(1):91–9.
11. Lauten A, Ferrari M, Goebel B, Rademacher W, Schumm J, Uth O, Kiehntopf M, Figulla HR, Jung C. Microvascular tissue perfusion is impaired in acutely decompensated heart failure and improves following standard treatment. Eur J Heart Fail. 2011;13:711–7.
12. Lim N, Dubois MJ, De Backer D, et al. Do all non survivors of cardiogenic shock die with a low cardiac index? Chest. 2003;124(5):1885–91.
13. Pries AR, Secomb TW, Gaehtgens P. The endothelial surface layer. Pflugers Arch. 2000;440(5):653–66.
14. Salgado DR, Favory R, De Backer D. Microcirculatory assessment in daily clinical practice – not yet ready but not too far! Einstein. 2010;8(1):107–16.
15. Moore JPR, Dyson A, Singer M, Fraser J. Microcirculatory dysfunction and resuscitation: why, when, and how. Br J Anaesth. 2015;115(3):366–75.
16. De Backer D, Ospina-Tascon G, Salgado D, Favory R, Creteur J, Vincent JL. Monitoring the microcirculation in the critically ill patient: current methods and future approaches. Intensive Care Med. 2010;36:1813–25.
17. Hainsworth R. Vascular capacitance: its control and importance. Rev Physiol Biochem Pharmacol. 1986;105:101–73.
18. Vallet B. Endothelial cell dysfunction and abnormal tissue perfusion. Crit Care Med. 2002;30:S229–34.
19. Daly CJ, McGrath JC. Previously unsuspected widespread cellular and tissue distribution of β-adrenoceptors and its relevance to drug action. Trends Pharmacol Sci. 2011;32:219–26.
20. De Backer D, Donadello K, Taccone FS, Ospina-Tascon G, Salgado D, Vincent JL. Microcirculatory alterations: potential mechanisms and implications for therapy. Ann Intensive Care. 2011;1:27.
21. Jung C, Ferrari M, Roediger C, Fritzenwanger M, Goebel B, Lauten A, Pfeifer R, Figulla HR. Evaluation of the sublingual microcirculation in cardiogenic shock. Clin Hemorheol Microcirc. 2009;42:141–8.
22. den Uil CA, Lagrand WK, van der Ent M, Jewbali LS, Cheng JM, Spronk PE, Simoons ML. Impaired microcirculation predicts poor outcome of patients with acute myocardial infarction complicated by cardiogenic shock. Eur Heart J. 2010;31(24):3032–9.
23. Kirschenbaum LA, Astiz ME, Rackow EC, Saha DC Lin R. Microvascular response in patients with cardiogenic shock. Crit Care Med. 2000;28:1290–4.

24. Katz SD, Khan T, Zeballos GA, et al. Decreased activity of the L -arginine–nitric oxide metabolic pathway in patients with congestive heart failure. Circulation. 1999;99:2113–7.
25. Harjola VP, Mullens W, Banaszewski M, Bauersachs J, Brunner-La Rocca HP, Chioncel O, Collins SP, Doehner W, Filippatos GS, Flammer AJ, Fuhrmann V, Lainscak M, Lassus J, Legrand M, Masip J, Mueller C, Papp Z, Parissis J, Platz E, Rudiger A, Ruschitzka F, Schäfer A, Seferovic PM, Skouri H, Yilmaz M, Mebazaa A. Organ dysfunction, injury and failure in acute heart failure: from pathophysiology to diagnosis and management. A review on behalf of the Acute Heart Failure Committee of the Heart Failure Association (HFA) of the European Society of Cardiology (ESC). Eur J Heart Fail. 2017;19(7):821–36.
26. de Backer D, Hollenberg S, Boerma C, et al. How to evaluate the microcirculation: report of a round table conference. Crit Care. 2007;11:R101.
27. Donati A, Domizi R, Damiani E, Adrario E, Pelaia P, Ince C. From macrohemodynamic to the microcirculation. Crit Care Res Prac. 2013;2013:892710.
28. Gilbert-Kawai E, Coppel J, Bountziouka V, Ince C, Martin D, Caudwell Xtreme Everest and Xtreme Everest 2 Research Groups. A comparison of the quality of image acquisition between the incident dark field and side stream dark field video-microscopes. BMC Med Imaging. 2016;16(1):10.
29. Gomez H, Torres A, Polanco P, Kim HK, Zenker S, Puyana JC, Pinsky MR. Use of non-invasive NIRS during a vascular occlusion test to assess dynamic tissue O2 saturation response. Intensive Care Med. 2008;34:1600–7.
30. Levy B, Gawalkiewicz P, Vallet B, Briancon S, Nace L, Bollaert PE. Gastric capnometry with air automated tonometry predicts outcome in critically ill patients. Crit Care Med. 2003;31:474–80.
31. Thygesen K, Alpert JS, Jaffe AS, Chaitman BR, Bax JJ, Morrow DA, White HD, ESC Scientific Document Group. Fourth universal definition of myocardial infarction (2018). Circulation. 2018;138:e618–51.
32. Xue Y, Clopton P, Peacock WF, Maisel AS. Serial changes in high-sensitive troponin I predict outcome in patients with decompensated heart failure. Eur J Heart Fail. 2011;13:37–42.
33. Greene SJ, Butler J, Fonarow GC, Subacius HP, Ambrosy AP, Vaduganathan M, Triggiani M, Solomon SD, Lewis EF, Maggioni AP, Böhm M, Chioncel O, Nodari S, Senni M, Zannad F, Gheorghiade M. Pre-discharge and early post-discharge troponin elevation among patients hospitalized for heart failure with reduced ejection fraction: findings from the ASTRONAUT trial. Eur J Heart Fail. 2018;20(2):281–91.
34. Damman K, Valente MA, Voors AA, O'Connor CM, van Veldhuisen DJ, Hillege HL. Renal impairment, worsening renal function, and outcome in patients with heart failure: an updated meta-analysis. Eur Heart J. 2014;35:455–69.
35. Lemley KV, Kriz W. Anatomy of the renal interstitium. Kidney Int. 1991;39:370–81.
36. Mullens W, Abrahams Z, Francis GS, Sokos G, Taylor DO, Starling RC, Young JB, Tang WH. Importance of venous congestion for worsening of renal function in advanced decompensated heart failure. J Am Coll Cardiol. 2009;53:589–96.
37. Legrand M, Mebazaa A, Ronco C, Januzzi JL Jr. When cardiac failure, kidney dysfunction, and kidney injury intersect in acute conditions: the case of cardiorenal syndrome. Crit Care Med. 2014;42:2109–17.
38. Verbrugge FH, Dupont M, Steels P, et al. Abdominal contributions to cardiorenal dysfunction in congestive heart failure. J Am Coll Cardiol. 2013;62:485–95.
39. Nagatomo Y, Wilson Tang WH. Intersections between microbiome and heart failure: revisiting the gut hypothesis. J Card Fail. 2015;21(12):973–80.
40. Chioncel O, Ambrosy AP. Trimethylamine N-oxide and risk of heart failure progression: marker or mediator of disease. Eur J Heart Fail. 2019;21(7):887–90.
41. Sundaram V, Fang JC. Gastrointestinal and liver issues in heart failure. Circulation. 2016;133:1696–703.
42. van Deursen VM, Damman K, Hillege HL, van Beek AP, van Veldhuisen DJ, Voors AA. Abnormal liver function in relation to hemodynamic profile in heart failure patients. J Card Fail. 2010;16:84–90.

43. Fuhrmann V, Kneidinger N, Herkner H, Heinz G, Nikfardjam M, Bojic A, Schellongowski P, Angermayr B, Kitzberger R, Warszawska J, Holzinger U Schenk P, Madl C. Hypoxic hepatitis: underlying conditions and risk factors for mortality in critically ill patients. Intensive Care Med. 2009;35:1397–405.
44. Ambrosy AP, Gheorghiade M, Bubenek S, Vinereanu D, Vaduganathan M, Macarie C, Chioncel O, Romanian Acute Heart Failure Syndromes (RO-AHFS) study investigators. The predictive value of transaminases at admission in patients hospitalized for heart failure: findings from the RO-AHFS registry. Eur Heart J Acute Cardiovasc Care. 2013;2(2):99–108.
45. Wan Z, Ristagno G, Sun S, Li Y, Weil MH, Tang W. Preserved cerebral microcirculation during cardiogenic shock. Crit Care Med. 2009;37(8):2333–7.
46. Chioncel O, Collins SP, Ambrosy AP, Gheorghiade M, Filippatos G. Pulmonary Oedema-therapeutic targets. Card Fail Rev. 2015;1(1):38–45.
47. Hermans C, Bernard A. Lung epithelium-specific proteins: characteristics and potential applications as markers. Am J Respir Crit Care Med. 1999;159:646–78.
48. Pappas L, Filippatos G. Pulmonary congestion in acute heart failure: from hemodynamics to lung injury and barrier dysfunction. Rev Esp Cardiol. 2011;64(9):735–8.
49. Parissis JT, Venetsanou KF, Mentzikof DG, Ziras NG, Kefalas CG, Karas SM. Tumor necrosis factor-alpha serum activity during treatment of acute decompensation of cachectic and non-cachectic patients with advanced congestive heart failure. Scand Cardiovasc J. 1999;33:344–50.
50. Hogan CJ, Ward KR, Franzen DS, Rajendran B, Thacker LR. Sublingual tissue perfusion improves during emergency treatment of acute decompensated heart failure. Am J Emerg Med. 2012;30:872–80.
51. Singer M, De Santis V, Vitale D, Jeffcoate W. Multiorgan failure is an adaptive, endocrine-mediated, metabolic response to overwhelming systemic inflammation. Lancet. 2004;364:545–8.
52. TRIUMPH Investigators, Alexander JH, Reynolds HR, Stebbins AL, Dzavik V, Harrington RA, Van de Werf F, Hochman JS. Effect of tilarginine acetate in patients with acute myocardial infarction and cardiogenic shock: the TRIUMPH randomized controlled trial. JAMA. 2007;297:1657–66.
53. Chioncel O, Collins SP, Greene SJ, Ambrosy AP, Vaduganathan M, Macarie C, Butler J, Gheorghiade M. Natriuretic peptide-guided management in heart failure. J Cardiovasc Med (Hagerstown). 2016;17(8):556–68.
54. den Uil CA, Lagrand WK, Spronk PE, van der Ent M, Jewbali LS, Brugts JJ, Ince C, Simoons ML. Low-dose nitroglycerin improves microcirculation in hospitalized patients with acute heart failure. Eur J Heart Fail. 2009;11:386–90.
55. den Uil CA, Caliskan K, Lagrand WK, van der Ent M, Jewbali LSD, van Kuijk JP, Spronk PE, Simoons ML. Dose-dependent benefit of nitroglycerin on microcirculation of patients with severe heart failure. Intensive Care Med. 2009;35:1893–9.
56. Mebazaa A, Motiejunaite J, Gayat E, Crespo-Leiro MG, Lund LH, Maggioni AP, Chioncel O, Akiyama E, Harjola VP, Seferovic P, Laroche C, Julve MS, Roig E, Ruschitzka F, Filippatos G, ESC Heart Failure Long-Term Registry Investigators. Long-term safety of intravenous cardiovascular agents in acute heart failure: results from the European Society of Cardiology Heart Failure Long-Term Registry. Eur J Heart Fail. 2018;20(2):332–41.
57. De Backer D, Creteur J, Dubois MJ, et al. The effects of dobutamine on microcirculatory alterations in patients with septic shock are independent of its systemic effects. Crit Care Med. 2006;34:403–8.
58. Hernandez G, Bruhn A, Luengo C, Regueira T, Kattan E, Fuentealba A, Florez J, Castro R, Aquevedo A, Pairumani R, McNab P, Ince C. Effects of dobutamine on systemic, regionalvand microcirculatory perfusion parametersvin septic shock: a randomized, placebo v controlled, v double-blind, crossover study. Intensive Care Med. 2013;39:1435–43.
59. den Uil CA, Lagrand WK, van der Ent M, Nieman K, Struijs A, Jewbali LS, Constantinescu AA, Spronk PE, Simoons ML. Conventional hemodynamic resuscitation may fail to optimize tissue perfusion: an observational study on the effects of dobutamine, enoximone, and norepinephrine in patients with acute myocardial infarction complicated by cardiogenic shock. PLoS One. 2014;9(8):e103978.

60. Wimmer R. Effects of levosimendan onmicrocirculation in patients with cardiogenic shock. Circulation. 2008;118:s664–5.
61. Werdan K, Gielen S, Ebelt H, et al. Mechanical circulatory support in cardiogenic shock. Eur Heart J. 2014;35(3):156–67.
62. Ince C. Hemodynamic coherence and the rationale for monitoring the microcirculation. Crit Care. 2015;19(Suppl 3):S8.
63. Thiele H, Zeymer U, Neumann FJ, et al. Intra-aortic balloon counterpulsation in acute myocardial infarction complicated by cardiogenic shock (IABP-SHOCK II): final 12 month results of a randomised, open-label trial. Lancet. 2013;382(9905):1638–45.
64. Thiele H, Zeymer U, Neumann FJ, et al. Intraaortic balloon support for myocardial infarction with cardiogenic shock. N Engl J Med. 2012;367(14):1287–96.
65. Zheng XY, Wang Y, Chen Y, et al. The effectiveness of intra-aortic balloon pump for myocardial infarction in patients with or without cardiogenic shock: a meta-analysis and systematic review. BMC Cardiovasc Disord. 2016;16(1):148.
66. Ibanez B, James S, Agewall S, et al. 2017 ESC guidelines for the management of acute myocardial infarction in patients presenting with ST-segment elevation: the task force for the management of acute myocardial infarction in patients presenting with ST-segment elevation of the European Society of Cardiology (ESC). Eur Heart J. 2018;39(2):119–77.
67. Jung C, Lauten A, Rödiger C, et al. Effect of intra-aortic balloon pump support on microcirculation during high-risk percutaneous intervention. Perfusion. 2009;24(6):417–21.
68. Den Uil CA, Lagrand WK, Van Der Ent M, et al. The effects of intra-aortic balloon pump support on macrocirculation and tissue microcirculation in patients with cardiogenic shock. Cardiology. 2009;114(1):42–6.
69. Jung C, Fuernau G, de Waha S, et al. Intraaortic balloon counterpulsation and microcirculation in cardiogenic shock complicating myocardial infarction: an IABP-SHOCK II substudy. Clin Res Cardiol. 2015;104(8):679–87.
70. Munsterman LDH, Elbers PWG, Ozdemir A, et al. Withdrawing intra-aortic balloon pump support paradoxically improves microvascular flow. Crit Care. 2010;14(4):R161.
71. Lam K, Sjauw KD, Henriques JP, Ince C, de Mol BA. Improved microcirculation in patients with an acute ST-elevation myocardial infarction treated with the Impella LP2.5 percutaneous left ventricular assist device. Clin Res Cardiol. 2009;98(5):311–8.
72. Keebler ME, Haddad EV, Choi CW, et al. Venoarterial extracorporeal membrane oxygenation in cardiogenic shock. JACC Heart Fail. 2018;6(6):503–16.
73. Kara A, Akin S, Dos Reis MD, Struijs A, Caliskan K, van Thiel RJ, Dubois EA, de Wilde W, Zijlstra F, Gommers D, Ince C. Microcirculatory assessment of patients under VA-ECMO. Crit Care. 2016;20(1):344.
74. Yeh YC, Lee CT, Wang CH, Tu YK, Lai CH, Wang YC, Chao A, Huang CH, Cheng YJ, Chen YS. Investigation of microcirculation in patients with venoarterial extracorporeal membrane oxygenation life support. Crit Care. 2018;22(1):200.
75. Millar JE, Fanning JP, McDonald CI, McAuley DF, Fraser JF. The inflammatory response to extracorporeal membrane oxygenation (ECMO): a review of the pathophysiology. Crit Care. 2016;20:387.
76. Aissaoui N, El-Banayosy A, Combes A. How to wean a patient from veno-arterial extracorporeal membrane oxygenation. Intensive Care Med. 2015;41(5):902–5.
77. Akin S, Dos Reis Miranda D, Caliskan K, Soliman OI, Guven G, Struijs A, van Thiel RJ, Jewbali LS, Lima A, Gommers D, Zijlstra F, Ince C. Functional evaluation of sublingual microcirculation indicates successful weaning from VA-ECMO in cardiogenic shock. Crit Care. 2017;21(1):265.

78. Drakos SG, Kfoury AG, Hammond EH, et al. Impact of mechanical unloading on microvasculature and associated central remodeling features of the failing human heart. J Am Coll Cardiol. 2010;56(5):382–91.
79. Sansone R, Stanske B, Keymel S, et al. Macrovascular and microvascular function after implantation of left ventricular assist devices in end-stage heart failure: role of microparticles. J Heart Lung Transplant. 2015;34(7):921–32.
80. Witman MA, Garten RS, Gifford JR, Groot HJ, Trinity JD, Stehlik J, Nativi JN, Selzman CH, Drakos SG, Richardson RS. Further peripheral vascular dysfunction in heart failure patients with a continuous-flow left ventricular assist device. J Am Coll Cardiol Heart Fail. 2015;3:703–11.

Chapter 14
Coronary Microcirculation and Arrhythmias: The Two Faces of a Janus

Radu Vatasescu, Stefan Bogdan, and Alexandru Deaconu

Case Presentation

We present the case of a 64 year-old woman who presented to the emergency room complaining of irregular heartbeats.

History

2008: First episodes of atrial fibrillation (AF) (Fig. 14.1) as well as atypical and typical atrial flutter (AFl).

The arrhythmias were firstly attributed to a thyroid dysfunction. She had been suffering from hyperthyroidism, on the background of a multinodular goiter and aggravated by treatment with amiodarone. After interrupting amiodarone and adequate control of hyperthyroidism under thiamazole treatment, she receved Propafenone 450 mg/day and Sotalol 160 mg/day in an attempt to control her arrhythmias.

2015: Our patient developed chest pain. She was admitted for stable angina associated with mild shortness of breath. She underwent a ECG stress test which was positive for coronary ischaemia. Coronary angiography was performed and found normal coronary arteries with no spontaneous or provoked epicardial coronary artery spasm. Therefore, our patient was diagnosed with coronary microvascular dysfunction and abnormal cardiac pain sensitivity—microvascular angina.

2016: She was also diagnosed with a bradycardia-tachycardia syndrome. Based on two episodes of syncope (each time preceded by hours of palpitations) and a 24 h

R. Vatasescu (✉) · S. Bogdan · A. Deaconu
University of Medicine and Pharmacy "Carol Davila", Bucharest, Romania

Emergency Hospital of Bucharest, Bucharest, Romania

M. Dorobantu, L. Badimon (eds.), *Microcirculation*,
https://doi.org/10.1007/978-3-030-28199-1_14

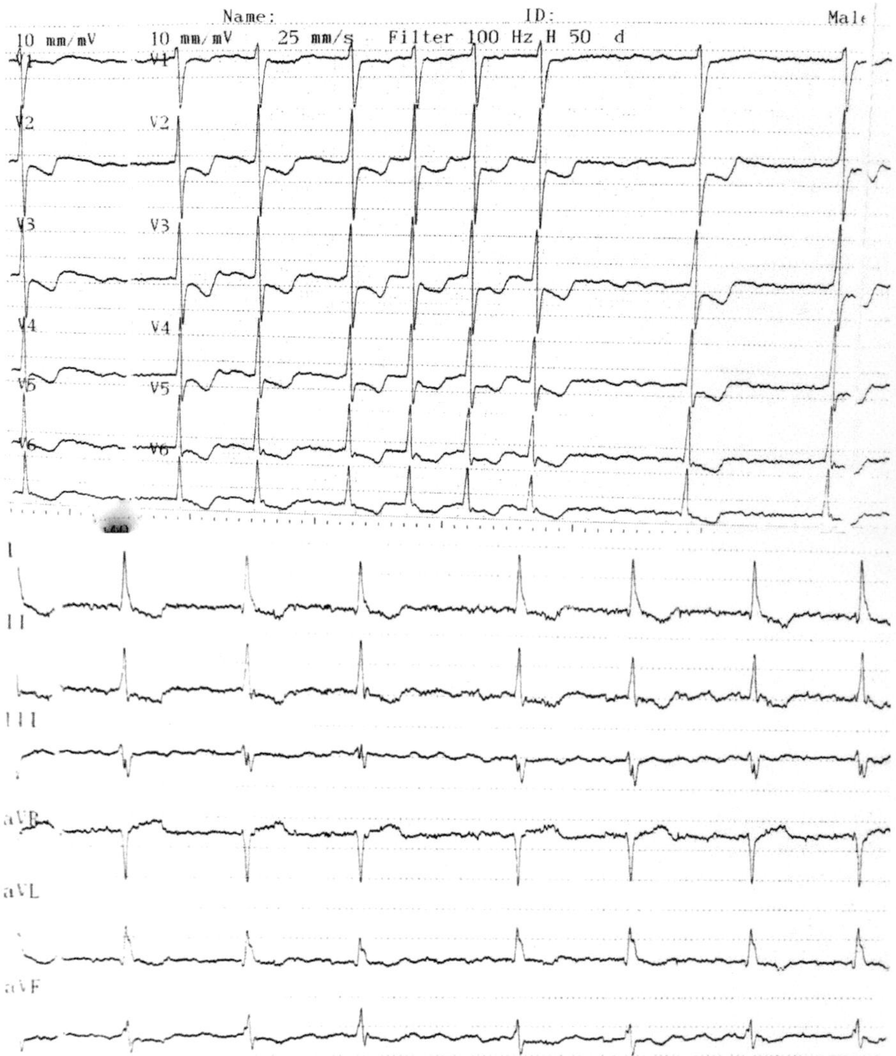

Fig. 14.1 Atrial fibrillation with significant ST depression

Holter ECG recording posttachycardic pauses, she was implanted with a permanent DDD pacemaker.

At the current admission we performed a work-up consisting of physical examination, ECG, routine lab tests, echocardiograhpy and pacemaker interrogation.

The physical examination was normal, her vital signs were stable and she was slightly hypertensive with a blood pressure (BP) of 155/100 mmHg. The ECG initially documented AF with high ventricular response which converted spontaneously to sinus rhythm.

In sinus rhythm, her electrocardiogram (ECG) showed left atrial enlargement, slightly wider QRS (100 ms), and anterior and lateral repolarization abnormalities: 2 mm downsloping ST segment depression in V2–V6, DI, aVL (Fig. 14.2).

Routine lab tests showed normal TSH levels and mild dyslipidemia.

Echocardiography documented a hypertrophic left ventricle (LV), with a interventricular septum (IVSd) of 14 mm, a posterior wall thickness (PWd) of 13 mm, a LV mass of 235 g and a LV mass index of 123 g/m^2 body surface area (BSA). Ejection fraction (EF) was normal with no wall motion abnormalities. Left atrium (LA) was severely enlarged with an area of 32 cm^2 and an indexed volume of 51 mL/m^2 BSA.

Pacemaker interrogation revealed a DDDR 60–130 bpm programmed device with a high percentage of atrial pacing (85%) and virtually no right ventricular pacing. In view of the patient's adequate sinus response to physical effort and emotions, the decision was made to reprogram the device to DDI 45 bpm.

A computerized tomography (CT) coronary angiogram was also performed, owing to the 3 years which had passed since the coronary angiography. It documented a calcium score of 151 with an equivalent mass of 26.34 mg/cm^3, which placed our patient within the 75 and 90 percentiles when adjusted for race, age and sex.

Polysomnography was performed and excluded obstructive sleep apnea syndrome.

On grounds of the unresponsiveness of the atrial arrhythmias to pharmacological treatment, electrophysiological study (EPS) and 3D assisted radiofrequency catheter ablation with isolation of the pulmonary veins for AF and radiofrequency ablation of the cavotricuspid isthmus for recurrent typical AFl were performed.

On a follow-up visit 6 months later our patient reported no recurrent angina, no palpitations and 24 h Holter ECG found no arrhythmias. PM interrogation revealed

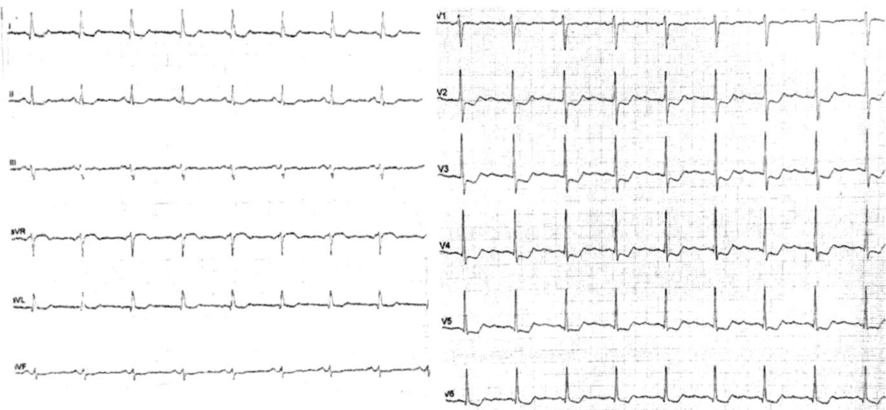

Fig. 14.2 Sinus rhythm with significant ST depression—prior to AF ablation

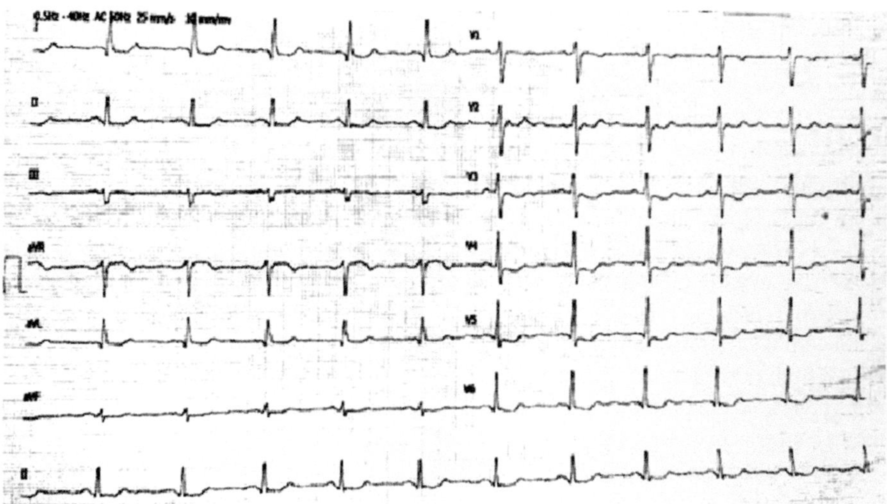

Fig. 14.3 Sinus rhythm with reduced ST depression—following AF ablation

no episode of AHR withAP% and VP% almost zero. She reported better control of her blood pressure, with home BP monitoring values of <130/80 mmHg. Her ECG retained the anterior and lateral abnormalities, but with less ST segment depression (Fig. 14.3).

Furthermore, echocardiography showed a reduction of the dimensions of the LA, with a indexed volume of 39 mL/m^2 BSA as well as a regress of the hypertrophy of the LV to a IVSd of 13 mm, a PWd of 12 mm and LV mass index of 112 g/m^2.

Coronary Microcirculation Disease: Background

Ischaemic heart disease, characterized by chest pain and ECG abnormalities and/or positive stress tests for ischaemia, may frequently occur in the absence of significant coronary atherosclerosis, especially in women [1]. The assumption is that the reduction of coronary perfusion in the absence of coronary artery stenosis would reflecta dysfunction at the level of coronary microcirculation. The coronary microcirculation disease (CMD) is usually related to endothelial dysfunction [2]. Coronary microcirculation is the major determinant of vascular resistance—80% of total resistance is due to coronary microcirculation—and so its dysfunction may compromise myocardial perfusion.

The presence of angina and an abnormal response to stress test in the absence of epicardial coronary disease has been referred to as cardiac syndrome X (CSX) [2]. In published studies the terms CSX and microvascular angina are sometimes superposable. However, some authors make a clear distinction between the two entities. For instance, Shaw et al. define CSX as chest pain in the absence of coronary lesions and proof of ischemic changes on non-invasive testing. Microvascular angina is a narrower term as it refers to patients with positive provocative testing during angiography or a myocardial perfusion reserve defect detected on positron emission tomography (PET) or cardiovascular magnetic resonance (CMR) [3].

The onset of chest pain in patients without any coronary lesions can be divided into two categories: ischaemia and non-ischaemia [3]. The recurrence of chest pain without any ischaemic explanation may be related to an increased proprioceptor sensitivity [4].

There are several entities of CMD discussed in a review in by Pries et al. in 2008 [2]:

1. Ischaemic heart disease in the absence of coronary lesions
2. Inadequate post-PCI and/or post-thrombolysis coronary reperfusion entailing an early phase referred to as 'microvascular obstruction'
3. Microvascular dysfunction in the context of epicardial vessel disease.

The prognosis of patients with chest pain and normal epicardial coronary arteries is less favorable than asymptomatic patients. Several studies demonstrate that this category of patients present an increased risk of major adverse cardiac events (MACE) and all-cause mortality compared to a normal population without ischaemic heart disease even after adjusting for traditional cardiac risk factors [5]. Especially among women with signs and symptoms of ischemia, non-obstructive CAD is common and associated with adverse outcomes over the longer term [6].

Coronary Microcirculation Disease and Arrhythmias: The Chicken or the Egg?

A common clinical setting that has been poorly addressed in literature is the occurrence of various arrhythmias in patients with CMD in the absence of coronary lesions (CSX). This clinical scenario is frequently seen in women, as discussed in the clinical case presented above.

The mechanisms underlying CMD can also be triggered by arrhythmias. Conversely, underlying CMD can lead to arrhythmias. Depending on the arrhythmia, either one or both causal relations can be true. In most clinical settings, the subgroup of patients with CMD often associates other comorbidities such as hypertension, arrhythmias, diabetes or dyslipidemia.

There are several arrhythmias related to the presence of CMD: supraventricular arrhythmias (e.g. atrial fibrillation) and ventricular arrhythmias. Furthermore,tachycardia-induced cardiomyopathies promote coronary microvascular dysfunction. Patients with pacemaker may also present pacing-induced CMD.

Atrial Fibrillation and CMD

Atrial fibrillation (AF) is the most common arrhythmia and its incidence is associated with the presence of comorbidities and increased age [7]. It is not seldom seen that patients with AF develop chest pain in the absence of coronary disease. Recent studies report that patients with AF have ventricular-flow abnormalities and higher incidence of cardiac events [8]. Moreover, coronary artery resistance is markedly elevated (by 62%), whereas myocardial blood flow is substantially reduced in AF patients [8].

In the presence of a coronary stenosis the flow reserve distal to the stenosis is decreased and leads to an impaired endothelial coronary blood flow regulation [2]. In addition to the effects of a stenosis on flow reserve within its own bed, coronary stenosis and occlusion also decrease flow reserve in adjacent non-stenotic beds in both experimental animal models and clinical populations [9]. This pathopysiological pathway explains the presence of arrhythimas in patients with epicardial coronary artery disease.

Furthermore, patients with normal epicardial coronary arteries and AF may present with clinical signs of ischaemia such as chest pain, ST-depression and even troponine release [10]. These findings suggest that there may be a relation between the AF and the myocardial ischaemia in the absence of coronary lesions, related to other mechanisms than decreased flow due to the coronary stenosis.

In practice, the presence of CMD may be documented by several investigations. The diagnosis is established in a patient with angina pectoris, a positive stress test and normal coronary angiography. The stress test may be an ECG stress test or Holter ECG dynamic monitoring which documents ST-segment depression in a patient complaining of chest pain. Stress echocardiography is less used because of the small and random distribution of perfusion defects which makes the abnormalities macroscopically undetectable. Ischaemic areas may be also detected by stress scintigraphy, which show stress induced perfusion defects, or by magnetic resonance and positron emission tomography.

The mechanism of myocardial ischaemia may be either the microvascular coronary dysfunction or arrhythmia induced coronary spasm [7]. In some studies performed on pigs, rapid atrial pacing with a duration of 6 h led to a substantial reduction in coronary flow reserve (CFR) [11], which supports the hypothesis that AF can adversely affect coronary vascular function [7].

A study performed by Range et al. demonstrates an impairment of myocardial perfusion and hyperemic perfusion reserve associated with an increase of coronary resistance in male patients suffering from idiopathic persistent AF [9]. Perfusion abnormalities were not acutely and completely reversible after restoration of stable sinus rhythm, but it was shown that in the subgroup of patients that maintain sinus rhythm following cardioversion, myocardial blood flow at rest normalized and hyperemic flow and coronary vascular resistance were significantly improved from baseline [9].

Another mechanism that can determine impaired coronary flow in patients with AF is the irregular pulse interval, even when the overall ventricular rate is adequately controlled [7]. One possible explanation is that irregular ventricular contraction may cause coronary vasoconstriction by increasing the release of angiotensin II or endothelin [7]. In addition to oxidative stress, a study by Goette and al showed that a relatively brief episode of AF with a moderate increase in ventricular response may enhance the systemic cTn-I levels demonstrating discrete cardiac ischaemia [12]. This can be explained by the induction of oxidative stress-induced microvascular flow abnormalities in the LV [12]. The same study showed that oxidative stress and microvascular flow abnormalities occur immediately after new-onset AF likely and this may represent key initiator mechanisms of AF-related ventricular remodelling [12]. In this setting, angiotensin receptor blocker therapy may attenuate most of the functional and molecular changes in the left ventricle [12].

Impaired coronary flow in patients with AF can also be the result of inflammation. Lim et al. studied the effect of atrial fibrillation on atrial thrombogenesis by analyzing patients with AF during catheter ablation and comparing thrombosis and inflammation markers to a control group. It was shown that a very short time period of 15 min rapid atrial rate (AF or rapid atrial pacing) was associated with increased platelet activation and thrombin generation. However, AF and not rapid atrial pacing led to local and systemic endothelial dysfunction and inflammation [13].

Ventricular Arrhythmias and CMD

Left Ventricular Hypertrophy Secondary to Hypertension

Left ventricular hypertrophy (LVH) leads to myocardial ischaemia due to the mismatch of oxygen supply and demand [14]. CMD with myocardial ischaemia has also been documented in the early stages of hypertension, even in the absence of LVH, particularly in patients treated with thiazide diuretics [14]. Such myocardial ischemia may be a trigger of ventricular arrhythmias and sudden cardiac death [14, 15].

Hypertrophic Cardiomyopathy

Microvascular dysfunction is a defining feature of hypertrophic cardiomyopathy and is caused by multiple mechanisms such as fibrosis, reduced arteriolar density and elevated left ventricular diastolic pressure [16].

In hypertrophic cardiomyopathy, CMD measured by myocardial blood flow (MBF) response to dipyridamole robustly predicts life-threatening ventricular arrhythmias [17]. The failure of myocardial blood flow to increase adequately on demand in these patients predisposes them to myocardial ischemia, which may lead to ventricular arrhythmias and sudden death [16]. Severe CMD was found in patients with mild or no symptoms and may precede left ventricular systolic dysfunction by years [17].

Arrhythmic events in patients with TS are diverse including a systole, pulseless electrical activity, complete sinoatrial and atrioventricular block but also ventricular tachycardia and ventricular fibrillation. Ventricular arrhythmias represent an important factor for morbidity and mortality in patients with TS [18]. The predominant mechanisms underlying most ventricular arrhythmia are reentry, triggered activity, and abnormal automaticity. Triggered activity may be related to the myocardial edema which is correlated with the repolarization abnormalities [18]. Furthermore, microcirculatory dysfunction might contribute, to some extent, to repolarization changes [18]. These changes lead to QT prolongation and early after depolarization-induced triggered activity in the setting of prolonged action potentials is a mechanism of arrhythmias in TS, particularly polymorphic ventricular tachycardia [18].

Tachycardiomyopathy and CMD

Tachycardia-induced cardiomyopathy refers to a decrease in LV function secondary to chronic tachycardia, which is partially or completely reversible after normalization of heart rate and rhythm irregularity [19].

The overwhelming evidence in the case of tachycardiomyopathy seems to suggest that it promotes and sustains coronary microvascular dysfunction. Tachycardia-induced cardiomyopathy may lead to changes in myocardial structure and function which include microcirculatory dysfunction by means of reduced myocardial capillaries and reduced blood flow, increased capillary-myocyte distance and impaired coronary reserve [20]. Coronary vascular resistance is also increased in tachycardiomyopathy [21]. These changes decrease myocardial blood flow (MBF) resulting in myocardial injury and impaired LV function [22].

One of the landmarks of tahycardiomyopathy is reversibility of LV dysfunction following treatment of the tachycardia. Available data refers to improvement of LV contractility, assessed by cardiac imaging. Microscopic alterations reverse slowly or are irreversible [20]. Tomita et al. [23] demonstrated that 1 year after radiofrequency ablation of ectopic atrial tachycardia resulting in dilated cardiomyopathy, histology revealed areas of myocardial fibrosis, although LV function was normal. The improved LV contractility occurs at the expense of increased wall thickness and a probable secondary chronic background ongoing supply demand mismatch of MBF and oxygen demand [20]. This leads to disease progression at the microscopic level in spite of apparent improvement at the clinical level [20]. Gradual resolution over time implies that improvement at the microscopic level takes place after a lag period [20]. Evidence of microscopic and molecular changes in the recovery phase of tachycardia-induced cardiomyopathy are currently scarce in the literature.

Microscopic and molecular changes including microvascular dysfunction also occur in tachycardia-induced atrial cardiomyopathy but have been shown to differ from its ventricular analogue [20]. Cellular changes at atrial level consist of increased angiotensin II concentration, tissue apoptosis, inflammatory cell infiltration and cell death [20]. This results in early atrial fibrosis which in turn leads to a tendency for recurrence of atrial arrhythmias. Consequently, prompt recognition and treatment of the underlying arrhythmia will improve prognosis and decrease risk of reccurence [20].

Left Bundle Branch Block and CMD

Left bundle branch block (LBBB) is found in 12% of the cases in patients with no heart disease [24].

The effects of CMD in the etiology of the LBBB in these patients remains unclear. There is evidence that LBBB leads to microvascular dysfunction rather than the other way around. Koepfli et al. found that LBBB generates a shift of septal to lateral myocardial blood flow during exercise [25]. This finding is explained by the reduced contribution of the interventricular septum to the left ventricular global performance, due to the asynchronous contraction [25]. This leads to a higher oxygen demand in the lateral wall, which supports a higher than normal workload [25]. However, a reversible LBBB induced by RV pacing would generate a similar but reversible pattern [25]. This findings support a functional mechanism of septal underperfusion, thus challenging the hypothesis of underlying septal microvascular dysfunction as a contributing to the development of non-ischaemic LBBB [25].

Cardiac Pacing and CMD

Patients with a permanent cardiac pacemaker (PM) frequently develop symptoms suggestive of ischemic heart disease in the absence of epicardial coronary lesions. These symptoms can be attributed to CMD.

A study performed by Skalidis et al. analyzed the myocardial perfusion in patients with permanent ventricular pacing and normal coronary arteries. Results show that permanent ventricular pacing from the right ventricular apex is associated with alteration in regional myocardial perfusion. Impairment of microvascular flow is the underlying mechanism for the perfusion defects during either exercise and dipyridamol myocardial scintigraphy [26].

Bradyarrhythmias and CMD

In an experimental model on pig hearts, bradycardia was shown to possibly improve microvascular supply by increasing capillary density [27].

Bradycardia may promote capillary growth in the absence of cardiac hypertrophy by prolonging diastolic perfusion, and/or mechanical stretch of vessels due to increased stroke volume capacity [27]. In these hemodynamic conditions, capillaries are subject to increased wall tension which could trigger angiogenesis [27].

Case Presentation Discussion

Our patient is a female suffering from documented coronary microvascular dysfunction. The diagnosis of coronary microvascular dysfunction was established on the association of typical angina, ECG changes consistent with myocardial ischaemia, positive ECG stress test and normal coronary arteries.

In her case, CMD induced microvascular angina as well as recurrent atrial fibrillation. In turn, frequent episodes of atrial fibrillation also aggravated CMD.

Atrial fibrillation ablation led to clinical improvements, with our patient reporting only occasional mild chest pain and no irregular heartbeats. ECG traces also ameliorated, with ST-T changes have significantly diminished 6 months after ablation (Figs. 14.2 and 14.3), probably owing to the improved coronary microcirculation. These findings support the hypothesis of atrial fibrillation worsened coronary microvascular dysfunction, thus confirming the bidirectional relationship between the two entities.

Conclusions

Both supraventricular arrhythmias (e.g. atrial fibrillation) and ventricular arrhythmias can be related to coronary microvascular dysfunction, in patients with no epicardial artery disease and no other significant comorbidities. The relationship between arrhythmias and coronary microcirculation appears to be bidirectional. In atrial fibrillation, the arrhythmia seems to promote microvascular dysfunction, while ventricular arrhythmias appear to be triggered by relative myocardial ischemia in the setting of CMD. One the other hand, tachycardiomyopathy facilitates and sustains CMD, further linking the two entities. There is need for future studies which would include patients with cardiac syndrome X and specific arrhythmias in order to clearly establish the causal relationship.

References

1. Kaski JC. Pathophysiology and management of patients with chest pain and normal coronary arteriograms (cardiac syndrome X). Circulation. 2004;109(5):568–72. https://doi.org/10.1161/01.CIR.0000116601.58103.62.
2. Pries AR, Habazettl H, Ambrosio G, et al. A review of methods for assessment of coronary microvascular disease in both clinical and experimental settings. Cardiovasc Res. 2008;80(2):165–74. https://doi.org/10.1093/cvr/cvn136.
3. Shaw J, Anderson T. Coronary endothelial dysfunction in non-obstructive coronary artery disease: risk, pathogenesis, diagnosis and therapy. Vasc Med. 2016;21(2):146–55. https://doi.org/10.1177/1358863X15618268.
4. Di Franco A, Di Monaco A, Lamendola P, et al. Evidence of exclusively silent microvascular ischemia: role of differences in nociceptive function compared to symptomatic microvascular ischemia. Eur Heart J. 2011;32:569.
5. Jespersen L, Hvelplund A, Abildstrøm SZ, et al. Stable angina pectoris with no obstructive coronary artery disease is associated with increased risks of major adverse cardiovascular events. Eur Heart J. 2012;33(6):734–44. https://doi.org/10.1093/eurheartj/ehr331.
6. Sharaf B, Wood T, Shaw L, et al. Adverse outcomes among women presenting with signs and symptoms of ischemia and no obstructive coronary artery disease: findings from the National Heart, Lung, and Blood Institute-sponsored women's ischemia syndrome evaluation (WISE) angiographic core lab. Am Heart J. 2013;166(1):134–41. https://doi.org/10.1016/j.ahj.2013.04.002.
7. Wijesurendra RS, Casadei B. Atrial fibrillation: effects beyond the atrium? Cardiovasc Res. 2015;105(3):238–47. https://doi.org/10.1093/cvr/cvv001
8. Range FT, Schäfers M, Acil T, et al. Impaired myocardial perfusion and perfusion reserve associated with increased coronary resistance in persistent idiopathic atrial fibrillation. Eur Heart J. 2007;28(18):2223–30. https://doi.org/10.1093/eurheartj/ehm246.
9. Range FT, Paul M, Schafers KP, et al. Myocardial perfusion in nonischemic dilated cardiomyopathy with and without atrial fibrillation. J Nucl Med. 2009;50(3):390–6. https://doi.org/10.2967/jnumed.108.055665.
10. Van Den Bos EJ, Constantinescu AA, Van Domburg RT, Akin S, Jordaens LJ, Kofflard MJM. Minor elevations in troponin i are associated with mortality and adverse cardiac events in patients with atrial fibrillation. Eur Heart J. 2011;32(5):611–7. https://doi.org/10.1093/eurheartj/ehq491.
11. Bukowska A, Hammwöhner M, Sixdorf A, et al. Dronedarone prevents microcirculatory abnormalities in the left ventricle during atrial tachypacing in pigs. Br J Pharmacol. 2012;166(3):964–80. https://doi.org/10.1111/j.1476-5381.2011.01784.x.
12. Goette A, Bukowska A, Dobrev D, et al. Acute atrial tachyarrhythmia induces angiotensin II type 1 receptor-mediated oxidative stress and microvascular flow abnormalities in the ventricles. Eur Heart J. 2009;30(11):1411–20. https://doi.org/10.1093/eurheartj/ehp046.
13. Lim HS, Willoughby SR, Schultz C, et al. Effect of atrial fibrillation on atrial thrombogenesis in humans: impact of rate and rhythm. J Am Coll Cardiol. 2013;61(8):852–60. https://doi.org/10.1016/j.jacc.2012.11.046.
14. Lip GYH, Coca A, Kahan T, et al. Hypertension and cardiac arrhythmias: executive summary of a consensus document from the European Heart Rhythm Association (EHRA) and ESC council on Hypertension, endorsed by the Heart Rhythm Society (HRS), Asia-Pacific Heart Rhythm Society (APHRS), and Sociedad Latinoamericana de Estimulación Cardíaca y Electrofisiología (SOLEACE). Eur Hear J Cardiovasc Pharmacother. 2017;3(4):235–50. https://doi.org/10.1093/ehjcvp/pvx019.
15. Kahan T, Bergfeldt L. Left ventricular hypertrophy in hypertension: its arrhythmogenic potential. Heart. 2005;91(2):250–6. https://doi.org/10.1136/hrt.2004.042473.

16. Cecchi F, Olivotto I, Gistri R, Lorenzoni R, Chiriatti G, Camici PG. Coronary microvascular dysfunction and prognosis in hypertrophic cardiomyopathy. N Engl J Med. 2003;349(11):1027–35. https://doi.org/10.1056/NEJMoa025050.
17. Herrmann J, Kaski JC, Lerman A. Coronary microvascular dysfunction in the clinical setting: from mystery to reality. Eur Heart J. 2012;33(22):2771–82. https://doi.org/10.1093/eurheartj/ehs246.
18. Möller C, Eitel C, Thiele H, Eitel I, Stiermaier T. Ventricular arrhythmias in patients with Takotsubo syndrome. J Arrhythm. 2018;34(4):369–75.
19. Gallagher JJ. Tachycardia and cardiomyopathy: the chicken-egg dilemma revisited. J Am Coll Cardiol. 1985;6(5):1172–3. https://doi.org/10.1016/S0735-1097(85)80328-4.
20. Khasnis A, Jongnarangsin K, Abela G, Veerareddy S, Reddy V, Thakur R. Tachycardia-induced cardiomyopathy: a review of literature. Pacing Clin Electrophysiol. 2005;28(7):710–21. https://doi.org/10.1111/j.1540-8159.2005.00143.x.
21. Spinale FG, Tanaka R, Crawford FA, Zile MR. Changes in myocardial blood flow during development of and recovery from tachycardia-induced cardiomyopathy. Circulation. 1992;85(2):717–29. https://doi.org/10.1161/01.CIR.85.2.717.
22. Spinale FG, Grine RC, Tempel GE, Crawford FA, Zile MR. Alterations in the myocardial capillary vasculature accompany tachycardia-induced cardiomyopathy. Basic Res Cardiol. 1992;87(1):65–79. https://doi.org/10.1007/BF00795391.
23. Tomita M, Ikeguchi S, Kagawa K, et al. Serial histopathologic myocardial findings in a patient with ectopic atrial tachycardia-induced cardiomyopathy. J Cardiol. 1997;29(1):37–42.
24. Jain AC, Mehta MC. Etiologies of left bundle branch block and correlations with hemodynamic and angiographic findings. Am J Cardiol. 2003;91(11):1375–8. https://doi.org/10.1016/S0002-9149(03)00337-0.
25. Koepfli P, Wyss CA, Gaemperli O, et al. Left bundle branch block causes relative but not absolute septal underperfusion during exercise. Eur Heart J. 2009;30(24):2993–9. https://doi.org/10.1093/eurheartj/ehp372.
26. Skalidis EI, Kochiadakis GE, Koukouraki SI, et al. Myocardial perfusion in patients with permanent ventricular pacing and normal coronary arteries. J Am Coll Cardiol. 2001;37(1):124–9. https://doi.org/10.1016/S0735-1097(00)01096-2.
27. Brown MD, Davies MK, Hudlicka O, et al. Cell Mol Biol Res. 1994;40(2):137–42.

Part III
Therapeutical Considerations

Chapter 15
Management of No-Reflow

Danijela Trifunovic, Jelena Dudic, Natalija Gavrilovic, and Olivia Manfrini

The goal of myocardial reperfusion is not just to achieve an open epicardial artery, but to restore the normal blood flow to cardiac tissues. Classically, the"no-reflow phenomenon" (NR) is defined as a lack of myocardial perfusion despite thesuccessful opening of the occluded epicardialartery [1]. It most frequently happens in the setting of primary percutaneous coronary intervention (pPCI), but it can also be seen during elective PCI. No-reflow is evident by the slowing of the coronary flow, a higher TIMI frame count, and an abnormal or absent myocardial blush. The frequency of NR varies with the methodology used to assess it, ranging from 5% to 60% in the published data [2].

The pathophysiology of NR is still not fully elucidated, and several mechanisms are proposed. The main mechanism is the microvascular injury that can be caused both by *intrinsic* and by*extrinsic* vascular processes [3]. The intrinsic phenomena leading to microvascular obstruction (MVO) include microvascular thrombosis, the distal embolization of a thrombus/atheroma, vasospasm and endothelial damage. The extrinsic problems include microvascular compression due to edema and inflammation. Endothelial damage harms capillary integrity causing edema and the hemorrhagic transformation of the infarct core. Microvascular obstruction precedes myocardial hemorrhage. While MVO can be reversible, myocardial hemorrhage is not because iron deposition within the infarcted myocardium drives inflammation, increasing the likelihood of ventricular arrhythmias, adverse remodeling and

D. Trifunovic (✉)
Department of Cardiology, Clinical Center of Serbia, Belgrade, Serbia

Faculty of Medicine, Belgrade University, Belgrade, Serbia

J. Dudic · N. Gavrilovic
Faculty of Medicine, Belgrade University, Belgrade, Serbia

O. Manfrini
Department of Experimental, Diagnostic and Specialty Medicine, University of Bologna, Bologna, Italy
e-mail: olivia.manfrini@unibo.it

M. Dorobantu, L. Badimon (eds.), *Microcirculation*,
https://doi.org/10.1007/978-3-030-28199-1_15

adverse cardiac events [4]. Management strategies, at least theoretically, should be focused on preventing or modulating those mechanisms in order to avert the consequences of NR.

Sometimes, the term NR is also used to describe a sudden loss of epicardial flow, typically after ballooning a lesion or placing a stent. In this setting, NR might be secondary to incomplete lesion dilation, epicardial spasm, or epicardial dissection with or without *in situ* thrombosis. In these cases, the first step would be to use intravascular ultrasound to distinguish a dissection and a spasm from a microvascular phenomenon [5].

Despite considerable progress in the identification of the risks to NR development and the improvement of the management strategies for NR, no specific therapies have been developed so far. Unquestionably, those patients with NR who have received therapy and who succeed to improve coronary flow have a better prognosis [6]. These observations strongly suggest the importance of the recognition and appropriate management of NR.

Prevention of No-Reflow

Many classical risk factors for cardiovascular diseases are also the well-defined risk factors for NR, including hypertension, smoking, dyslipidemia, diabetes, and other inflammatory processes. The general measures taken in order to control these factors can reduce the occurrence of NR. Optimal blood glucose control before PCI reduce the occurrence of NR [7], both presumably improving the coronary microcirculation and avoiding the poor effects of acute hyperglycemia on reperfusion injury [8]. Similarly, intensive statin therapy before PCI in individuals with hyperlipidemia is advantageous in reducing NR. A meta-analysis of seven studies with pre-procedural statin therapy in 3086 patients has demonstrated the complete prevention of NR in 4.2% and the attenuation of no-reflow in the additional 5% of the patients treated with statins, compared with the control patients receiving a placebo, usual care, or lower-dose statin therapy [9].

Prediction of No-Reflow

The risk awareness of NR development is important. In the case of a patient at risk for NR, certain techniques might have some potential to reduce the degree of NR: primary stenting, the avoidance of high-pressure stent deployment and thrombectomy before the intervention [2].

The *patient-specific* features carrying a high risk for NR in STEMI patients include the following: a delayed presentation to the catheterization laboratory [6], hyperglycemia, and hypercholesterolemia, the female gender, hypertension, mild-to-moderate renal insufficiency, and elevated inflammatory markers [10–13].

The *lesion-specific* features affecting the risk for NR include plaque composition and a thrombus burden detected by intravascular ultrasound [14, 15]. However, any time-consuming procedure that might delay the door-to-balloon time is not recommended in the management of STEMI patients because a prolonged ischemic time is one of the strongest factors leading to a microcirculatory damage and the consequent development of NR [1].

The possible treatment modalities of NR include: (1) pharmacological therapy, (2) interventional treatment, and (3) non-invasive treatments.

Pharmacotherapy

Pharmacotherapy includes vasodilatators, antiplatelet drugs and fibrinolytic drugs. Basically, no significant difference was demonstrated between various pharmacological intervention strategies, but a significant clinical benefit was observed when NR was resolved [6].

Vasodilatators

In the majority of centers, the current standard of care when NR happens during PCI first includes checking whether the epicardial artery is optimally treated, only to be followed by the initiation of the intracoronary injection of a vasodilatator such as *adenosine*, at a dose of 100–200 mcg [16] *nicardipine*, at a median dose of 400 mcg [17], or *nitroprusside*, at doses ranging from 50 to 300 mcg [18]. Other vasodilators include *nicorandil* (used in some laboratories). Frequent consecutive doses of the previously mentioned vasodilators may be repeated as long as they are well-tolerated by blood pressure. Distal coronary administration using a micro-infusion catheter is preferred over injection through the guiding catheter because the latter may have significant systemic effects and because only a small amount of the agent is likely to actually reach the distal coronary bed [2].

Adenosine is a purine nucleoside that binds to adenosine receptors and exerts effects both on cardiac myocytes and on blood vessels. In ischemic cardiomycites within a few seconds of ischemia, the levels of endogen interstitial adenosine increase and cause arteriolar vasodilatation. In addition to vasodilatation, in experimental studies, adenosine had an inhibitory (protective) effect on many other mechanisms involved in myocardial ischemia and infarction, such as platelet aggregation, inflammatory cell activation, the generation of oxygen free radicals, and decreasing the cellular calcium overload [19]. Adenosine also has negative chronotropic and dromotropic effects.

Initial larger clinical trials investigating the use of adenosine to improve outcomes following intervention for STEMI were AMISTAD (Acute Myocardial Infarction Study of Adenosine) [20] and AMISTAD II [21]. In the AMISTAD trial, the investigators examined if a continuous adenosine infusion [70 mcg/kg/min for 3 h or a placebo given before thrombolytic therapy) would reduce the myocardial infarct size as measured by SPECT imaging. In the AMISTAD II trial, the patients were randomized to a placebo or one of the two doses of intravenous adenosine (50 mcg/kg/min or 70 mcg/kg/min) in adjunction to either thrombolysis or PCI. In both trials, adenosine was shown to reduce the infarct size (if the dose of adenosine was 70 mcg/kg/min), but they failed to show improvements in clinical outcomes unless the patients had achieved early reperfusion with either thrombolysis (60%) or primary PCI (40%).

Vijayalakshmi et al. compared the use of intracoronary adenosine or verapamil in patients with STEMI and NSTEMI, thus showing that the use of either of the two agents was correlated with an improvement in coronary blood flow and, subsequently, in the wall motion index. Although both drugs had similar benefits, verapamil was associated with hypotension and complete heart block lasting up to 3 h in 18% of the cases [22]. The REOPENAMI (Intracoronary Nitroprusside Versus Adenosine in Acute Myocardial Infarction) trial published by Niccoli et al. investigated the effect of intracoronary adenosine or nitroprusside in 240 patients with STEMI following intracoronary thrombus aspiration and showed a better ST-segment resolution at 90 min, as well as the more favorable remodeling of the left ventricle in the adenosine groupat 1 year of follow-up [23]. This positive effect was also translated into a lower incidence of the composite events that included myocardial infarction, heart failure, and death. These favorable effects were not seen in the nitroprusside group.

Multiple meta-analyses were performed regarding adenosine efficacy in preventing NR [24–28]. Although there was an overlap, the studies included in each meta-analysis varied, and their ultimate conclusions differed. The first conclusion of the meta-analysis performed by Su et al. [26] published in 2015 that included 11 randomized clinical trials with 1027 patients was that the quality and quantity of available research studies were insufficient and that the overall risk of the bias of the included studies was moderate. Secondly, they concluded that adenosine as a treatment for NR during pPCI could, on the one hand, reduce angiographic no-reflow (TIMI flow grade <3) (a relative risk 0.62, 95% CI 0.42–0.91, p value = 0.01), whereas on the other, it could also increasethe occurrence of adverse events such as: bradycardia (RR 6.32, 95% CI 2.98–13.41, p value <0.00001), hypotension (RR 11.43, 95% CI 2.75–47.57, p value = 0.0008) and atrioventricular (AV) block (RR 6.78, 95% CI 2.15–21.38, p value = 0.001). Indeed, Su et al. were unable to find supportive pieces of evidence suggesting that adenosine reduced all-cause mortality, non-fatal myocardial infarction or the incidence of the myocardial blush grade from 0 to 1. However, an updated meta-analysis performed by Bulluck et al. in 2016 including 13 randomized controlled trials investigating adenosine as an adjunct to reperfusion in 4273 STEMI patients revealed less heart failure (the risk ratio of 0.44 [95% CI 0.25–0.78], p = 0.005) and alower incidence of coronary no-reflow (the risk ratio for TIMI flow <3 post-reperfusion 0.68 [95% CI 0.47–0.99], p = 0.04) in patients given adenosine intracoronary, but not intravenously, compared to the control [28].

The dose of adenosine for NR treatment is obviously important. High-dose intracoronary adenosine (2–3 mg in total) and sodium nitroprusside (500 µg in total) during pPCI in a REFLO-STEMI study did not reduce the infarct size or the MVO measured by cardiac magnetic resonance. Furthermore, in this study, adenosine adversely affected the mid-term clinical outcome [29].

Adenosine has a very short half-life, which is its limitation. Data from animal models showed that a 2-h intracoronary adenosine infusion is superior to an adenosine bolus in ameliorating no-reflow [30]. However, adenosine infusion into the arterial bed may result in atrioventricular block. Summarizing the data, adenosine is not currently routinely used during PCI, but it may be used to treat no-reflow, preferably by intracoronary administration at a dose up to 2 mg.

Several *calcium channel blockers (CCB)* have been investigated for the efficacy in the treatment of NR, these including verapamil, diltiazem, and nicardipine.

Verapamil is an L-type CCB inhibiting the calcium ion influx through *slow channels* into the myocardium and the coronary arteries. Consequently, it relieves coronary vasospasm and improves myocardial perfusion. Indeed, this CCB agent has proven to be very efficient in relieving the anginal symptoms caused by coronary vasospasm. Intracoronary administered verapamil injection was associated with a reduction incoronary NR and short-term MACEs in the patients undergoing pPCI, whereas it had no impact on improving the ejection fraction [31]. Kaplan et al. compared intracoronary verapamil (100–500 g) with nitroglycerin for the treatment of NR in degenerated vein grafts and demonstrated an improved TIMI flow in all the patients treated with verapamil [32]. The meta-analyses assessing the efficacy of verapamil and diltiazem or verapamil alone for the treatment of NR have demonstrated a significant benefit over the standard of care with respect to NR [26, 33]. *Nicardipine* was beneficial in the studies of NR prevention during rotational atherectomy [34] and percutaneous interventions in vein grafts [35] with a minimal myocardial depressant effect [36]. At present, some interventionalists are using intracoronary verapamil, nicardipine, or diltiazem with a variable success for the treatment of NR. However, the present data are not sufficient to allow for definitive conclusions regarding CCB efficacy, but rather suggest the need for a large, randomized, controlled trial.

Nicorandile is a hybrid of the mitochondrial potassium-channel opener and nitrate, with a potential to mitigate NR. When isolated after reperfusion, mitochondria are structurally altered, contain large quantities of Ca2+, and produce an excess of oxygen free radicals. Their membrane pores are stimulated and the capacity for oxidative phosphorylation is irreversibly disrupted [37]. Nicorandil reduces intracellular calcium and leads to a relief from coronary vasospasm. Although therapy with nicorandil prior to reperfusion in the meta-analysis performed by Wu et al. in 2013 [38] was associated with the improvement of coronary reflow, as well as with the suppression of ventricular arrhythmia, and further improved the left ventricular function in the patients who underwent pPCI, the definite clinical benefits of nicorandil were not found due to the small sample size of the selected studies.

Sodium nitroprusside releases the nitric oxide (NO) that activates guanylate cyclase in the vascular smooth muscle. This leads to the increased production of intracellular cGMP, which stimulates calcium ion movement from the cytoplasm to the endoplasmic reticulum, thus reducing the level of the available calcium ions that can bind to calmodulin. This ultimately results in the vascular smooth muscle relaxation and the vessel dilation. Intracoronary nitroprusside at the doses of 50–300 mcg was demonstrated to be quite effective in the treatment of no-reflow [2], especially so when injected distally in thecoronary artery. In this manner, it has a negligible systemic effect (on blood pressure), but induces a marked improvement of the coronary flow and the myocardial tissue blush. Nitroprusside combined with tirofiban was more effective compared to tirofiban alone in 162 STEMI patients who underwent pPCI with thrombus aspiration, including a more rapid ST-segment elevation resolution, fewer major adverse cardiac events, and a higher left ventricular ejection fraction [39]. However, the TIMI flow grade did not differ between the groups (rather suggesting that the TIMI flow grade is not the most sensitive method for defining coronary blood flow). In a small study assessing NR in STEMI patients, both nitroprusside and nicorandil improved coronary blood flow; however, nitroprusside was more effective when the TIMI frame count was measured [40]. Compared to the other drugs used for NR, nitroprusside appears to have a more sustained effect, especially when compared to adenosine [39], with which it may be combined in order to prolong adenosine effects [41]. There are also negative studies dedicated to the application of nitroprusside in the treatment of NR. In a study concerning the role of nitroprusside in the prevention of NR, nitroprusside failed to improve the coronary flow and myocardial tissue reperfusion, but it did improve the clinical outcomes at 6 months [42]. In order to overcome the limitations of small studies, two meta-analyses have been conducted with nitroprusside, both confirming a clear benefit of nitroprusside in the management of no-reflow during PCI [43, 44]. The total dose of nitroprusside given for NR is important. The high dose of intracoronary delivered nitroprusside (500 mcg total) immediately following thrombectomy and again following the stenting did not reduce the infarct size or the MVO measured by CMR (the REFLO-STEMI study) [29].

Anisodamine, a belladonna alkaloid employed in traditional Chinese medicine, is a non-subtype-selective muscarinic, and a nicotinic cholinoceptor antagonist, which has antioxidant, antithrombotic and antiarrhytmicproperties [45]. Like atropine and scopolamine, anisodamine exhibits the usual spectrum of the pharmacological effects of this drug class, although being less potent and less toxic than atropine. It also has a relatively weak alpha (1) adrenergic antagonistic activity, which may explain its vasodilatation capacity. It also interacts with and disruptsthe liposome structure which may reflect its effects on cellular membranes. The mechanism of the action of anisodamine implies the blockage of the intracelular Ca overload, which is one of the main apoptoic mehanisms due to the membrane protein damage by reactive oxygen species (ROS). Animal and clinical studies have shown that *anisodamine* can increase blood pressure and coronary perfusion pressure, and improve the microcirculation, thus making it a potentially useful drug for preventing NR. Recent meta-analysis comprising 41 RCTs involving 4069 patients showed that, when compared to the standardly used vasodilatators (verapamil, adenosine, diltiazem and nicorandil), anisodamine is associated with higher LVEF and a lower risk from MACEs [46]. However, the authors of this meta-analysis suggested that, given the limited quality and quantity of the included studies, more rigorous randomized trials are needed to verify the role of this regimen.

Glycoprotein IIb/IIIa Inhibitors

Glycoprotein IIb/IIIa inhibitors (GP IIb/IIIa inhibitors) are powerful antiplatelet drugs proven to lower the thrombus burden in patients with myocardial infarction. According to the current ESC guidelines for the management of STEMI and NSTEMI [47, 48] GP IIb/IIIa inhibitors are the only drugs officially recommended as bailout therapy in the case of the angiographic evidence of a slow- or no-reflow, as reasonable (the class of recommendation IIa, the level of recommendation C) although this strategy has not been tested in a randomized trial. The AIDA AMI trial compared intracoronary to intravenous abciximab and found that the intracoronary abciximab bolus administration could possibly be related to the reduced rates of congestive heart failure at 90 days, but there were no differences in the combined endpoint of death, reinfarction, or congestive heart failure [49]. Unfortunately, there are no studies comparing the relative efficacy of a prolonged intravenous infusion compared to a single or multiple intracoronary boluses of abciximab. A small study of 49 patients compared anintracoronary bolus-only with an intravenous bolus plus the infusion of tirofiban, but found no superiority in either of the two [50]. According to a recent meta-analysis, the intralesional administration of IIb/IIIa compared to intracoronary administration yielded favorable outcomes in terms of myocardial tissue reperfusion as evidenced by the improved TIMI flow grade, a complete ST-segment resolution, and decreased MACE without increasing in-hospital major bleeding events [51]. The targeted strategy combining adjunctive IIb/IIIa platelet receptor antagonist administration with aspiration and prolonged balloon inflation was described in a series of 71 patients undergoing PCI for the ST-segment elevation, and this combination of therapies appeared to prevent NR [52].

Glucagon-Like Peptide (GLP)-1 Analog

A potentialof the *glucagon-like peptide (GLP)-1 analog*liraglutide to reduce NR was shown in a small, randomized, controlled trial conducted in 210 subjects [53]. The proposed mechanisms include the modulation of the glucose levels, reduced inflammation and the improved endothelial function, and a further study has been proposed.

Intracoronary Fibrinolytic Therapy

Intracoronary fibrinolytic therapy as an adjunct to pPCI in patients with a large intracoronary thrombus burden was tested only in few RCTs and registry studies [54]. The majority of the data suggested that fibrinolytic therapy as an adjunct to PCI is not useful in everyday clinical practice including the treatment of NR, and that a critical reappraisal of this therapy is needed. The studies of adjunctive fibrinolytic therapy to pPCI have multiple limitations; nevertheless, several of them demonstrate a positive effect on myocardial perfusion [55–57]. It is not known at present how much of this improvement may translate into a prognostic benefit.

Invasive Treatment

Deferred Stenting

The important mechanism behind NR is the embolization of the atherothrombotic debris during the manipulation of the culprit vessel and stent deployment is identified as a step with the highest risk of distal embolization. A deferred or delayed stenting strategy might be a feasible alternative to the conventional approach with immediate stenting in the selected STEMI patients undergoing pPCI. By delaying a stent implantation after mechanical flow restoration, vasodilators, antithrombotic drugs (GP IIb/IIIa inhibitors) and statins might be initiated, which can remove vasospasm, dissolve an intracoronary thrombus and stabilize an atherosclerotic plaque. Also, as the acute phase is resolved, this strategy allows the simultaneous intervention of the IRA and non-IRA vessels in patients with a multivessel disease. In the meta-analysis that included eight studies with 744 patients, deferred stenting satisfactorily improved the TIMI flow grade, TMBG, and a complete ST-segment resolution, and decreased MACEs without increasing the major bleeding events in patients with STEMI and a high thrombus burden [58].

Postconditioning

Postconditioning consists of brief, repeatedly induced coronary occlusions immediately after prolonged myocardial ischemia. Some evidences suggested that it is associated with a reduction in the myocardial infarct size compared with sudden reperfusion. The protection mechanism involves the activation of extracellular signal-regulated kinase, the production of nitric oxide, the opening of the mitochondrial potassium channels and the inhibition of the opening of the mitochondrial permeability transition pore. Staat et al. performed a study of 30 patients, in which the patients in the experimental group were submitted to the repeated inflation and deflation of the angioplasty balloon (four times) immediately after coronary flow had been obtained. Compared to the control group, in the experimental group there was a significant decrease in the creatine kinase peak, the infarct size (as assessed by the level of creatine kinase) was lower (by 36%), and the blush grade was significantly higher [59].

Distal Embolic Protection Devices

There are two distal protection devices to capture embolic debris during PCI that have proven to be clinically beneficial for the PCI of saphenous vein graft lesions [60, 61]. However, the Protection Devices in PCI-Treatment of Myocardial Infarction for Salvage of Endangered Myocardium (the PROMISE study) by the FilterWire was announced as a negative one [62]. Nevertheless, the second generation of the FilterWire EZ System was further examined in the treatment of an acute myocardial infarction in the FLAME study and compared with aspiration alone by using the Export or Rescue catheter. This study showed that a combination of distal embolic protection with aspiration vs aspiration alone was significantly more efficient regarding the capture of embolic debris. However, despite those encouraging results seen in the combined group, no effect on the infarct size, or a clinical benefit was demonstrable [63]. There are currently no data to support the routine use of distal protection in the routine cases of pPCI.

Thrombus Aspiration

Manipulating the occluded area with balloons and stents might result in the distal embolization of a thrombus, thus contributing to the development of NR. Therefore, the prevention of distal embolization by thrombus aspiration before PCI should lessen the degree of NR and the results in better clinical outcomes. Indeed, this concept was initially confirmed in the ATTEMPT (Analysis of Trials on Thrombectomy in Acute Myocardial Infarction Based on Individual Patient Data) study [64], and thrombus aspiration has since become an integral part of the intervention, particularly when a visible thrombus is present. Thrombus aspiration must begin with forward aspiration starting proximal to the occlusion, making multiple passes, until the canalization of the vessel with an improved anterograde flow is demonstrated. However, a meta-analysis published by Mongeon et al. [65] failed to show a long-term benefit of thrombus aspiration in STEMI patients. Of note, it included many different studies applying various techniques, including rheolyticthrombectomy, which may increase NR in some patients [66].

In a more recent meta-analysis [67], large ($n \geq 1000$), randomized, controlled trials comparing manual thrombectomy and pPCI alone in STEMI patients were included (TAPAS, TASTE and TOTAL). The prespecified primary efficacy outcome was cardiovascular mortality within 30 days, and the primary safety outcome was a stroke or a transient ischemic attack within 30 days. The authors concluded that routine thrombus aspiration during PCI for STEMI did not improve the clinical outcomes. However, in the high-risk subgroup (i.e. the one with a high thrombus burden), the trends toward reduced cardiovascular death, although coupled with an increased risk for a stroke or a transient ischemic attack, provide a rationale for future trials of improved thrombus aspiration.

The other complementary techniques that may help prevent distal embolization include the avoidance of high-pressure stent deployment and the full coverage of the diseased segment in the coronary artery [2].

Nonpharmacological Interventions

In addition to the procedures described in the preceding text, otherless well-supported, nonpharmacological treatment strategies for no-reflow have been described.

Hypothermia

There is some evidence that therapeutic hypothermia, given after initial reperfusion, can be beneficial in reducing the infarct size and the prevention of NR [68]. By using the rat model, Dai et al. showed that late hypothermia (performed by initiating a room-temperature saline solution 60 min after reperfusion) reduced the extent of the no-reflow size, but had no effect on the infarct size, suggesting that no-reflow is a true form of the reperfusion injury and is likely due to damage done to the microvasculature by reactive oxygen radicals.

The recently published COOL AMI EU pilot trial [69] investigated the rapid induction of therapeutic hypothermia (20 min of endovascular cooling at 33.6 °C) by using the ZOLL Proteus Intravascular Temperature Management System in 50 patients with anterior STEMI without cardiac arrest. Except for self-terminating atrial fibrillation, there was no excess of adverse events and no clinically important cooling-related delay to reperfusion. A statistically non-significant numerical 7.1% absolute and 30% relative reduction in the infarct size (measured by CMR) was reported, warranting a pivotal trial powered for efficacy.

Ischemic Postconditioning

Ischemic postconditioninghas been shown to reduce no-reflow in small trials, but similar larger studies failed to find such an effect [70, 71]. Long-term clinical follow-up and conduct of phase III trials are currently lacking.

Conclusion

No-reflow is a frequent occurrence during PCI in the setting of STEMI. Prevention and treatment are of supreme importance because NR is associated with a larger infarct size, a reduced ejection fraction, and higher mortality. The prevention of NR necessitates shorter door-to-balloon times and the avoidance of long stents and high-pressure stent development. When there is angiographic evidence of a thrombus burden, intracoronary thrombectomy might be used. Distal protection devices have less proven long-term benefits. When NR is recognized, pharmacological intervention proves to be beneficial (according to the current knowledge, preferably the distal intracoronary infusion of adenosine or nitroprusside with a repetition if needed). The problem of NR has not yet been solved and further work in this field is needed.

References

1. Kloner RA, Ganote CE, Jennings RB. The “no-reflow” phenomenon after temporary coronary occlusion in the dog. J Clin Invest. 1974;54(6):1496–508
2. Rezkalla SH, Stankowski RV, Hanna J, Kloner RA. Management of no-reflow phenomenon in the catheterization laboratory. JACC Cardiovasc Interv. 2017;10(3):215–23.
3. Berry C, Maznyczka AM, McCartney P. Failed myocardial reperfusion during primary PCI: an unmet therapeutic need. EuroIntervention. 2019;14(16):1528–30.
4. Carrick D, Haig C, Ahmed N, et al. Myocardial hemorrhage after acute reperfused ST-segment-elevation myocardial infarction: relation to microvascular obstruction and prognostic significance. Circ Cardiovasc Imaging. 2016;9(1):e004148.
5. Bouleti C, Mewton N, Germain S. The no-reflow phenomenon: state of the art. Arch Cardiovasc Dis. 2015;108:661–74.
6. Rezkalla SH, Dharmashankar KC, Abdalrahman IB, Kloner RA. No-reflow phenomenon following percutaneous coronary intervention for acute myocardial infarction: incidence, outcome, and effect of pharmacologic therapy. J Interv Cardiol. 2010;23(5):429–36.
7. Malmberg K, Rydén L, Efendic S, et al. Randomized trial of insulin-glucose infusion following by subcutaneous insulin treatment in diabetic patients with acute myocardial infarction (DIGAMI study): effects on mortality at 1 year. J Am Coll Cardiol. 1995;26:57–65.
8. Di Carli NF, Janisse J, Grunberger G, Ager J. Role of chronic hyperglycemia in the pathogenesis of coronary microvascular dysfunction in diabetes. J Am Coll Cardiol. 2003;41(8):1387–93.
9. Li XD, Yang YJ, Hao YC, et al. Effects of pre-procedural statin therapy on myocardial no-reflow following percutaneous coronary intervention: a meta analysis. Chin Med J. 2013;126(9):1755–60.
10. Pantsios C, Kapelios C, Vakrou S, et al. Effect of elevated reperfusion pressure on “no reflow” area and infarct size in a porcine model of ischemia-reperfusion. J Cardiovasc Pharmacol Ther. 2016;21(4):405–11.
11. Ipek G, Onuk T, Karatas MB, et al. CHA2DS2-VASc score is a predictor of no-reflow in patients with ST-segment elevation myocardial infarction who underwent primary percutaneous intervention. Angiology. 2016;67(9):840–5.
12. Kurtul A, Murat SN, Yarlioglues M, et al. Mild to moderate renal impairment is associated with no-reflow phenomenon after primary percutaneous coronary intervention in acute myocardial infarction. Angiology. 2015;66(7):644–51.
13. Kurtul A, Yarlioglues M, Celik IE, et al. Association of lymphocyte-to-monocyte ratio with the no-reflow phenomenon in patients who underwent a primary percutaneous coronary intervention for ST-elevation myocardial infarction. Coron Artery Dis. 2015;26(8):706–12.

14. Amano H, Ikeda T, Toda M, et al. Plaque composition and no-reflow phenomenon during percutaneous coronary intervention of low-echoic structures in grayscale intravascular ultrasound. Int Heart J. 2016;57(3):285–91.
15. Suda A, Namiuchi S, Kawaguchi T, et al. A simple and rapid method for identification of lesions at high risk for the no-reflow phenomenon immediately before elective coronary stent implantation. Heart Vessel. 2016;31(12):1904–14.
16. Grygier M, Araszkiewicz A, Lesiak M, Grajek S. Role of adenosine as an adjunct therapy in the prevention and treatment of no-reflow phenomenon in acute myocardial infarction with ST segment elevation: review of the current data. Kardiol Pol. 2013;71(2):115–20.
17. Fischell TA, Maheshewari A. Current applications for nicardipine in invasive and interventional cardiology. J Invasive Cardiol. 2004;16(8):428–32.
18. Wang HJ, Lo PH, Lin JJ, et al. Treatment of slow/no-reflow phenomenon with intracoronary nitroprusside injection in primary coronary intervention for acute myocardial infarction. Catheter Cardiovasc Interv. 2004;63(2):171–6.
19. Johnson-Cox HA, Yang D, Ravid K. Physiological implications of adenosine receptor-mediated platelet aggregation. J Cell Physiol. 2011;226(1):46–51.
20. Mahaffey KW, Puma JA, Barbagelata NA, et al. Adenosine as an adjunct to thrombolytic therapy for acute myocardial infarction: results of a multicenter, randomized, placebo-controlled trial: the Acute Myocardial Infarction STudy of adenosine(AMISTAD) trial. J Am Coll Cardiol. 1999;34(6):1711–20.
21. Ross AM, Gibbons RJ, Stone GW, AMISTAD-II Investigators, et al. A randomized, double-blinded, placebo controlled multicenter trial of adenosine as an adjunct to reperfusion in the treatment of acute myocardial infarction (AMISTAD-II). J Am Coll Cardiol. 2005;45(11):1775–80.
22. Vijayalakshmi K, Whittaker VJ, Kunadian B, et al. Prospective, randomised, controlled trial to study the effect of intracoronary injection of verapamil and adenosine on coronary blood flow during percutaneous coronary intervention in patients with acute coronary syndromes. Heart. 2006;92(9):1278–84.
23. Niccoli G, Rigattieri S, De Vita MR, et al. Open label, randomized, placebo-controlled evaluation of intracoronary adenosine or nitroprusside after thrombus aspiration during primary percutaneous coronary intervention for the intervention of microvascular obstruction in acute myocardial infarction: the REOPEN-AMI study (Intracoronary Nitroprusside Versus Adenosine in Acute Myocardial Infarction). JACC Cardiovasc Interv. 2013;6(6):580–9.
24. Navarese EP, Buffon A, Andreotti F, et al. Adenosine improves post-procedural coronary flow but not clinical outcomes in patients with acute coronary syndrome: a meta-analysis of randomized trials. Atherosclerosis. 2012;222(1):1–7.
25. Gao Q, Yang B, Guo Y, Zheng F. Efficacy of adenosine in patients with acute myocardial infarction undergoing primary percutaneous coronary intervention: a PRISMA-compliant meta-analysis. Medicine (Baltimore). 2015;94(32):e1279.
26. Su Q, Nyi TS, Li L. Adenosine and verapamil for no-reflow during primary percutaneous coronary intervention in people with acute myocardial infarction. Cochrane Database Syst Rev. 2015;5:CD009503.
27. Polimeni A, De Rosa S, Sabatino J, et al. Impact of intracoronary adenosine administration during primary PCI: a meta-analysis. Int J Cardiol. 2016;203:1032–41.
28. Bulluck H, Sirker A, Loke YK, et al. Clinical benefit of adenosine as an adjunct to reperfusion in ST-elevation myocardial infarction patients: an updated meta-analysis of randomized controlled trials. Int J Cardiol. 2016;202:228–37.
29. Nazir SA, McCann GP, Greenwood JP. Strategies to attenuate micro-vascular obstruction during P-PCI: the randomized reperfusion facilitated by local adjunctive therapy in ST-elevation myocardial infarction trial. Eur Heart J. 2016;37:1910–9.
30. Yetgin T, Uitterdijk A, te Lintel HM, et al. Limitation of infarct size and no-reflow by intracoronary adenosine depends critically on dose and duration. JACC Cardiovasc Interv. 2015;8(15):1990–9.

31. Su Q, Li L, Liu Y. Short-term effect of verapamil on coronary no-reflow associated with percutaneous coronary intervention in patients with acute coronary syndrome: a systematic review and meta-analysis of randomized controlled trials. Clin Cardiol. 2013;36(8):E11–6.
32. Kaplan BM, Benzuly KH, Kinn JW, et al. Treatment of no-reflow in degenerated saphenous vein graft intervention: comparison of intracoronary verapamil and nitroglycerin. Catheter Cardiovasc Diagn. 1996;39(2):113–8.
33. Wang L, Cheng Z, Gu Y, Peng D. Short-term effects of verapamil and diltiazem in the treatment of no reflow phenomenon: a meta-analysis of randomized controlled trials. Biomed Res Int. 2015;2015:382086.
34. Fischell TA, Haller S, Pulukurthy S, Virk IS. Nicardipine and adenosine "flush cocktail" to prevent no-reflow during rotational atherectomy. Cardiovasc Revasc Med. 2008;9(4):224–8.
35. Fischell TA, Subraya RG, Ashraf K, et al. "Pharmacologic" distal protection sing prophylactic, intragraft nicardipine to prevent no-reflow and non-Q wave myocardial infarction during elective saphenous vein graft intervention. J Invasive Cardiol. 2007;19(2):58–62.
36. Lambert CR, Pepine CJ. Effects of intravenous and intracoronary nicardipine. Am J Cardiol. 1989;64(15):8H–15H.
37. Ferrari R. The role of mitochondria in ischemic heart disease. J Cardiovasc Pharmacol. 1996;28:1–10.
38. Wu M, Huang Z, Xie H, Zhou Z. Nicorandil in patients with acute myocardial infarction undergoing primary percutaneous coronary intervention: a systematic review and meta-analysis. PLoS One. 2013;8(10):e78231.
39. Parham WA, Bouhasin A, Ciaramita JP, et al. Coronary hyperemic dose responses of intracoronary sodium nitroprusside. Circulation. 2004;109(10):1236–43.
40. Kobatake R, Sato T, Fujiwara Y, et al. Comparison of the effects of nitroprusside versus nicorandil on the slow/no-reflow phenomenon during coronary interventions for acute myocardial infarction. Heart Vessel. 2011;26(4):379–84.
41. Parikh KH, Chag MC, Shah KJ, et al. Intracoronary boluses of adenosine and sodium nitroprusside in combination reverses slow/no-reflow during angioplasty: a clinical scenario of ischemic preconditioning. Can J Physiol Pharmacol. 2007;85(3–4):476–82.
42. Su Q, Li L, Naing KA, Sun Y. Safety and effectiveness of nitroprusside in preventing no-reflow during percutaneous coronary intervention: a systematic review. Cell Biochem Biophys. 2014;68(1):201–6.
43. Zhao S, Qi G, Tian W, et al. Effect of intracoronary nitroprusside in preventing no reflow phenomenon during primary percutaneous coronary intervention: a meta-analysis. J Interv Cardiol. 2014;27(4):356–64.
44. Amit G, Cafri C, Yaroslavtsev S, et al. Intracoronary nitroprusside for the prevention of the no-reflow phenomenon after primary percutaneous coronary intervention in acute myocardial infarction. A randomized, double-blind, placebo-controlled clinical trial. Am Heart J. 2006;152(5):887.
45. Poupko JM, Baskin SI, Moore E. The pharmacological properties of anisodamine. J Appl Toxicol. 2007;27(2):116–21.
46. Niu X, Zhang J, Bai M, et al. Effect of intracoronary agents on the no-reflow phenomenon during primary percutaneous coronary intervention in patients with ST-elevation myocardial infarction: a network meta-analysis. BMC Cardiovasc Disord. 2018;18(1):3.
47. Ibanez B, James S, Agewall S, ESC Scientific Document Group, et al. 2017 ESC Guidelines for the management of acute myocardial infarction in patients presenting with ST-segment elevation: The Task Force for the management of acute myocardial infarction in patients presenting with ST-segment elevation of the European Society of Cardiology (ESC). Eur Heart J. 2018;39(2):119–77.
48. Roffi M, Patrono C, Collet JP, ESC Scientific Document Group, et al. 2015 ESC Guidelines for the management of acute coronary syndromes in patients presenting without persistent ST-segment elevation: Task Force for the Management of Acute Coronary Syndromes in Patients Presenting without Persistent ST-Segment Elevation of the European Society of Cardiology (ESC). Eur Heart J. 2016;37(3):267–315.

49. Thiele H, Wöhrle J, Hambrecht R, et al. Intracoronary versus intravenous bolus abciximab during primary percutaneous coronary intervention in patients with acute ST-elevation myocardial infarction: a randomised trial. Lancet. 2012;379(9819):923–31.
50. Kirma C, Erkol A, Pala S, et al. Intracoronary bolus-only compared with intravenous bolus plus infusion of tirofiban application in patients with ST-elevation myocardial infarction undergoing primary percutaneous coronary intervention. Catheter Cardiovasc Interv. 2012;79(1):59–67.
51. Sun B, Liu Z, Yin H, et al. Intralesional versus intracoronary administration of glycoprotein IIb/IIIa inhibitors during percutaneous coronary intervention in patients with acute coronary syndromes: a meta-analysis of randomized controlled trials. Medicine (Baltimore). 2017;96(40):e8223.
52. Potdar A, Sharma S. The 'MAP strategy' (maximum aspiration of atherothrombus and adjunctive glycoprotein IIb/IIIa inhibitor utilization combined with prolonged inflation of balloon/stent) for preventing no-reflow in patients with ST-segment elevation myocardial infarction undergoing percutaneous coronary intervention: a retrospective analysis of seventy-one cases. Indian Heart J. 2015;67(Suppl 3):S43–6.
53. Chen WR, Tian F, Chen YD, et al. Effects of liraglutide on no-reflow in patients with acute ST-segment elevation myocardial infarction. Int J Cardiol. 2016;208:109–14.
54. Agarwal SK, Agarwal S. Role of intracoronary fibrinolytic therapy in contemporary PCI practice. Cardiovasc Revasc Med. 2018. https://doi.org/10.1016/j.carrev.2018.11.021.
55. Sezer M, Oflaz H, Gören T, et al. Intracoronary streptokinase after primary percutaneous coronary intervention. N Engl J. 2007;356(18):1823–34.
56. Sezer M, Çimen A, Aslanger E, et al. Effect of intracoronary streptokinase administered immediately after primary percutaneous coronary intervention on long-term left ventricular infarct size, volumes, and function. J Am Coll Cardiol. 2009;54(12):1065–71.
57. Geng W, Zhang Q, Liu J, et al. A randomized study of prourokinase during primary percutaneous coronary intervention in acute ST segment elevation myocardial infarction. J Interv Cardiol. 2018;31(2):136–43.
58. Sun B, Liu J, Yin H, et al. Delayed vs. immediate stenting in STEMI with a high thrombus burden: a systematic review and meta-analysis. Herz. 2018. https://doi.org/10.1007/s00059-018-4699-x.
59. Staat P, Rioufol G, Piot C, et al. Postconditioning the human heart. Circulation. 2005;112(14):2143–8.
60. Grube E, Schofer JJ, Webb J, et al. Evaluation of a balloon occlusion and aspiration system for protection from distal embolization during stenting in saphenous vein grafts. Am J Cardiol. 2002;89(8):941–5.
61. Grube E, Gerckens U, Yeung AC, et al. Prevention of distal embolisation during coronary angioplasty in saphenous vein grafts and native vessels using porous filter protection. Circulation. 2001;104(20):2436–41.
62. Gick M, Jander N, Bestehorn HP, et al. Randomized evaluation of the effects of filter-based distal protection on myocardial perfusion and infarct size after primary percutaneous catheter intervention in myocardial infarction with and without st-segment elevation. Circulation. 2005;112(10):1462–9.
63. Chollet F, Tardy J, Albucher JF, et al. Fluoxetine for motor recovery after acute ischaemic stroke (FLAME): a randomised placebo-controlled trial. Lancet Neurol. 2011;10(2):123–30.
64. De Vita M, Burzotta F, Biondi-Zoccai GG, et al. Individual patient-data meta-analysis comparing clinical outcome in patients with ST-elevation myocardial infarction treated with percutaneous coronary intervention with or without prior thrombectomy. ATTEMPT study: a pooled Analysis of Trials on ThrombEctomy in acute Myocardial infarction based on individual PatienT data. Vasc Health Risk Manag. 2009;5(1):243–7.
65. Mongeon FP, Bélisle P, Joseph L, et al. Adjunctive thrombectomy for acute myocardial infarction: a bayesian meta-analysis. Circ Cardiovasc Interv. 2010;3(1):6–16.

66. Awadalla H, Salloum J, Moustapha A, et al. Rheolytic thrombectomy does not prevent slow-, no-reflow during percutaneous coronary intervention in acute myocardial infarction. Int J Angiol. 2003;12(3):183–7.
67. Jolly SS, James S, Džavík V, et al. Thrombus aspiration in ST-segment-elevation myocardial infarction: an individual patient meta-analysis: thrombectomy trialists collaboration. Circulation. 2017;135(2):143–52.
68. Herring MJ, Dai W, Hale SL, Kloner RA. Rapid induction of hypothermia by the ThermoSuit system profoundly reduces infarct size and anatomic zone of no reflow following ischemia-reperfusion in rabbit and rat hearts. J Cardiovasc Pharmacol Ther. 2015;20(2):193–202.
69. Noc M, Erlinge D, Neskovic AN. COOL AMI EU pilot trial: a multicentre, prospective, randomised controlled trial to assess cooling as an adjunctive therapy to percutaneous intervention in patients with acute myocardial infarction. EuroIntervention. 2017;13(5):e531–9.
70. Mewton N, Thibault H, Roubille F, et al. Postconditioning attenuates no-reflow in STEMI patients. Basic Res Cardiol. 2013;108(6):383.
71. Ovize M, Baxter GF, Di Lisa F, Working Group of Cellular Biology of Heart of European Society of Cardiology, et al. Postconditioning and protection from reperfusion injury: where do we stand? Position paper from the Working Group of Cellular Biology of the Heart of the European Society of Cardiology. Cardiovasc Res. 2010;87(3):406–23.

Chapter 16
Hypercholesterolemia, Lipid-Lowering Strategies and Microcirculation

Teresa Padró, Gemma Vilahur, and Lina Badimon

Introduction

Elevated levels of blood lipids is a well-documented risk factor for cardiovascular disease (CVD), the major underlying cause for clinical events such as myocardial infarction and ischemic stroke worldwide. As such, hyperlipidemias, mainly defined as isolated elevation of total cholesterol (TC), isolated elevation of triglyceride (TG) or mixed patterns with elevations of both TC and TG are widely recognized as common metabolic disorders associated with increased atherosclerosis and ischemic heart disease [1]. Hypercholesterolemia, with a prevalence of 39% in males and 40% in females in the western countries [2], is the most common form of hyperlipidemia, thereby largely contributing to the major cause of morbidity and mortality worldwide. According to the World Health Organization (WHO), more than 50% of the ischemic heart disease and 18% of the ischemic strokes are associated with increased cholesterol levels [3].

There is a growing body of experimental and clinical studies suggesting that myocardial ischemia may occur as consequence of abnormal changes in the microvascular structure and function either in the absence of obstructive epicardial

T. Padró (✉) · G. Vilahur
Cardiovascular Program-ICCC, Research Institute Hospital de la Santa Creu i Sant Pau, IIB-Sant Pau, Barcelona, Spain

CIBERCV Instituto de Salud Carlos III, Barcelona, Spain
e-mail: tpadro@santpau.cat; gvilahur@santpau.cat

L. Badimon
Cardiovascular Program-ICCC, Research Institute Hospital de la Santa Creu i Sant Pau, IIB-Sant Pau, Barcelona, Spain

CIBERCV Instituto de Salud Carlos III, Barcelona, Spain

UAB, Barcelona, Spain
e-mail: lbadimon@santpau.cat

M. Dorobantu, L. Badimon (eds.), *Microcirculation*,
https://doi.org/10.1007/978-3-030-28199-1_16

coronary artery disease (reviewed in [4, 5]). Indeed, intra-myocardial microcirculatory disturbances are already apparent at early stages of atherosclerosis preceding any angiographically visible epicardial coronary stenosis [6]. In this respect, experimental studies using a swine model of familial hypercholesterolemia have convincingly shown the relevance of coronary microvascular dysfunction (CMD) in cardiac ischemia and impaired cardiac function before the development of critical coronary stenosis [7]. The iPowers Study aimed to investigate the association between reduced coronary flow velocity reserve (CFVR) and cardiovascular risk factors in 3568 women (27% of them with angina-like chest pain diagnostic). The authors found that women with impaired CFVR had significantly lower high-density lipoprotein cholesterol (HDL-C) levels and suggested coronary CMD as the main cause for clinical evidence of angina pectoris in the absence of obstructive coronary artery disease (<50% stenosis by coronary angiography) [8]. In addition, a cohort of 1439 patients, presenting to the catheterization laboratory with chest pain and non-obstructive coronary artery disease (>40% stenosis), revealed 64% prevalence of CMD, irrespective of sex [9].

Coronary microcirculation refers to different anatomically and functionally vascular compartments (arterioles, capillaries, and venules) with a critical role for the physiological regulation of myocardial perfusion. Typically, microvessels or "resistance vessels" such as arterioles (<100 μm diameter) are composed by an endothelial layer surrounded by smooth muscle cells. Resistance vessels have a primary function that includes the regulation of blood flow distribution to cover the metabolic demands of the heart and modulate peripheral vascular resistance playing an important role in maintaining the blood pressure [10]. Unlike large epicardial conduit arteries, arterioles respond to local metabolites rather than being under endothelial vasomotor control [11, 12]. This might facilitate a fine autonomic regulation of the coronary blood flow to match increased myocardial oxygen demand and therefore contribute to mitigate ischemia when myocardial perfusion is threatened by the progression of atherosclerosis in epicardial coronary arteries (reviewed in [5, 13]). In this respect, several studies have convincingly shown an increased risk of suffering cardiovascular events in association with CMD regardless of the degree of epicardial disease [14–16]. These observations suggest that abnormal coronary microcirculation might have prognostic value as the early sub-clinical culprit in the pathogenesis and progression of heart disease in the setting of dyslipidemia. As such, impaired function of resistance vessels, rather than conduit arteries, have predicted 5-year CVD risk in the population-based PIVUS (Prospective Study of the Vasculature in Uppsala Seniors) study [17]. Pathological processes affecting macro- and micro-vessels are closely related. Thus, current scientific evidence support the coexistence of CMD with atherosclerosis and suggest CMD as a relevant mechanism contributing to the level of cardiovascular mortality associated to the presence of cardiovascular risk factors-related comorbidities such as hypercholesterolemia (reviewed in [17, 18]).

The mechanisms by which CMD might cause cardiovascular events in the absence of epicardial artery disease are still not fully understood. However, different studies suggest that common cardiovascular risk factors such as hyperlipidemia, diabetes mellitus, hypertension, and smoking are implicated in abnormal microvascular dilatation leading to impaired coronary flow reserve (CFR), a surrogate hallmark of CMD, even in individuals without evidence of obstructive atherosclerosis (reviewed [19]).Thus, a large cohort study including 1063 participants (63% women) with <30% narrowing on coronary angiography has shown that coronary risk based on the Framingham prediction score is independently associated with the myocardial blood flow assessed by CFR [20]. Also the sub-cohort study of the Multi-Ethnic Study of Atherosclerosis (MESA) trial carried out on 222 asymptomatic middle-aged, and older men and women, supported an inverse association between the Framingham risk score and the vasodilator function of the coronary microcirculation at rest and during adenosine-induced hyperemia [21]. By these findings, Cha et al. [22] have recently demonstrated an inverse association between increasing number of cardiovascular risk factors (hypertension, diabetes, hyperlipidemia, and smoking) and reduced values of myocardial perfusion reserve index suggesting impaired coronary microcirculation in 134 self-referred as asymptomatic participants undergoing cardiac magnetic resonance analysis.

The following chapter provides an overview of the current clinical and scientific evidence regarding the presence of hyperlipidemias, particularly high LDL-cholesterol levels, and its pathological implication on the microcirculation both in the myocardium and other microvascular beds. Furthermore, the chapter highlights the pathophysiological mechanisms linking hyperlipidemia and microvascular dysfunction and discusses on the response of microvascular integrity and function to therapeutic strategies targeted to prevent and treat hypercholesterolemia.

Hypercholesterolemia and Microvascular Dysfunction

A tight relationship between serum lipids and microcirculatory changes is supported by epidemiologic evidence and observational studies as well as by prospective interventional trials. Myocardial, cerebral and retinal microvasculature share enough anatomical and physiological similarities to allow the extrapolation of the results between the different vascular compartments. Comparable to the macrovascular disease, several studies focusing on the retinal microvascular bed suggest an effect of dyslipidemia on the microcirculatory function. Thus, the results of a recently published study, including 950 participants between 7 and 19 years, supports the view that the elevation of atherogenic lipids in adolescents older than 12 years significantly associates with narrower retinal arterioles [23]. Retinal arteriolar narrowing has been documented as an independent predictor for stroke [24], metabolic syndrome [25] and coronary heart disease [26] among other cardiovascular-related comorbidities. These results point out the retinal arteriole response as a surrogate marker for peripheral vascular resistance and as such for the systemic microcirculation. In addition, early changes in the geometry of the retinal vasculature have been suggested as preclinical markers of systemic cardiovascular diseases in young individuals at high cardiovascular risk [27, 28]. In a recently published observational study, Nägele et al. [29] have reported retinal microvascular dysfunction before any clinical evidence of cardiovascular disease and any decrease in flow-mediated dilatation (brachial artery) as a measure of macrovascular function in hypercholesterolemic patients when compared to healthy controls. Studies in other microvascular territories, such as the cutaneous microcirculation, have also proven a direct association between hypercholesterolemia and microvascular dysfunction in preclinical-state diseases. In this regard, Kenney et al. [30], based on a healthy cohort with serum lipid concentrations in a broad range, found LDL-C as the best lipid-related predictor of NO-dependent cutaneous microvascular dilatation. This differs from studies in the conduit circulation where oxLDL is strongly associated with changes in the flow-mediated vasodilatation response [31] supporting the currently accepted opinion that microvascular dysfunction precedes functional changes in larger vessels during the progression of atherosclerosis disease. Expanding these findings, Bender et al. [7], using the swine model of familial hypercholesterolemia (FH), the most common monogenic disorder associated to LDL metabolism resulting in severe lifetime hypercholesterolemia, revealed that FH-derived coronary microvascular dysfunction plays a key role in limiting the myocardial oxygen balance at rest and during exercise, and thereby the cardiac efficiency in the absence of severe coronary stenosis.

Clinical Insights on the Association Between Hypercholesterolemia and Coronary Microvascular Disfunction

Reduced levels of coronary flow reserve (CFR) assessed by positron emission tomography (PET) have been documented in hypercholesterolemic asymptomatic patients with normal coronary arteries [32]. More recently, Kaufmann et al. [33], using similar PET technique in a study aimed to specifically evaluate the contribution of TC and different lipoprotein-cholesterol subfractions to CFR in hypercholesterolemic asymptomatic subjects, found that LDL-C inversely correlates with CFR in asymptomatic patients with hypercholesterolemia, whereas changes in CFR did not relate to TC and only weakly with HDL-C levels, supporting the pathogenic relevance of the LDL-C subfraction on coronary microvascular dysfunction. In addition, Mangiacapra et al. [34], using an invasive method to measure FFR and the index of microvascular resistance (IMR) in a group of hypercholesterolemic middle-age patients undergoing elective coronary angiography for CAD detection, further supported the pathogenic role of high LDL-C levels on microvascular function. The authors demonstrated a significant correlation between TC and LDL-C levels and coronary microvascular dysfunction which, in turn, was independent on the severity of epicardial coronary atherosclerosis and the number of diseased vessels, underlining the relevance of considering the microcirculatory function to better diagnose and triage asymptomatic patients at high cardiovascular risk (i.e. hypercholesterolemia). In line with these observations, Behrenbeck et al. [35], by using myocardial perfusion computed tomography (CT), convincingly showed significant changes in the spatial subresolution distribution at the intramyocardial microcirculatory blood volume in hypercholesterolemic subjects before they developed any significant change in conventional perfusion parameters.

LDL- and HDL- lipoprotein fractions comprise a spectrum of particles with different size, floatation characteristics, and function. Although risk management relies on LDL-C measurement, increasing evidence suggests that the number of LDL- particles (LDL-P) measured by nucleic magnetic resonance (NMR) is more closely related to future cardiovascular disease than levels of lipoprotein-cholesterol either in men as in women [36]. Similarly to LDL, the number of HDL particles (HDL-P) has been suggested to more accurately reflect HDL-function than HDL-cholesterol levels [37]. As such, Narang et al. [38] have shown, in a group of 24 patients with LDL-C levels below 100 mg/dL undergoing vasodilator stress cardiovascular magnetic resonance (CMR), that the number of large-HDL-P was the only lipid subfraction, among other conventional lipid variables (TC, LDL-C, HDL-C, TG) and novel lipid parameters measured by NMR, that remained associated with myocardial perfusion reserve index after multivariable adjustment.

Hypercholesterolemia plays a key pathophysiological role in the development of acute ST-elevation myocardial infarction (STEMI) [39], and microvascular injury (MVI) is a main determinant of clinical outcome after STEMI [40–43]. A substantial proportion of STEMI patients undergoing percutaneous coronary intervention (PCI) for mechanical reperfusion, despite presenting a successful epicardial coronary artery recanalization, do not achieve satisfactory myocardial reperfusion, a pathological phenomenon commonly identified as "no reflow" or as microvascular obstruction [44]. As such, several studies have proven the relationship between microvascular injury, electrocardiographic signs of no-reflow and clinical outcome [45, 46]. Thus, Van Kranenburg et al. [40] by pooling data from 1025 reperfused STEMI patients, found microvascular obstruction as an independent predictor of MACE and cardiac death at two years after infarction. Regarding hypercholesterolemia, a recent sub-analysis from *the International Survey of Acute Coronary Syndromes in Transitional Countries* registry (ISACS-TC) in 5997 patients undergoing percutaneous coronary intervention (PCI) due to myocardial infarction reported that those patients with no-reflow (2.1% of the total) were more likely to have a history of hypercholesterolemia (OR: 1.95, 95% CI: 1.31–2.91), [47]. Supporting this observation, Dobrzycki et al. [48] has demonstrated a direct association between high TC-and LDL-C levels and persistent ST-segment elevation, as assessed by ECG in STEMI patients subjected to successful primary angioplasty after MI. In a recent prospective observational study including 235 revascularized STEMI-patients, Reindl et al. [49] have proven that LDL-C levels at admission are independently associated with microvascular injury and predict the occurrence of MACE and clinical outcome after PCI in a MVI dependent manner.

Microvascular Responses to Hypercholesterolemia: Mechanistic Insights

The link between hypercholesterolemia and microvascular dysfunction mostly resides in changes associated with endothelial cell activation in both arterioles and postcapillary venules as well as impaired endothelium-dependent vasodilatation in the arteriole compartment [50, 51]. There is consistent evidence that hypercholesterolemia goes along with the creation of an inflammatory condition that may end in a severe impairment of vascular reactivity [52], enhanced leukocyte-and platelet- endothelial cell adhesion, impaired endothelial barrier function [53], enhanced thrombosis [54], and vasomotor dysfunction [55] (Fig. 16.1).

Microvascular endothelial dysfunction in response to high cholesterol levels is, at least in part, due to high oxidative stress resulting in the elevated generation of reactive oxygen species (ROS) and a consequent decline innitric oxide (NO) bioavailability [56]. Evidence of *in vivo* increased oxidative stress in the microvasculature under hypercholesterolemic conditions has been reported in hypercholesterolemic mice, in which high oxidative levels were detected by using intravital microscopy in postcapillary cremaster muscle venules [57]. The exacerbated production of ROS refers to different species including superoxide anions, hydrogen peroxides, and hydroxyl radicals. As such, it has been reported an enhanced generation of superoxide products derived from xanthineoxidases in large arteries of

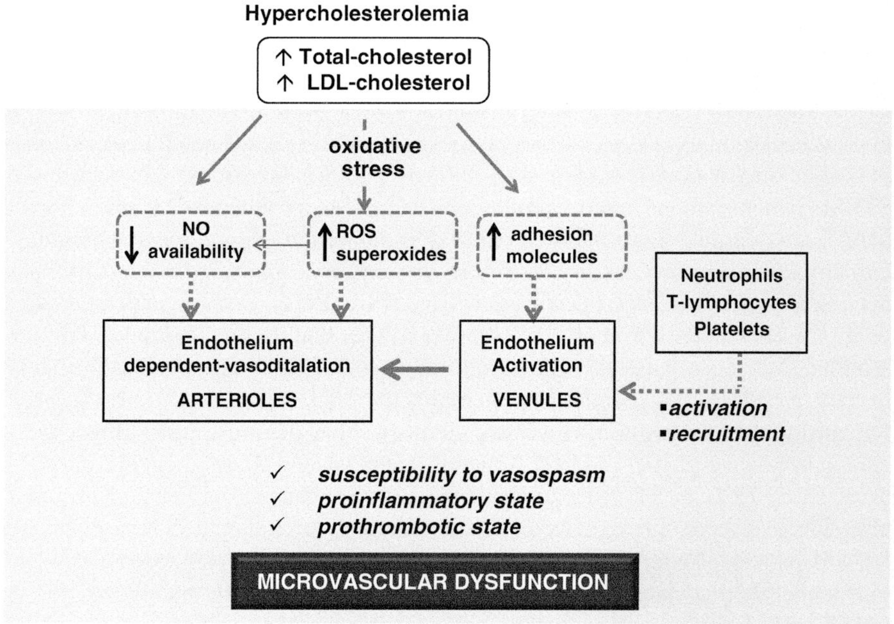

Fig. 16.1 Microvasculature responses to elevated cholesterol levels. *ROS* reactive oxygen species, *NO* endothelial nitric oxide

hypercholesterolemic animals which in turn were associated with impaired NO bioavailability [58]. Increased oxidative stress and generation of ROS species may also contribute to increased levels of oxidized forms of LDL-C (oxLDL), which are implicated in atherosclerosis-related vascular-dysfunction and inflammation [59]. Unlike results of studies performed in conduit arteries neither oxLDL or the lectin-like oxLDL (LOX-1) show an independent predictor value in cutaneous vasodilatation [30]. These observations suggest a different sensitivity for the macro- and micro- vascular compartments to signaling mechanisms induced by the specific LDL-forms.

In the arterioles, hypercholesterolemia-induced endothelial dysfunction is manifested as reduced secretion of endothelium-derived relaxing factors such as NO in response to agents that under physiological conditions stimulate NO production in the endothelial cell. A decrease in the endothelium-dependent vasodilatation is evident in the cutaneous microcirculation of hypercholesterolemic subjects in response to local skin heating [60], a stimulus associated with higher NO synthase (NOs) levels and increased NO production [61]. In agreement with these findings, Kenney et al. [30] reported an inverse correlation between LDL-C levels and eNOS-dependent cutaneous vasodilatation, a model for microvascular function, in a healthy cohort of subjects with a broad spectrum of serum cholesterol concentrations. Also, Sorop et al. [62], using an experimental high-fat diet model in swine, demonstrated reduced basal NO production and a concomitant trend toward lower eNOS expression levels in the microvessels of the heart in association with increased TC- and LDL-C plasma levels. In addition, the same authors have recently demonstrated that chronic hypercholesterolemia, when combined with other common cardiovascular comorbidities such as diabetes mellitus and hypertension, leads to left ventricular diastolic dysfunction, in the absence of major geometrical alterations in the heart, but in association with perturbed myocardial NO production and oxidative stress, endothelium-dependent microvascular dysfunction and systemic inflammation [63]. Two other findings further support the relevance of the ROS/NO imbalance for hypercholesterolemia induced microvascular dysfunction. As such, Nellore et al. [64] proved that administration of the NOS substrate, L-arginine, reverses the impaired perfusion of the microvasculature in a rat model of acute hypercholesterolemia, and Mugge et al. [65] demonstrated that supplementation with endogenous superoxide scavengers such as superoxide dismutase (SOD) restores normal function of arteries in cholesterol-fed rabbits.

The high capacity of superoxides to interact with NO may account for the low NO-availability detected when microvessels are exposed to hypercholesterolemia. However, according to Holowatz et al. [60], the detrimental effects of hypercholesterolemia in the skin microcirculation are mainly a consequence of low L-arginine bioavailability due to upregulation of arginase-activity, increase in ascorbate sensitive oxidants [66], and decrease in the eNOS cofactor tetrahydrobiopterin [67]. Furthermore, hypercholesterolemia goes along with increased levels of the eNOS inhibitor ADMA (asymmetric dimethylarginine), which might result in part by a concomitant decrease in its degradation enzyme dimethylarginine dimethylaminohydrolase [68]. In addition, adenosine-mediated relaxation is shown to be significantly impaired in coronary arterioles of diet-induced hypercholesterolemic swine, an effect that has been associated with impaired adenosine-activation of Kv channels in both endothelium-intact and -denuded coronary arterioles [69].

Over recent years, it has become increasingly recognized that micro vessels also display inflammatory and thrombogenic properties in response to hypercholesterolemia, involving pathophysiological mechanisms similar to those occurring in macrovascular disease (*reviewed in* [70]). Yet, under hypercholesterolemic conditions, there is an increased and diffuse leukocyte adhesion in venular segments of the microcirculation in contrast to the local leukocyte recruitment that occurs at sites of damaged large-arteries. In the microvasculature, inflammatory cells are primarily recruited to post-capillary venules from where they perfuse and exert detrimental effects in other areas of the microvascular bed [64]. Thus, the venular endothelium rapidly upregulates the expression of adhesion molecules such as P-selectin and ICAM-1 upon exposure to high cholesterol levels favoring leukocyte rolling and further recruitment [71]. More recently, Lubrano et al. [72] have suggested a direct link between LDL-dependent microvascular inflammation, oxidative stress, and up-regulation of LOX-1-, in a process mediated by cytokines such as interleukin-6.

Interestingly, interleukin-6 has also been associated with microvascular thrombosis in other inflammatory-related pathologies [73]. Neutrophils represent the predominant type of inflammatory cells recruited at the postcapillary venules as an early response to hypercholesterolemia.

Recruited neutrophils support platelet adhesion into the post-capillary venules favoring a pro-thrombotic state [74]. In turn, soluble factors released into the blood from leucocytes and platelets recruited to nearby venules further contribute to expanding arteriolar dysfunction [75]. T-lymphocytes and the release of inflammatory cytokines such as interferon-γ (IFN- γ) and the CD40/CD40L dyad have also been reported as being relevant components contributing to the oxidative stress and vasomotor dysfunction that occurs in the microcirculation in response to hypercholesterolemia [75–77].

Effect of Lipid-Lowering Treatments on Microvascular Dysfunction

Current classification schemes and interventional strategies for the treatment of hyperlipidemia are based on the National Cholesterol Education Panel's (NCEP) Adult Treatment Program-3 (ATP-III) guidelines. Concerning microcirculation, no large studies have been conducted so far to investigate the effects of lipid-lowering therapies on abnormal microvascular function. Most studies are small and not always randomized. In addition, the high variability in the clinical data does not allow drawing solid conclusions regarding the potential link between lowering LDL-C levels and the modulation of microvessel function.

Supporting the association between LDL-cholesterol levels and microvascular dysfunction, the use of lipoprotein apheresis, as an interventional strategy to remove LDL-C or other lipoproteins from plasma [78], has consistently proved to improve microvascular function by reducing the detrimental effects of high-cholesterol levels. Thus, myocardial blood perfusion, assessed as CFR by stress echocardiography on the left anterior descending coronary artery, is increased as compared to baseline in patients with severe FH regularly treated with lipid-apheresis on top of maximally tolerated lipid-lowering therapy. As such, CFR values in these patients are found to be significantly higher than those in the control group which only receive lipid-lowering drugs during a follow-up period of 24 months [79]. Several other studies have also reported an improvement of the cardiac microcirculation in patients undergoing lipid-apheresis therapy by increasing CFR and minimal coronary resistance [80, 81]. Recently, Wu et al. [82] demonstrated, by using myocardial contrast echocardiography (MCE) and skeletal muscle contrast-microvascular perfusion (CEU), that resting coronary microvascular function is immediately restored to normal levels in patients with a diagnosis of FH after being subjected to lipoprotein apheresis.

Interestingly, this study observes that changes in microvascular flux rate do not correlate with any of the lipid variables despite their substantial reduction after lipoprotein-apheresis. Accordingly, the authors suggest that the benefits of lipoprotein apheresis in the microvasculature mostly relies on the improvement of hypercholesterolemia-induced effects, such as reduced bioavailability of endothelial-derived vasodilators, increased oxidative signaling, or levels of circulating inflammatory markers. In line with these findings, the study by Rossenbach et al. [83] on peripheral microcirculation supports that beneficial effects after a single LA-session are directly related to changes in vasoconstrictory and dilatative mediators in blood viscosity and erythrocyte aggregation.

To date, statins are the first-line therapy according to the guidelines to lower elevated LDL-C levels and their use has shown to be highly effective in both reducing plasma LDL-C levels and preventing cardiovascular clinical events [84]. Key clinical trials have clearly demonstrated the value of statins in primary and secondary prevention of coronary heart disease [85]. However, studies investigating the effects of statins on the microcirculation are limited and mainly focus on the clinical benefit of statins in improving microvascular function in the infarcted area of patients with acute MI after -PCI [86]. In this regard, Paraskevaidis et al. [87] reported that statin therapy prior revascularization improves coronary microcirculation in patients with acute coronary syndromes, with and without STEMI, as assessed by contrast echocardiography in a 30 days follow-up period.

Statins act by inhibiting 3-hydroxy-3-methylglutaryl-CoA reductase (HMGCR), which results in the reduction of intracellular cholesterol through inhibition of the hepatic cholesterol biosynthesis and thereby in the upregulation of hepatic low-density lipoprotein (LDL) receptors, consequently increasing the clearance of LDL-C from the bloodstream. Whether the benefits of statins on microvascular-function occur via their lipid-lowering effect or through the so-called pleiotropic properties is still under debate. As such, Magiacapra et al. [34] have reported, in hypercholesterolemic patients with different degree of disease severity and treated with various patterns of lipid-lowering therapy, a direct correlation between LDL-C levels and the index of microvascular resistance, independently of statin intake and dosage, –, suggesting that the benefits of statins on microvascular function mainly occur through lipid-lowering rather pleiotropic-related effects. In contrast, Bonetti et al. [88], have proved, in a pig model of diet-induced hypercholesterolemia that simvastatin prevents attenuation of the myocardial perfusion response and the increase in coronary microvascular permeability during cardiac stress associated with hypercholesterolemia, independently of any lipid-lowering effect. Similarly, 12-week atorvastatin treatment in subjects with FH and no obstructive coronary artery disease has shown to normalize the myocardial blood flow reserve before achieving the optimal target for LDL-C [89]. In agreement with these observations, a 4-week treatment with statins in patients with a newly diagnosed hypercholesterolemia resulted in a consistent improvement in the vasodilatation of retinal arterioles and venules through a mechanism that seems to involve the NO-mediated pathway [90]. Besides, statins have demonstrated to attenuate platelet adhesion to intestinal venules in a diet-induced hypercholesterolemic mice model through a NO-mediated mechanism rather than by a cholesterol-lowering effect [91].

Statin-induced reduction of microvascular injury in the setting of cardiac interventions seems to occur through pleiotropic effects as well. By using a Western-diet fed pig model, we have provided evidence that acute HMG-CoA-reductase inhibition during total ischemia and prior reperfusion limits reperfusion injury and that oral maintenance with simvastatin for 42 days improves cardiac healing post-myocardial infarction at the time that suppresses cardiac RhoA mobilization and triggers the protective Akt/eNOS signaling pathway [92]. In the clinical setting, a prospective study in 74 patients undergoing percutaneous transluminal coronary angioplasty (PTCA) has demonstrated that pravastatin administration increased microvascular perfusion in normocholesterolemic patients with single-vessel coronary disease [93]. By using radionuclide exercise stress testing by myocardial perfusion single-photon emission computed tomography (SPECT), the authors concluded that 3% of patients receiving statins showed reversible perfusion defects confined to the microvasculature after 6 months from the PCTA, whereas this pathological response referred to 29% of patients receiving placebo. In agreement with these experimental and clinical findings, the ARMYDA (Atorvastatin for Reduction of Myocardial Damage) trial evidenced that pretreatment with atorvastatin for 7 days prior to elective PCI prevented peri-procedural myocardial injury [94]. The authors attributed this benefit to statin-related anti-inflammatory properties likely contributing to reducing microembolization during coronary intervention. Interestingly, a clinical benefit in terms of 30-day MACE was reported in either stable angina patients already on statin treatment [95] as well as in ACS patients [96].

Regulation of the hepatic LDL-R activity is primarily mediated by two mechanisms involving the sterol regulatory element-binding protein 2 (SREBP-2) during transcription and PCSK9 (convertase subtilisin/kexin type 9) post-transcriptionally. Over recent years, PCSK9 inhibitors have emerged as a promising new target in the field of lipid management [98, 99]. PCSK9 reduces the number of LDLR in hepatocytes by promoting their metabolism, thereby, targeting and inactivating PCSK9 results in a marked reduction in LDL-C levels [97], Interestingly, a prospective cohort study with 4232 participants and 491 incident events during 15-years follow-up, has proved that baseline serum PCSK9 concentrations associate with future risk of CVD independently of established risk factors [100]. Moreover, the FOURIER (Further Cardiovascular Outcomes Research With PCSK9 Inhibition in Patients With Elevated Risk) study, a placebo-control trial involving 27,564 patients with atherosclerotic cardiovascular disease confirmed the concept that PCSK9 inhibition might provide protection against atherosclerotic cardiovascular diseases and improve cardiovascular outcomes beyond the existing conventional therapy [101]. Although, little information is available about potential effects other that LDL-lowering involved in athero protection by PCSK9 inhibition, recently published experimental studies suggest that PCSK9 inhibition attenuates oxidative stress and induces anti-inflammatory effects in atherosclerotic vessels (revised in [102]). However, no studies so far have reported on the effects of PCSK9 inhibition on hypercholesterolemia-associated microcirculation dysfunction.

Conclusions

Detrimental effects of hypercholesterolemia on coronary microcirculation refer to a combination of structural and functional abnormalities with a causative role for cardiovascular disease, both in early stages of the atherosclerotic process prior the development of coronary stenosis as well in the setting of acute ischemic coronary event, contributing to enlarge the extent of myocardial damage. While the mechanisms underlying microvascular dysfunction in response to hypercholesterolemia are not fully understood, the available evidence reveals a plethora of events resulting in a severe pro-inflammatory condition, endothelial cell dysfunction in association with enhanced oxidative stress, and reduced NO bioavailability and higher platelet susceptibility, predisposing to a prothrombotic condition and further worsening microvascular damage. To date, the benefits of lipid-lowering therapies on coronary microcirculation have mostly focused on statins and patients undergoing cardiac intervention. However, given the similarity of pathological responses induced by chronic and abnormal lipid levels on macro- and micro- vessels, novel interventional strategies to treat hypercholesterolemia and related cardiovascular diseases need to be urgently addressed in the microcirculation.

Sources of Funding This work was supported by FIS [PI16/01915 to T.P.] from Instituto de Salud Carlos II; Plan Nacional de Salud (PNS) [PNS 2015-71653-R (to G.V.) and 2013-42962-R to L.B.] from the Spanish Ministry of Science and Innovation; CIBERCV (L.B.) and; FEDER "Una Manera de Hacer Europa". We thank the continuous support of the Generalitat of Catalunya (Secretaria d'Universitats i Recerca del Departament d'Economia i Coneixement de la Generalitat; 2014SGR1303) and the Fundación Investigación Cardiovascular.

References

1. Ramasamy I. Update on the molecular biology of dyslipidemias. Clin Chim Acta. 2016;454:143–85. https://doi.org/10.1016/j.cca.2015.10.033.
2. World Health Organization. Rapport sur la Situation Mondiale des Maladies non Transmissibles (Résumé d'Orientation). Geneva: OMS; 2010. https://www.who.int/nmh/publications/ncd_report-summary_fr.pdf.
3. World Health Organization. Global Health Observatory. Raised Cholesterol: observations trends 2011. 2011. http://www.who.int/gho/ncd/risk_factors/cholesterol_text/en/WHO.
4. Herrmann J, Kaski JC, Lerman A. Coronary microvascular dysfunction in the clinical setting: from mystery to reality. Eur Heart J. 2012;33:2771–2782b. https://doi.org/10.1093/eurheartj/ehs246.
5. Pries AR, Habazettl H, Ambrosio G, et al. A review of methods for assessment of coronary microvascular disease in both clinical and experimental settings. Cardiovasc Res. 2008;80(2):165–74.
6. van den Heuvel M, Sorop O, Koopmans S-J, et al. Coronary microvascular dysfunction in a porcine model of early atherosclerosis and diabetes. Am J Physiol Heart Circ Physiol. 2012;302:H85–94. https://doi.org/10.1152/ajpheart.00311.2011.
7. Bender SB, de Beer VJ, Tharp DL, et al. Severe familial hypercholesterolemia impairs the regulation of coronary blood flow and oxygen supply during exercise. Basic Res Cardiol. 2016;111:61. https://doi.org/10.1007/s00395-016-0579-9.
8. Mygind ND, Michelsen MM, Pena A, et al. Coronary microvascular function and myocardial fibrosis in women with angina pectoris and no obstructive coronary artery disease: the iPOWER study. J Cardiovasc Magn Reson. 2016;18(1):76. https://doi.org/10.1186/s12968-016-0295-5.
9. Sara JD, Widmer RJ, Matsuzawa Y, et al. Prevalence of coronary microvascular dysfunction among patients with chest pain and nonobstructive coronary artery disease. JACC Cardiovasc Interv. 2015;8:1445–53. https://doi.org/10.1016/j.jcin.2015.06.017.
10. Camici PG, d'Amati G, Rimoldi O. Coronary microvascular dysfunction: mechanisms and functional assessment. Nat Rev Cardiol. 2015;12:48–62. https://doi.org/10.1038/nrcardio.2014.160.
11. Kuo L, Chilian WM, Davis MJ. Coronary arteriolar myogenic response is independent of endothelium. Circ Res. 1990;66:860–6. https://doi.org/10.1161/01.RES.66.3.860
12. Quyyumi AA, Dakak N, Andrews NP, et al. Nitric oxide activity in the human coronary circulation. Impact of risk factors for coronary atherosclerosis. J Clin Invest. 1995;95:1747–55. https://doi.org/10.1172/JCI117852.
13. Pries AR, Reglin B. Coronary microcirculatory pathophysiology: can we afford it to remain a black box? Eur Heart J. 2017;38(7):478–88. https://doi.org/10.1093/eurheartj/ehv760
14. Lerman A, Holmes DR, Herrmann J, Gersh BJ. Microcirculatory dysfunction in ST-elevation myocardial infarction: cause, consequence, or both? Eur Heart J. 2007;28:788–97. https://doi.org/10.1093/eurheartj/ehl501.
15. Pepine CJ, Anderson RD, Sharaf BL, et al. Coronary microvascular reactivity to adenosine predicts adverse outcome in women evaluated for suspected ischemia results from the National Heart, Lung and Blood Institute WISE (Women's Ischemia Syndrome Evaluation) study. J Am Coll Cardiol. 2010;55:2825–32. https://doi.org/10.1016/j.jacc.2010.01.054.
16. Britten MB, Zeiher AM, Schächinger V. Microvascular dysfunction in angiographically normal or mildly diseased coronary arteries predicts adverse cardiovascular long-term outcome. Coron Artery Dis. 2004;15:259–64. https://doi.org/10.1097/01.mca.0000134590.99841.81.
17. Lind L, Berglund L, Larsson A, Sundström J. Endothelial function in resistance and conduit arteries and 5-year risk of cardiovascular disease. Circulation. 2011;123:1545–51. https://doi.org/10.1161/CIRCULATIONAHA.110.984047.
18. Duncker DJ, Koller A, Merkus D, Canty JM. Regulation of coronary blood flow in health and ischemic heart disease. Prog Cardiovasc Dis. 2015;57:409–22. https://doi.org/10.1016/j.pcad.2014.12.002.

19. Crea F, Camici PG, Bairey Merz CN. Coronary microvascular dysfunction: an update. Eur Heart J. 2014;35:1101–11. https://doi.org/10.1093/eurheartj/eht513.
20. Rubinshtein R, Yang EH, Rihal CS, et al. Coronary microcirculatory vasodilator function in relation to risk factors among patients without obstructive coronary disease and low to intermediate Framingham score. Eur Heart J. 2010;31:936–42. https://doi.org/10.1093/eurheartj/ehp459.
21. Wang L, Jerosch-Herold M, Jacobs DR, et al. Coronary risk factors and myocardial perfusion in asymptomatic adults. J Am Coll Cardiol. 2006;47:565–72. https://doi.org/10.1016/j.jacc.2005.09.036.
22. Cha MJ, Kim SM, Kim HS, et al. Association of cardiovascular risk factors on myocardial perfusion and fibrosis in asymptomatic individuals: cardiac magnetic resonance study. Acta Radiol. 2018;59:1300–8. https://doi.org/10.1177/0284185118757274.
23. Xiao W, Guo X, Ding X, He M. Serum lipid profiles and dyslipidaemia are associated with retinal microvascular changes in children and adolescents. Sci Rep. 2017;7:44874. https://doi.org/10.1038/srep44874.
24. Yatsuya H, Folsom AR, Wong TY, et al. Retinal microvascular abnormalities and risk of lacunar stroke. Stroke. 2010;41:1349–55. https://doi.org/10.1161/STROKEAHA.110.580837.
25. Saito K, Kawasaki Y, Nagao Y, Kawasaki R. Retinal arteriolar narrowing is associated with a 4-year risk of incident metabolic syndrome. Nutr Diabetes. 2015;5:e165. https://doi.org/10.1038/nutd.2015.15.
26. Wong TY, Klein R, Sharrett AR, et al. Retinal arteriolar narrowing and risk of coronary heart disease in men and women. The atherosclerosis risk in communities study. JAMA. 2002;287:1153–9. https://doi.org/10.1001/jama.287.9.1153.
27. Broe R, Rasmussen ML, Frydkjaer-Olsen U, et al. Retinal vascular fractals predict long-term microvascular complications in type 1 diabetes mellitus: the Danish Cohort of Pediatric Diabetes 1987 (DCPD1987). Diabetologia. 2014;57:2215–21. https://doi.org/10.1007/s00125-014-3317-6.
28. Benitez-Aguirre PZ, Sasongko MB, Craig ME, et al. Retinal vascular geometry predicts incident renal dysfunction in young people with type 1 diabetes. Diabetes Care. 2012;35:599–604. https://doi.org/10.2337/dc11-1177.
29. Nägele MP, Barthelmes J, Ludovici V, et al. Retinal microvascular dysfunction in hypercholesterolemia. J Clin Lipidol. 2018;12:1523–1531.e2. https://doi.org/10.1016/j.jacl.2018.07.015.
30. Kenney WL, Cannon JG, Alexander LM. Cutaneous microvascular dysfunction correlates with serum LDL and sLOX-1 receptor concentrations. Microvasc Res. 2013;85:112–7. https://doi.org/10.1016/j.mvr.2012.10.010.
31. van der Zwan LP, Teerlink T, Dekker JM, et al. Circulating oxidized LDL: determinants and association with brachial flow-mediated dilation. J Lipid Res. 2009;50:342–9. https://doi.org/10.1194/jlr.P800030-JLR200.
32. Yokoyama I, Ohtake T, Momomura S, et al. Reduced coronary flow reserve in hypercholesterolemic patients without overt coronary stenosis. Circulation. 1996;94:3232–8. https://doi.org/10.1161/01.cir.94.12.3232.
33. Kaufmann PA, Gnecchi-Ruscone T, Schäfers KP, et al. Low density lipoprotein cholesterol and coronary microvascular dysfunction in hypercholesterolemia. J Am Coll Cardiol. 2000;36:103–9. https://doi.org/10.1016/s0735-1097(00)00697-5.
34. Mangiacapra F, De Bruyne B, Peace AJ, et al. High cholesterol levels are associated with coronary microvascular dysfunction. J Cardiovasc Med (Hagerstown). 2012;13:439–42. https://doi.org/10.2459/JCM.0b013e328351725a.
35. Behrenbeck TR, McCollough CH, Miller WL, et al. Early changes in myocardial microcirculation in asymptomatic hypercholesterolemic subjects: as detected by perfusion CT. Ann Biomed Eng. 2014;42:515–25. https://doi.org/10.1007/s10439-013-0934-z.
36. Cromwell WC, Otvos JD, Keyes MJ, et al. LDL particle number and risk of future cardiovascular disease in the Framingham offspring study - implications for LDL management. J Clin Lipidol. 2007;1:583–92. https://doi.org/10.1016/j.jacl.2007.10.001.

37. Tan HC, Tai ES, Sviridov D, et al. Relationships between cholesterol efflux and high-density lipoprotein particles in patients with type 2 diabetes mellitus. J Clin Lipidol. 2011;5:467–73. https://doi.org/10.1016/j.jacl.2011.06.016.
38. Narang A, Mor-Avi V, Bhave NM, et al. Large high-density lipoprotein particle number is independently associated with microvascular function in patients with well-controlled low-density lipoprotein concentration: a vasodilator stress magnetic resonance perfusion study. J Clin Lipidol. 2016;10:314–22. https://doi.org/10.1016/j.jacl.2015.12.006.
39. Catapano AL, Graham I, De Backer G, et al. 2016 ESC/EAS guidelines for the management of dyslipidaemias. Atherosclerosis. 2016;253:281–344. https://doi.org/10.1016/j.atherosclerosis.2016.08.018.
40. van Kranenburg M, Magro M, Thiele H, et al. Prognostic value of microvascular obstruction and infarct size, as measured by CMR in STEMI patients. JACC Cardiovasc Imaging. 2014;7:930–9. https://doi.org/10.1016/j.jcmg.2014.05.010.
41. Hamirani YS, Wong A, Kramer CM, Salerno M. Effect of microvascular obstruction and intramyocardial hemorrhage by CMR on LV remodeling and outcomes after myocardial infarction: a systematic review and meta-analysis. JACC Cardiovasc Imaging. 2014;7:940–52. https://doi.org/10.1016/j.jcmg.2014.06.012.
42. de Waha S, Desch S, Eitel I, et al. Impact of early vs. late microvascular obstruction assessed by magnetic resonance imaging on long-term outcome after ST-elevation myocardial infarction: a comparison with traditional prognostic markers. Eur Heart J. 2010;31:2660–8. https://doi.org/10.1093/eurheartj/ehq247.
43. Eitel I, de Waha S, Wöhrle J, et al. Comprehensive prognosis assessment by CMR imaging after ST-segment elevation myocardial infarction. J Am Coll Cardiol. 2014;64:1217–26. https://doi.org/10.1016/j.jacc.2014.06.1194.
44. Rezkalla SH, Kloner RA. Coronary no-reflow phenomenon: from the experimental laboratory to the cardiac catheterization laboratory. Catheter Cardiovasc Interv. 2008;72:950–7. https://doi.org/10.1002/ccd.21715.
45. Rommel KP, Baum A, Mende M, et al. Prognostic significance and relationship of worst lead residual ST segment elevation with myocardial damage assessed by cardiovascular MRI in myocardial infarction. Heart. 2014;100:1257–63. https://doi.org/10.1136/heartjnl-2013-305462.
46. Wu KC, Zerhouni EA, Judd RM, et al. Prognostic significance of microvascular obstruction by magnetic resonance imaging in patients with acute myocardial infarction. Circulation. 1998;97:765–72. https://doi.org/10.1161/01.cir.97.8.765.
47. Cenko E, Ricci B, Kedev S, et al. The no-reflow phenomenon in the young and in the elderly. Int J Cardiol. 2016;222:1122–8. https://doi.org/10.1016/j.ijcard.2016.07.209.
48. Dobrzycki S, Kozuch M, Kamiński K, et al. High cholesterol in patients with ECG signs of no-reflow after myocardial infarction. Rocz Akad Med Bialymst. 2003;48:118–22.
49. Reindl M, Reinstadler SJ, Feistritzer H-J, et al. Relation of low-density lipoprotein cholesterol with microvascular injury and clinical outcome in revascularized ST-elevation myocardial infarction. J Am Heart Assoc. 2017;6(10):e006957. https://doi.org/10.1161/JAHA.117.006957.
50. Gould KL, Martucci JP, Goldberg DI, et al. Short-term cholesterol lowering decreases size and severity of perfusion abnormalities by positron emission tomography after dipyridamole in patients with coronary artery disease. A potential noninvasive marker of healing coronary endothelium. Circulation. 1994;89:1530–8. https://doi.org/10.1161/01.cir.89.4.1530.
51. Scalia R, Appel JZ, Lefer AM. Leukocyte-endothelium interaction during the early stages of hypercholesterolemia in the rabbit: role of P-selectin, ICAM-1, and VCAM-1. Arterioscler Thromb Vasc Biol. 1998;18:1093–100.
52. Stokes KY. Microvascular responses to hypercholesterolemia: the interactions between innate and adaptive immune responses. Antioxid Redox Signal. 2006;8:1141–51. https://doi.org/10.1089/ars.2006.8.1141.
53. Acharya NK, Qi X, Goldwaser EL, et al. Retinal pathology is associated with increased blood–retina barrier permeability in a diabetic and hypercholesterolaemic pig model: beneficial

effects of the $LpPLA_2$ inhibitor Darapladib. Diabetes Vasc Dis Res. 2017;14:200–13. https://doi.org/10.1177/1479164116683149.
54. Granger DN, Rodrigues SF, Yildirim A, Senchenkova EY. Microvascular responses to cardiovascular risk factors. Microcirculation. 2010;17:192–205. https://doi.org/10.1111/j.1549-8719.2009.00015.x.
55. Raman KG, Gandley RE, Rohland J, et al. Early hypercholesterolemia contributes to vasomotor dysfunction and injury associated atherogenesis that can be inhibited by nitric oxide. J Vasc Surg. 2011;53:754–63. https://doi.org/10.1016/j.jvs.2010.09.038.
56. Hein TW, Kuo L. LDLs impair vasomotor function of the coronary microcirculation: role of superoxide anions. Circ Res. 1998;83:404–14. https://doi.org/10.1161/01.res.83.4.404.
57. Stokes KY, Clanton EC, Clements KP, Granger DN. Role of interferon-gamma in hypercholesterolemia-induced leukocyte-endothelial cell adhesion. Circulation. 2003;107:2140–5. https://doi.org/10.1161/01.CIR.0000062687.80186.A0.
58. Ohara Y, Peterson TE, Sayegh HS, et al. Dietary correction of hypercholesterolemia in the rabbit normalizes endothelial superoxide anion production. Circulation. 1995;92:898–903. https://doi.org/10.1161/01.CIR.92.4.898.
59. Weber C, Erl W, Weber KS, Weber PC. Effects of oxidized low density lipoprotein, lipid mediators and statins on vascular cell interactions. Clin Chem Lab Med. 1999;37:243–51. https://doi.org/10.1515/CCLM.1999.043.
60. Holowatz LA, Santhanam L, Webb A, et al. Oral atorvastatin therapy restores cutaneous microvascular function by decreasing arginase activity in hypercholesterolaemic humans. J Physiol. 2011;589:2093–103. https://doi.org/10.1113/jphysiol.2010.203935.
61. Bruning RS, Santhanam L, Stanhewicz AE, et al. Endothelial nitric oxide synthase mediates cutaneous vasodilation during local heating and is attenuated in middle-aged human skin. J Appl Physiol. 2012;112:2019–26. https://doi.org/10.1152/japplphysiol.01354.2011.
62. Sorop O, van den Heuvel M, van Ditzhuijzen NS, et al. Coronary microvascular dysfunction after long-term diabetes and hypercholesterolemia. Am J Physiol Heart Circ Physiol. 2016;311:H1339–51. https://doi.org/10.1152/ajpheart.00458.2015.
63. Sorop O, Heinonen I, van Kranenburg M, et al. Multiple common comorbidities produce left ventricular diastolic dysfunction associated with coronary microvascular dysfunction, oxidative stress, and myocardial stiffening. Cardiovasc Res. 2018;114:954–64. https://doi.org/10.1093/cvr/cvy038.
64. Nellore K, Harris NR. L-arginine and antineutrophil serum enable venular control of capillary perfusion in hypercholesterolemic rats. Microcirculation. 2002;9:477–85. https://doi.org/10.1038/sj.mn.7800162.
65. Mügge A, Elwell JH, Peterson TE, et al. Chronic treatment with polyethylene-glycolated superoxide dismutase partially restores endothelium-dependent vascular relaxations in cholesterol-fed rabbits. Circ Res. 1991;69:1293–300. https://doi.org/10.1161/01.res.69.5.1293.
66. Holowatz LA, Kenney WL. Oral atorvastatin therapy increases nitric oxide-dependent cutaneous vasodilation in humans by decreasing ascorbate-sensitive oxidants. Am J Physiol Regul Integr Comp Physiol. 2011;301:R763–8. https://doi.org/10.1152/ajpregu.00220.2011.
67. Holowatz LA, Kenney WL. Acute localized administration of tetrahydrobiopterin and chronic systemic atorvastatin treatment restore cutaneous microvascular function in hypercholesterolaemic humans. J Physiol. 2011;589:4787–97. https://doi.org/10.1113/jphysiol.2011.212100.
68. Landmesser U, Hornig B, Drexler H. Endothelial dysfunction in hypercholesterolemia: mechanisms, pathophysiological importance, and therapeutic interventions. Semin Thromb Hemost. 2000;26:529–38. https://doi.org/10.1055/s-2000-13209.
69. Heaps CL, Tharp DL, Bowles DK. Hypercholesterolemia abolishes voltage-dependent K+ channel contribution to adenosine-mediated relaxation in porcine coronary arterioles. Am J Physiol Heart Circ Physiol. 2005;288:H568–76. https://doi.org/10.1152/ajpheart.00157.2004.
70. Vitiello L, Spoletini I, Gorini S, et al. Microvascular inflammation in atherosclerosis. IJC Metab Endocr. 2014;3:1–7. https://doi.org/10.1016/j.ijcme.2014.03.002.

71. Ishikawa M, Stokes KY, Zhang JH, et al. Cerebral microvascular responses to hypercholesterolemia: roles of NADPH oxidase and P-selectin. Circ Res. 2004;94:239–44. https://doi.org/10.1161/01.RES.0000111524.05779.60.
72. Lubrano V, Balzan S. Roles of LOX-1 in microvascular dysfunction. Microvasc Res. 2016;105:132–40. https://doi.org/10.1016/j.mvr.2016.02.006.
73. Hozumi H, Russell J, Vital S, Granger DN. IL-6 mediates the intestinal microvascular thrombosis associated with experimental colitis. Inflamm Bowel Dis. 2016;22:560–8. https://doi.org/10.1097/MIB.0000000000000656.
74. Tailor A, Granger DN. Hypercholesterolemia promotes leukocyte-dependent platelet adhesion in murine postcapillary venules. Microcirculation. 2004;11:597–603. https://doi.org/10.1080/10739680490503393.
75. Stokes KY, Granger DN. Platelets: a critical link between inflammation and microvascular dysfunction. J Physiol. 2012;590:1023–34. https://doi.org/10.1113/jphysiol.2011.225417.
76. Stokes KY, Clanton EC, Bowles KS, et al. The role of T-lymphocytes in hypercholesterolemia-induced leukocyte-endothelial interactions. Microcirculation. 2002;9:407–17. https://doi.org/10.1038/sj.mn.7800148.
77. Stokes KY, Gurwara S, Granger DN. T-cell derived interferon-gamma contributes to arteriolar dysfunction during acute hypercholesterolemia. Arterioscler Thromb Vasc Biol. 2007;27:1998–2004. https://doi.org/10.1161/ATVBAHA.107.146449.
78. Wang A, Richhariya A, Gandra SR, et al. Systematic review of low-density lipoprotein cholesterol apheresis for the treatment of familial hypercholesterolemia. J Am Heart Assoc. 2016;5(7):e003294. https://doi.org/10.1161/JAHA.116.003294.
79. Sampietro T, Sbrana F, Pasanisi EM, et al. LDL apheresis improves coronary flow reserve on the left anterior descending artery in patients with familial hypercholesterolemia and chronic ischemic heart disease. Atheroscler Suppl. 2017;30:135–40. https://doi.org/10.1016/j.atherosclerosissup.2017.05.038.
80. Mellwig KP, Van Buuren F, Schmidt HK, et al. Improved coronary vasodilatatory capacity by H.E.L.P. apheresis: comparing initial and chronic treatment. Ther Apher Dial. 2006;10(6):510–7. https://doi.org/10.1111/j.1744-9987.2006.00441.x.
81. Nishimura S, Sekiguchi M, Kano T, et al. Effects of intensive lipid lowering by low-density lipoprotein apheresis on regression of coronary atherosclerosis in patients with familial hypercholesterolemia: Japan low-density lipoprotein apheresis coronary atherosclerosis prospective study (L-CAPS). Atherosclerosis. 1999;144(2):409–17. https://doi.org/10.1016/S0021-9150(98)00328-1.
82. Wu MD, Moccetti F, Brown E, et al. Lipoprotein apheresis acutely reverses coronary microvascular dysfunction in patients with severe hypercholesterolemia. JACC Cardiovasc Imaging. 2018;12(8 Pt 1):1430–1440. https://doi.org/10.1016/j.jcmg.2018.05.001.
83. Rossenbach J, Mueller GA, Lange K, et al. Lipid-apheresis improves microcirculation of the upper limbs. J Clin Apher. 2011;26(4):167–73. https://doi.org/10.1002/jca.20285.
84. Baigent C, Blackwell L, Emberson J, et al. Efficacy and safety of more intensive lowering of LDL cholesterol: a meta-analysis of data from 170 000 participants in 26 randomised trials. Lancet. 2010;376(9753):1670–81. https://doi.org/10.1016/S0140-6736(10)61350-5.
85. Hsia J, MacFadyen JG, Monyak J, Ridker PM. Cardiovascular event reduction and adverse events among subjects attaining low-density lipoprotein cholesterol. J Am Coll Cardiol. 2011;57(16):1666–75. https://doi.org/10.1016/j.jacc.2010.09.082.
86. Ishida K, Geshi T, Nakano A, et al. Beneficial effects of statin treatment on coronary microvascular dysfunction and left ventricular remodeling in patients with acute myocardial infarction. Int J Cardiol. 2012;155(3):442–7. https://doi.org/10.1016/j.ijcard.2011.11.015.
87. Paraskevaidis IA, Iliodromitis EK, Ikonomidis I, et al. The effect of acute administration of statins on coronary microcirculation during the pre-revascularization period in patients with myocardial infraction. Atherosclerosis. 2012;223(1):184–9. https://doi.org/10.1016/j.atherosclerosis.2012.04.002.

88. Bonetti PO, Wilson SH, Rodriguez-Porcel M, et al. Simvastatin preserves myocardial perfusion and coronary microvascular permeability in experimental hypercholesterolemia independent of lipid lowering. J Am Coll Cardiol. 2002;40(3):546–54. https://doi.org/10.1016/S0735-1097(02)01985-X.
89. Lario FC, Miname MH, Tsutsui JM, et al. Atorvastatin treatment improves myocardial and peripheral blood flow in familial hypercholesterolemia subjects without evidence of coronary atherosclerosis. Echocardiography. 2013;30(1):64–71. https://doi.org/10.1111/j.1540-8175.2012.01810.x.
90. Terai N, Spoerl E, Fischer S, et al. Statins affect ocular microcirculation in patients with hypercholesterolaemia. Acta Ophthalmol. 2011;89(6):e500–4. https://doi.org/10.1111/j.1755-3768.2011.02154.x.
91. Tailor A, Lefer DJ, Granger DN. HMG-CoA reductase inhibitor attenuates platelet adhesion in intestinal venules of hypercholesterolemic mice. Am J Physiol Hear Circ Physiol. 2004;286(4):H1402–7. https://doi.org/10.1152/ajpheart.00993.2003.
92. Vilahur G, Casani L, Peña E, et al. HMG-CoA reductase inhibition prior reperfusion improves reparative fibrosis post-myocardial infarction in a preclinical experimental model. Int J Cardiol. 2014;175(3):528–38. https://doi.org/10.1016/j.ijcard.2014.06.040.
93. Manfrini O, Pizzi C, Morgagni G, et al. Effect of pravastatin on myocardial perfusion after percutaneous transluminal coronary angioplasty. Am J Cardiol. 2004;93(11):1391–3, A6. https://doi.org/10.1016/j.amjcard.2004.02.037.
94. Pasceri V, Patti G, Nusca A, et al. Randomized trial of atorvastatin for reduction of myocardial damage during coronary intervention: results from the ARMYDA (Atorvastatin for Reduction of MYocardial Damage during Angioplasty) study. Circulation. 2004;110(6):674–8. https://doi.org/10.1161/01.CIR.0000137828.06205.87.
95. Patti G, Pasceri V, Colonna G, et al. Atorvastatin pretreatment improves outcomes in patients with acute coronary syndromes undergoing early percutaneous coronary intervention. Results of the ARMYDA-ACS randomized trial. J Am Coll Cardiol. 2007;49(12):1272–8. https://doi.org/10.1016/j.jacc.2007.02.025.
96. Di Sciascio G, Patti G, Pasceri V, et al. Efficacy of atorvastatin reload in patients on chronic statin therapy undergoing percutaneous coronary intervention. Results of the ARMYDA-RECAPTURE (atorvastatin for reduction of myocardial damage during angioplasty) randomized trial. J Am Coll Cardiol. 2009;s(6):558–65. https://doi.org/10.1016/j.jacc.2009.05.028.
97. Yadav K, Sharma M, Ferdinand KC. Proprotein convertase subtilisin/kexin type 9 (PCSK9) inhibitors: present perspectives and future horizons. Nutr Metab Cardiovasc Dis. 2016;26(10):853–62. https://doi.org/10.1016/j.numecd.2016.05.006.
98. Robinson JG, Farnier M, Krempf M, et al. Efficacy and safety of alirocumab in reducing lipids and cardiovascular events. N Engl J Med. 2015;372:1489–99. https://doi.org/10.1056/NEJMoa1501031.
99. Sabatine MS, Giugliano RP, Wiviott SD, et al. Efficacy and safety of evolocumab in reducing lipids and cardiovascular events. N Engl J Med. 2015;372:1500–9. https://doi.org/10.1056/NEJMoa1500858.
100. Leander K, Mälarstig A, van't Hooft FM, et al. Circulating proprotein convertase subtilisin/kexin type 9 (PCSK9) predicts future risk of cardiovascular events independently of established risk factorsclinical perspective. Circulation. 2016;133:1230–9. https://doi.org/10.1161/CIRCULATIONAHA.115.018531.
101. Sabatine MS, Giugliano RP, Keech AC, et al. Evolocumab and clinical outcomes in patients with cardiovascular disease. N Engl J Med. 2017;376:1713–22. https://doi.org/10.1056/NEJMoa1615664.
102. Karagiannis AD, Liu M, Toth PP, et al. Pleiotropic anti-atherosclerotic effects of PCSK9 inhibitorsfrom molecular biology to clinical translation. Curr Atheroscler Rep. 2018;20(4):20. https://doi.org/10.1007/s11883-018-0718-x.

Chapter 17
Proangiogenic and Proarteriogenic Therapies in Coronary Microvasculature Dysfunction

Lina Badimon, Gemma Vilahur, and Maria Borrell-Pages

Introduction

Heart failure following myocardial infarction (MI) remains one of the major causes of death and disability worldwide [1]. Primary percutaneous coronary intervention (PCI), early reperfusion in patients with acute MI has demonstrated to decrease mortality. Indeed, 80% of patients following PCI within the first 90 min after medical contact achieve perfusion of the occluded epicardial coronary artery [2]. However, a significant amount of patients undergoing primary PCI experience inadequate myocardial perfusion owing to dysfunction of the microcirculation in a process known as "no reflow". Alternative approaches to restore blood flow to the myocardium at risk for these patients and for patients with untreatable coronary lesions or contraindications to bypass surgery are urgently needed.

The ability to develop a collateral circulation (a process termed arteriogenesis) is an important factor that determines the outcome of an acute coronary event as reduced long-term cardiac mortality is associated with well developed coronary collateral arteries [3, 4]. About one-third of patients with coronary artery disease (CAD) and about one-fifth of patients without CAD show sufficiently developed collateral arteries that

L. Badimon (✉)
Cardiovascular Program ICCC, Institut de Recerca de l'Hospital de la Santa Creu i Sant Pau, Barcelona, Spain

Cardiovascular Research Chair, UAB, Barcelona, Spain

CIBER-CV, Instituto de Salud Carlos III, Madrid, Spain
e-mail: lbadimon@santpau.cat

G. Vilahur · M. Borrell-Pages
Cardiovascular Program ICCC, Institut de Recerca de l'Hospital de la Santa Creu i Sant Pau, Barcelona, Spain

CIBER-CV, Instituto de Salud Carlos III, Madrid, Spain
e-mail: GVilahur@santpau.cat; MBorrellPa@santpau.cat

M. Dorobantu, L. Badimon (eds.), *Microcirculation*,
https://doi.org/10.1007/978-3-030-28199-1_17

prevent signs of myocardial ischaemia during brief vascular occlusion [4]. Indeed, clinicians frequently encounter cardiovascular patients with few or no ischemic symptoms despite a significant stenosis or even occlusion of the main coronary vessel. This is mostly the case in patients with slowly progressing vascular occlusions, where an

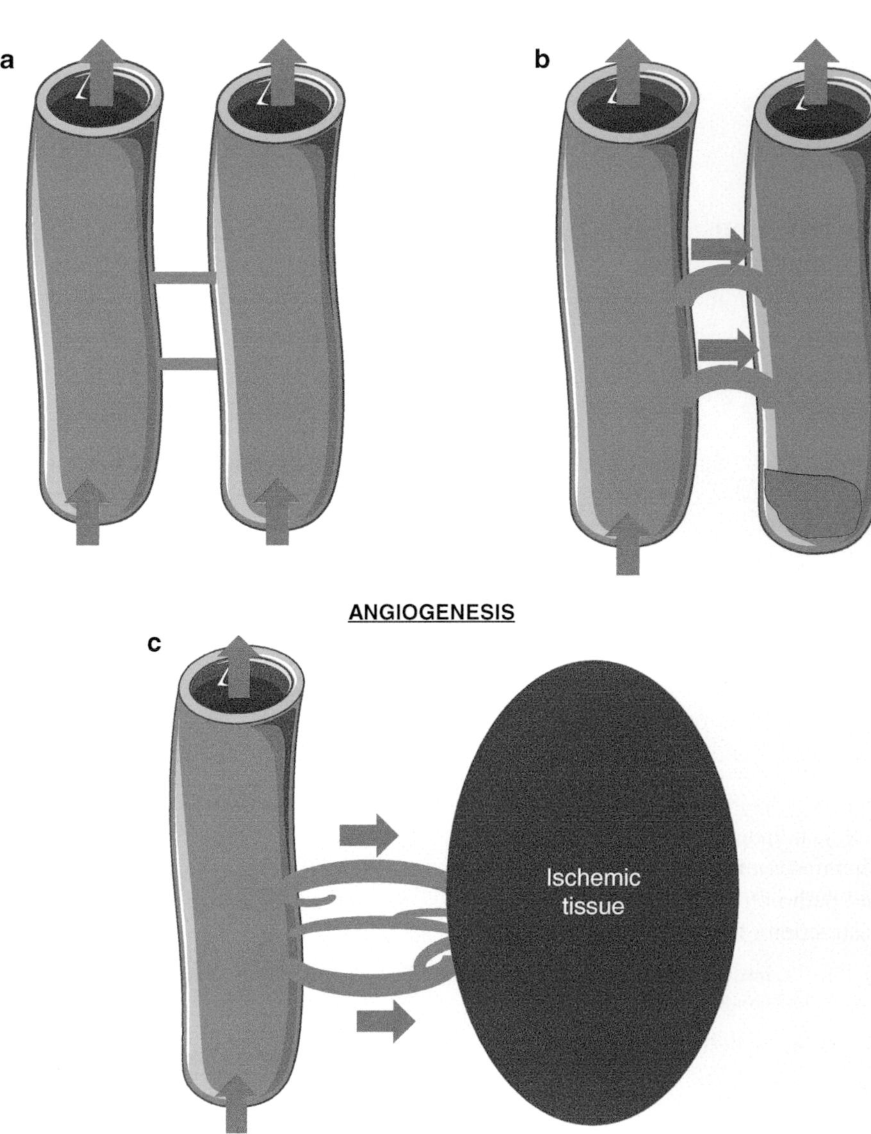

Fig. 17.1 (**a**) Blood flow (arrows) in healthy arteries in the absence of arterial stenosis. (**b**) Arteriogenesis is induced after occlusion or stenosis (grey patch) of a major artery. Fluid shear stress initiates the remodeling of preexisting collateral anastomoses to functional arteries. (**c**) Angiogenesis involves sprouting of new blood vessels from preexisting capillaries

endogenous collateral circulation has had sufficient time to develop, bypassing the site of stenosis and protecting the downstream tissue from ischemic injury (Fig. 17.1) [5].

In patients where coronary occlusion takes place, a key factor for an adequate post-ischemic repair is the formation of new blood vessels from existing ones that restore nutrient and oxygen supply to the infarcted tissue. This process is called angiogenesis, is induced by ischemia and has the potential to salvage ischemic myocardium at early stages after MI. It also plays a crucial role in preventing adverse left ventricular remodeling and the consequent development of heart failure (Fig. 17.1) [6]. In summary, strategies that promote the recovery of dysfunctional microvasculature and therapeutic options to prevent microvascular dysfunction are eagerly searched in the settings of MI.

Pathogenesis of the Dysfunctional Microvasculature

The coronary microvasculature is composed of small vessels including arterioles, capillaries and venules. The endothelial lining of blood vessels in their inner surface acts as a selective barrier between the lumen and its surrounding tissue and regulates hemostatic, vasomotor and inflammatory responses. Loss of these vital physiological endothelial cell functions, caused by prolonged myocardial ischemia, finally impairs myocardial perfusion. Reperfusion induces an additional damage not detected during ischemia, the so-called reperfusion injury. Myocardial cell injury, induced by the burst of oxygen free radicals [7–10], upregulates the expression of adhesion molecules in endothelial cells, platelet activation and the release of inflammatory mediators. These effects will subsequently enhance the inflammatory response and will trigger the coagulation cascade [11]. In turn, leukocyte recruitment to the vascular wall will plug small vessels compromising the integrity of the microvasculature that, in combination with vasoconstriction and cellular and interstitial edema will lead to capillary occlusion. Myocardial perfusion may be further hampered by the distal embolization of atheromatous and thrombotic debris, either spontaneously or after primary PCI [12, 13]. Paradoxically, reperfusion therapies, which aim to salvage viable myocardial tissue, augment vasoconstriction, cell injury, inflammatory and coagulation responses, and leukocyte plugging [14–16]. Therefore, microvascular dysfunction is caused by a series of molecular, cellular and patho-physiological responses that finally result in the obstruction and partial destruction of the coronary microvasculature.

Arteriogenesis and Angiogenesis in the Recovery of the Dysfunctional Microvasculature

A key factor for adequate postischemic tissue repair is the formation of new blood vessels from the ischemic border zone into the infarcted area, restoring oxygen and nutrient supply to the infarcted tissue [17]. This can be achieved by two different processes: arteriogenesis and angiogenesis. Arteriogenesis is initiated by the pressure deficit from a donor artery to an occluded artery triggering the transformation of small arteriolar anastomosis into large functional arteries. Angiogenesis is characterized by the sprouting of new blood vessels from preexisting capillaries. In the initial stage, endothelial cells loosen and detach from the vascular wall when exposed to angiogenic stimulus such as growth factors resulting in increased vascular permeability. Then, the degradation of the basement membrane and the extracellular matrix allows the formation of a provisional matrix onto which endothelial cells migrate. Finally a vessel lumen is formed, coated with perycytes to ensure neovessel stability and integrated into the circulation [18]. Although triggering of arteriogenesis in MI patients treated with primary PCI does not occur as there is no pressure deficit, in non-reperfused acute MI patients and in patients with chronic obstructive CAD arteriogenesis is much more efficient in the restoration of myocardial perfusion than angiogenesis [19].

Stimulation of Arteriogenesis

Arteriogenesis takes place in a non-hypoxic environment distant from the ischemic area; therefore, for the initiation of arteriogenesis, hypoxia is not required. Indeed, an experimental rabbit model of femoral artery occlusion showed that arteriogenesis occurred at the level of occlusion where there is no rise in ischemic markers [20]. Also, zebra fish studies support that arteriogenesis occurs without ischemia, as the zebra fish gains sufficient oxygen through diffusion to prevent ischemia [21].

Smooth muscle cell proliferation constitutes the most important process in arteriogenesis [22]. During arteriogenic processes, smooth muscle cells proliferate, secrete extracellular matrix components and digest the internal elastic lamina, facilitating the remodeling of pre-existing arterioles and the proliferation and invasion of circulating cells [23].

Blood vessels regress when not constantly perfused and their walls become thicker swith high pressures. After arterial occlusion mechanical forces activate endothelial cells of preexisting arteriolar anastomoses, which increase blood flow and fluid shear stress. The initiating role of shear stress in arteriogenesis is under debate. Indeed, cellular proliferation and remodeling of collateral arteries is induced by short period of femoral artery occlusion in mice but mostly developed during the reperfusion of the femoral artery after the increase of shear stress is no longer present [24]. Also, collateral flow has been shown to be undiminished in patients 24 h after opening of a chronic total occlusion of a coronary artery. In the following hours, functional collateral support subsequently declined but did not regress completely [25]. Contrarily, Zimarino et al. showed that collateral circulation in patients with chronic total occlusion started to decline 10 min after successful stent implantation and the restoration of antegrade flow. However, this rapid decrease of collaterals may likely put these patients at risk of future ischemic events [26].

Similarly, collateral function was decreased by 23% after PCI and by another 23% after 5 months in patients with chronic total coronary occlusion because collateral arteries were not recruited after acute occlusion had occurred. However, collaterals had the potential to recover in the case of chronic occlusion [27].

Circulating cells play a key role in mediating arteriogenesis. Indeed, upon endothelial activation by shear stress, monocytes are recruited to the site of collateral artery growth. The Monocyte Chemoattractant Protein 1 (MCP-1) is upregulated in collateral arteries and arteriogenesis is significantly reduced in mice lacking MCP-1 or its receptor [28]. Circulating monocytes are recruited and adhere to endothelial cells via their CD11b/CD18 (Mac1) receptor. Indeed, blocking Mac1 via antibody infusion has shown to significantly reduce collateral artery formation [29]. Perivascular macrophages are also important as they secrete Tumour Necrosis Factor α (TNFα) that is essential for arterial remodeling. Indeed, mice devoid of TNFα show delayed arteriogenesis, and the inhibition of TNFα signalling using the TNFαantagonists etanercept and infliximab also resulted in attenuated arteriogenesis [30]. CD44, a cell surface glycoprotein involved in cell-cell interactions, is of importance for the interaction of transmigrating monocytes with the extravascular matrix and is differentially regulated in monocytes from patients with sufficiently and insufficiently developed coronary collateral arteries [31]. CD8+T lymphocytes are also thought to contribute to arteriogenesis, attracting CD4+ mononuclear cells to sites of collateral artery growth [32]. Similar to other regenerative processes such as angiogenesis or myocardial regeneration the recruitment of progenitor cells leads to enhanced collateral artery growth [33].

Stimulation of Angiogenesis

The mechanisms involved in angiogenesis in reperfused myocardium after MI have not been fully described. Angiogenesis after MI reperfusion seems to be stimulated by two families of growth factors: vascular endothelial growth factor (VEGF) and fibroblast growth factor (FGF) [34]. Hepatocyte growth factor (HGF) can also be an inducer of angiogenesis post MI [35].

Hypoxia Inducible Factor (HIF) proteins are activated immediately upon ischemia and induce the release of VEGFA. VEGFA can bind to VEGF receptor 1 (VEGFR1) and VEGFR2 promoting the migration and proliferation of endothelial cells for blood vessels formation [36] (Fig. 17.2). The administration of VEGFA in rat and pig models of experimentally induced MI has been associated to the proangiogenic activity of VEGFA with a benefit on cardiac function [37, 38]. Also, increased plasma VEGFA levels have been found in patients with reperfused MI [39]. However, VEGFA can also inhibit vessel maturation by binding to and inhibiting platelet derived growth factor receptor β (PDGFRβ) signaling [40]. Therefore, for the formation of a stable microvascular network timely regulated angiogenic signals are indispensable. Another member of the VEGF family of growth factors is VEGFB that was initially demonstrated to exert a proangiogenic effect through its

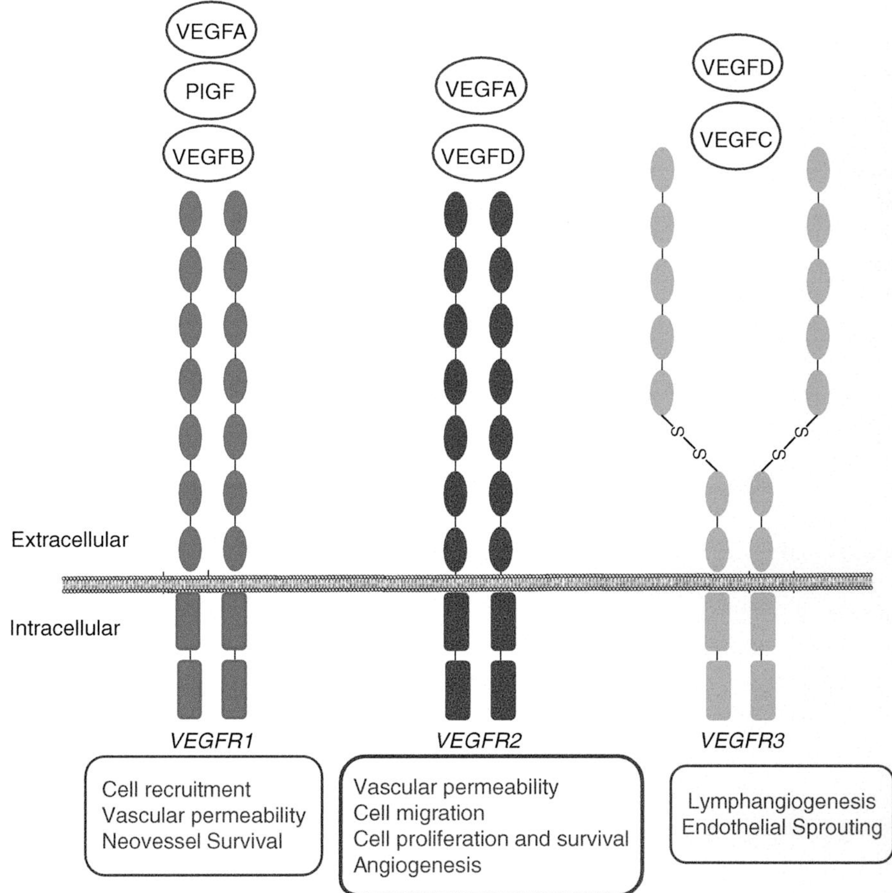

Fig. 17.2 VEGF family of growth factors. The VEGF family of growth factors and receptors has important roles in angiogenesis post MI as they participate in several processes including endothelial cell survival, vascular permeability, angiogenesis and recruitment of inflammatory and reparatory cells

binding to VEGFR1 in a murine model of hindlimb ischemia [41] and in the murine infarcted heart [42]. However experiments with cardiomyocytes overexpressing VEGFB in transgenic rat hearts have shown that VEGFB does not induce angiogenesis but coronary artery growth [43]. Furthermore, VEGFB has been shown not to be needed for vessel growth in mice, but to be essential for endothelial cells, pericytes and smooth muscle cells survival [44]. Therefore, it seems that VEGFB prosurvival actions allow newly formed vessels in the ischemic myocardium to mature and survive although it may not be necessary for the angiogenic process *per se*.

In addition to its well known role as lymphangiogenesis promoter, VEGFC has also been shown to induce angiogenesis after ischemia by its binding to VEGFR3

[45]. An indirect effect has been described as VEGFC induces vessel maturation in ischemic tissues through promotion of PDGFBB expression [46]. However VEGFC/VEGFR3 role in angiogenesis post-MI has not been properly studied yet. VEGFD is closely related to VEGFC because of the unique N- and C-terminal ends that other VEGF family members lack. The mature form can activate VEGFR2 and VEGFR3. Although, as VEGFC it is well known for its role in lymphangiogenesis, VEGFD is also able to induce angiogenesis in rabbit's hind limb muscles when delivered into their skeletal muscle [47]. Finally, placental growth factor (PlGF) also belongs to the VEGF family of growth factors and activates angiogenesis in ischemic tissues. It binds VEGFR1, induces VEGFR2 transphosphorylation and amplifies VEGFA dependent signaling [48] (Fig. 17.2).

Members of the FGF family of growth factors were amongst the first proteins described to induce angiogenesis, being FGF1 and FGF2 the most extensively characterized members. However, there are 22 FGF ligands (in human and mice), four tyrosine kinase receptors and a redundancy in the different FGF growth factor functions that complicates the comprehension of the mechanisms mediating the angiogenic effects of this family of growth factors. It is known that FGF1 and FGF2 promote the proliferation of endothelial cells and their organization into tubular structures [49]. Indeed, experiments performed in rabbits [50], dogs [51] and pigs [52] with FGF1 or FGF2 treatments showed that they promote angiogenesis in the ischemic heart and induce cardiac repair after MI. However, conflicting studies in rat models of ischemia/reperfusion showed that FGF2 treatments did not induce proliferation of endothelial cells [53] nor did they induce any changes in left ventricular function after myocardial ischemia/reperfusion injury [54]. Therefore, further studies are needed to understand the specific role of FGF2 in angiogenesis post-MI (Fig. 17.3).

Growth factor's coadministration studies have allowed proposing the existence of a synergy between angiogenic and arteriogenic signaling pathways. Indeed, FGF2 and PDGFBB treatments in porcine models of experimental MI lead to increased angiogenesis, perfusion of the ischemic myocardium an in consequence, improved cardiac outcome [55]. Similarly, in a mice model of hind limb ischemia FGF2 and PDGFBB coadministrationpromoted angiogenesis and vascular stability [56]. These results show that coadministration of FGF2 and PDGFBB increases blood vessel maturation and stability probably by inducing PDGFRβ (PDGFBB receptor) expression levels and intracellular signaling.

Other members of the FGF family of growth factors are also involved in the promotion of angiogenesis after MI. Indeed macrophages overexpressing FGF4 and injected into murine models of MI showed increased angiogenic response in the ischemic myocardium (Fig. 17.3). Furthermore, accumulation of the FGF4 injected macrophages was observed in the ischemic myocardium suggesting that macrophages are responsible for the enhanced angiogenic response [57]. Also, intracoronary administration of FGF5 promoted blood flow recovery and improved cardiac function in a porcine model of MI [58] and FGF9 treatments stimulated the formation of multilayered, perfused neovessels in a hindlimb ischemia model [59].

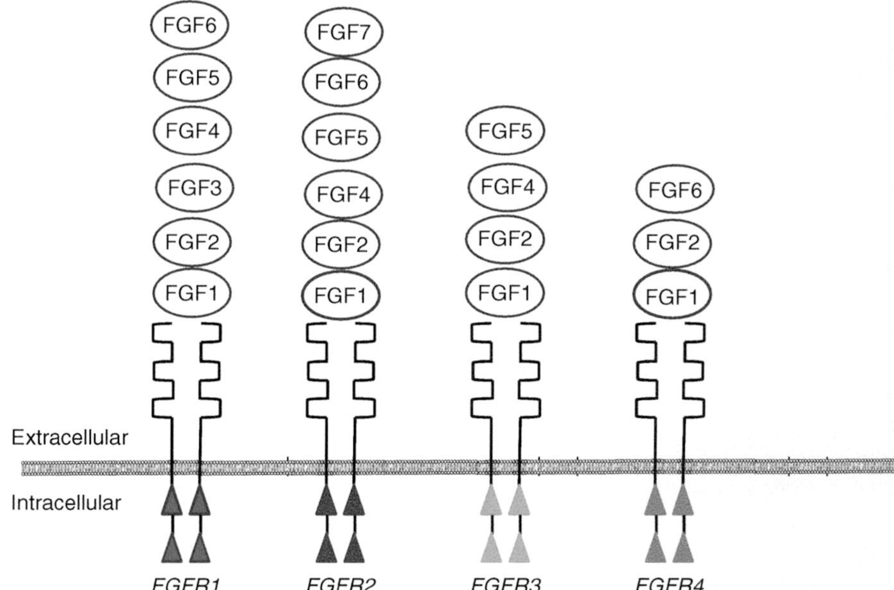

Fig. 17.3 FGF family of growth factors and their receptors. The FGF receptors consist of an extracellular domain with 3 immunoglobulin-like domains, a transmembrane domain, and intracellular domains with tyrosine kinase activity. They act as receptors for more than 20 FGF ligands

HGF can stimulate cellular angiogenesis by inducing endothelial cell proliferation, migration and the formation of tube-like vessels. In a rabbit model of MI, HGF gene transfer increased capillary density in the ischemic myocardium and preserved ventricular function [60]. Similar results were observed in a porcine model of MI [61]. In humans, elevated plasmatic HGF levels have been observed in reperfused MI patients [62] and in the cardiac vein draining the infarcted area, as opposed to the cardiac vein that drains non infarcted areas suggesting there is increased HGF production during MI [63].

Besides specific growth factors, different cell lineages including inflammatory monocytes and macrophages have also been shown to participate in angiogenesis stimulation post MI. Strikingly, monocytes were first described in ischemic tissues for their participation in arteriogenesis and promotion of collateral growth in ischemic tissues. Indeed monocyte circulating levels correlated with the extent of collateral growth in a rabbit model of hindlimb ischemia [64] and the presence of monocytes around collateral vessels correlates with endothelial cells progression [65]. Monocytes recruited into ischemic tissues can also regulate endothelial cell function. Certainly, monocytes and endothelial cells share surface markers and phenotypic features [66]. Furthermore, monocytes can function as angioblasts and obtain endothelial like properties after angiogenic stimulation [67]. Interestingly, we have demonstrated that monocytes can transdifferentiate into endothelial cell-like (ECL) through a tissue factor (TF)-dependant mechanism and promote angiogenesis [68]. Indeed, monocytes release WNT family member 5a (Wnt5a), which interacts with Frizzled 5 (FZD5) in microvascular endothelial cells and through the non-canonical pathway increase intracellular Ca^{2+} release and NF-κB activation upregulating TF expression and inducing angiogenesis [69].

Circulating monocytes are recruited to the target tissue, infiltrate and differentiate to macrophages. Depending on microenvironment signals human macrophages can be polarized into two different subtypes: M1 macrophages are the result of an inflammatory niche and are considered proinflammatory macrophages while M2 macrophages develop in response to anti-inflammatory conditions and are considered anti-inflammatory and repair macrophages. M2 macrophages show high expression levels of matrix metalloproteinase 9 (MMP9) and VEGF and are thought to promote angiogenic functions and induce tissue repair and vascular remodeling. Indeed, *in vivo* analyses of M2 macrophages show an improvement of postischemic cardiac neovascularization after being injected intravenously into mice immediately after coronary artery ligation [70]. However, in murine models of hindlimb ischemia the role of M2 macrophages seemed more prominent in arteriogenesis than in angiogenesis [71]. Inflammatory M1 macrophages are also thought to promote angiogenesis as M1 macrophages are able to form cell columns, which can support the construction of new vessels by EPCs in *in vivo* matrigel experiments [72]. Also, delivery of a small number of inflammatory monocytes in a mouse hind limb ischemia model inducedMCP1 release that associated with a second wave of monocyte recruitment to the ischemic tissue and subsequent stimulation of angiogenesis [73]. Furthermore, monocytes isolated from $SHIP^{-/-}$ mice (that induce M2 polarization preferentially) after ischemia, are not effective in promoting angiogenesis postischemia [74]. Therefore, the role of M1 and M2 macrophages in ischemia induced angiogenic processes needs further basic research before clinical trials can be considered.

Finally, endothelial progenitor cells (EPC), can adhere to the endothelium at sites of ischemia and participate in new vessel formation. Therefore, EPCs are a promising target of regenerative medicine research.

Issues to Be Resolved for Successful Angiogenic and Arteriogenic Clinical Trials

A number of problems hamper translation of successful stimulation of arteriogenesis and angiogenesis from experimental animal models to humans and sustain the disappointing outcomes of recent clinical trials. Stimulation of arteriogenesis or angiogenesis with growth factors is prone to potentially unwanted side effects since collateral vessel growth shares many common mechanisms with inflammatory diseases such as atherosclerosis. Both angiogenesis and arteriogenesis include endothelial activation, upregulation of adhesion molecules and recruitment of circulating cells into the vascular wall leading to a persistent trade-off between these two processes. Also it is important to note that the majority of data on angiogenesis and arteriogenesis is obtained from non-atherosclerotic animal models. And both angiogenesis and arteriogenesis are less susceptible to therapeutic stimulation under atherosclerotic conditions [75].

To date, all arteriogenic and angiogenic clinical trials have failed to demonstrate major benefits on myocardial left ventricular function. Several reasons including the selection of an appropriate patient population, the route of administration of the treatments, the therapeutic strategy and the choice of therapeutic end points may explain the mistrials. Indeed, most clinical trials have been performed in patients that are more resistant to stimulation of angiogenesis as they have failed or are not candidates for revascularization. Another challenge is the introduction of growth factors into ischemic tissues (by intracoronary, intramyocardial or intravenous delivery). Additionally, the choice of therapeutic strategy (gene, protein or cell therapy), the dosing plan (daily, weekly, single doses) and the selection of therapeutic end points and means of their assessment are also crucial. Therefore, several challenges need to be overcome to successfully translate the positive results of preclinical studies into clinical trials.

The therapeutic potential of bone marrow cells (BMC) has also been given a lot of attention in angiogenesis induction post-MI. Indeed, improved cardiac function, reduced MI recurrence, a decline in the need for revascularization procedures and reduced death has been observed after intracoronary BMCs deliver within the first week following MI [76]. However intracoronary delivery of autologous BMCs, 2–3 weeks of MI did not lead to improved benefit on left ventricular function at 3 weeks [77] or at 6 months follow-up [78]. Therefore, proangiogenic trials with BMCs remain disappointing. Although the different techniques of administration of the growth factor or the gene as well as the way in which mononuclear cells were isolated may partly explain such failures it seems that the induction of a single cell type or a single growth factor is not enough to promote cardiac angiogenesis.

CD34+ multipotent cells have been traditionally employed to reconstitute the hematopoietic system after radiation and/or chemotherapy in cancer patients. Yet, CD34+ cells have demonstrated to induce therapeutic angiogenesis in animal models of ischemic CVD. As such, these cells have shown to contribute to the formation of new vessels directly by incorporating into the developing vasculature structures and/or through the paracrine secretion of angiogenic factors which support the ischemia-induced angiogenic response [79]. The safety and effectiveness demonstrated upon the administration of CD34+ cells in multiple preclinical animal models of MI [80] encouraged their clinical application in patients who had recently experienced MI. There have been inconsistencies in phase II clinical trials, some reporting an improvement in left ventricular function (around 2.5%) and a reduction in infarct size upon intracoronary infusion of BMCs containing CD34+cells (TOPCARE-AMI, REPAIR-AMI, BOOST, pre-SERVE-AMI [76, 81–83] whereas others not (ASTAMI, REGENT [78, 84, 85]). Of note, except for the REGENT study, which assessed the efficacy of administering CD34+ selected cells, the other trials tested the safety/efficacy of administering BMC fractions that contained CD34+ cells (from 0.5% to 2.5%) not allowing to rule out the therapeutic contribution of non-CD34+ cells. Yet, a recent phase III clinical trial (PERFECT trial) has demonstrated that intramyocardial administration of autologous CD34+/

CD133+ BMCs as an adjunctive therapy in patients undergoing coronary artery bypass graft revascularization (CABG) leads to a marked improvement in LVEF (≈6%) in 60% of the patients ("the responders") which in turn also display lower scar damage [86]. Overall, several meta-analysis have shown that administration of BMCs is safe and improves left ventricular structure and function [87, 88]. Further research is needed to resolve the detected inconsistencies and the long term clinical outcomes.

The combinatorial therapy that simultaneously promotes angiogenesis and arteriogenesis seems to be a promising avenue. Indeed, the combined administration of FGF2 and PDGFBB enhanced angiogenesis in the ischemic heart [55] and co-administration of smooth muscle cells and EPCs induced the formation of mature blood vessels in ischemic tissues [89]. In this regard, we investigated in a pig model of MI using standard clinical procedures whether co-administration of adipose derived mesenchymal stem cells (ASCs) and their secreted products (secretomes) could recover myocardial rarefaction post-MI. We demonstrated that the co-administration of both ASCs and their secretomes synergistically contributed to improve neovascularization of the infarcted myocardium through the coordinated upregulation of the proangiogenic protein interactome [90].

Conclusions

Although primary PCI has dramatically improved patients survival after acute MI, still more than 30% of patients show microvascular dysfunction, adverse left ventricular remodeling and heart failure. The restoration of the microvascular network, which has been damaged during both ischemia and reperfusion, appears as a promising approach to prevent the deleterious effects triggered upon coronary obstruction. In rodents, growth factors can induce angiogenesis and arteriogenesis. However, human trials aimed to stimulate arteriogenesis or angiogenesis have failed. Better understanding of arteriogenic mechanisms leading to treatments that have a stimulatory effect on vascular growth while leaving atherosclerosis unaffected is urgently needed. Also, the identification of novel efficient therapeutic targets to promote angiogenesis in the ischemic heart is an unmet clinical need. Furthermore, experiments aimed to decipher the mechanism of endothelial cell-cardiomyocyte cross-talk in the ischemic heart, and a better understanding of how the delivery of gene and proteins affect therapeutically stimulated angiogenesis are immediately required.

Disclosures and Funding typos are different from Conclusions and References typo None.

Funding This work was supported by the Spanish Ministry of Economy and Competition and FEDER funds [SAF2016-76819-R to L.B. and SAF2015-71653-R to G.V.]; the Instituto de Salud Carlos III [CIBERCV CN16/11/00411 to L.B., TERCEL RD16/0011/018 to L.B. and FIS2016-02014 to M.B.P.]; the Generalitat of Catalunya-Secretaria d'Universitats i Recerca del Departament d'Economia i Coneixement de la Generalitat [2014SGR1303 to L.B.]; the Fundacion Investigación Cardiovascular to L.B.; and the Spanish Society of Cardiology [SEC2015 to M.B.P.].

References

1. Roger VL, Go AS, Lloyd-Jones DM, Adams RJ, Berry JD, Brown TM, et al. Heart disease and stroke statistics--2011 update: a report from the American Heart Association. Circulation. 2011;123:e18–e209. https://doi.org/10.1161/CIR.0b013e3182009701.
2. Keeley EC. Abciximab following clopidogrel reduces post-PCI complications in patients with acute coronary syndromes. Nat Clin Pract Cardiovasc Med. 2006;3:650–1. https://doi.org/10.1038/ncpcardio0706.
3. Sabia PJ, Powers ER, Ragosta M, Sarembock IJ, Burwell LR, Kaul S. An association between collateral blood flow and myocardial viability in patients with recent myocardial infarction. N Engl J Med. 1992;327:1825–31. https://doi.org/10.1056/NEJM199212243272601.
4. Meier P, Gloekler S, Zbinden R, Beckh S, de Marchi SF, Zbinden S, et al. Beneficial effect of recruitable collaterals. A 10- year follow-up study in patients with stable coronary artery disease undergoing quantitative collateral measurements. Circulation. 2007;116:975–83. https://doi.org/10.1161/CIRCULATIONAHA.107.703959.
5. Elsman P, van't Hof AW, de Boer MJ, Hoorntje JC, Suryapranata H, Dambrink JH, et al. Role of collateral circulation in the acute phase of ST-segment-elevation myocardial infarction treated with primary coronary intervention. Eur Heart J. 2004;25:854–8. https://doi.org/10.1016/j.ehj.2004.03.005.
6. van der Laan AM, Piek JJ, van Royen N. Targeting angiogenesis to restore the microcirculation after reperfused MI. Nat Rev Cardiol. 2009;6:515–23. https://doi.org/10.1038/nrcardio.2009.103.
7. Bonderman D, Teml A, Jakowitsch J, Adlbrecht C, Gyöngyösi M, Sperker W, et al. Coronary no-reflow is caused by shedding of active tissue factor from dissected atherosclerotic plaque. Blood. 2002;99:2794–800.
8. Hirata K, Matsuda Y, Akita H, Yokoyama M, Fukuzaki H. Myocardial ischaemia induced by endothelin in the intact rabbit: angiographic analysis. Cardiovasc Res. 1990;24:879–83.
9. Ma XL, Weyrich AS, Lefer DJ, Lefer AM. Diminished basal nitric oxide release after myocardial ischemia and reperfusion promotes neutrophil adherence to coronary endothelium. Circ Res. 1993;72:403–12.
10. Maxwell L, Gavin J. Anti-oxidant therapy improves microvascular ultrastructure and perfusion in postischemic myocardium. Microvasc Res. 1992;43:255–66.
11. Maier W, Altwegg LA, Corti R, Gay S, Hersberger M, Maly FE, et al. Inflammatory markers at the site of ruptured plaque in acute myocardial infarction: locally increased interleukin-6 and serum amyloid A but decreased C-reactive protein. Circulation. 2005;111:1355–61. https://doi.org/10.1161/01.CIR.0000158479.58589.0A.
12. Sheridan FM, Cole PG, Ramage D. Leukocyte adhesion to the coronary microvasculature during ischemia and reperfusion in an in vivo canine model. Circulation. 1996;93:1784–7.
13. Kotani J, Nanto S, Mintz GS, Kitakaze M, Ohara T, Morozumi T, et al. Plaque gruel of atheromatous coronary lesion may contribute to the no reflow phenomenon in patients with acute coronary syndrome. Circulation. 2002;106:1672–7.
14. Manciet LH, Poole DC, McDonagh PF, Copeland JG, Mathieu CO. Microvascular compression during myocardial ischemia: mechanistic basis for no-reflow phenomenon. Am J Phys. 1994;266:H1541–50. https://doi.org/10.1152/ajpheart.1994.266.4.H1541.
15. Maxwell L, Gavin JB. The role of postischaemic reperfusion in the development of microvascular incompetence and ultrastructural damage in the myocardium. Basic Res Cardiol. 1991;86:544–53.

16. Matsumura K, Jeremy RW, Schaper J, Becker LC. Progression of myocardial necrosis during reperfusion of ischemic myocardium. Circulation. 1998;97:795–804.
17. Reffelmann T, Kloner RA. Microvascular reperfusion injury: rapid expansion of anatomic no reflow during reperfusion in the rabbit. Am J Physiol Heart Circ Physiol. 2002;283:H1099–107. https://doi.org/10.1152/ajpheart.00270.2002.
18. Carmeliet P, Jain RK. Molecular mechanisms and clinical applications of angiogenesis. Nature. 2011;473:298–307. https://doi.org/10.1038/nature10144.
19. Simons M, Bonow RO, Chronos NA, Cohen DJ, Giordano FJ, Hammond HK, et al. Clinical trials in coronary angiogenesis: issues, problems, consensus: an expert panel summary. Circulation. 2000;102:e73–86.
20. Ito WD, Arras M, Scholz D, Winkler B, Htun P, Schaper W. Angiogenesis but not collateral growth is associated with ischemia after femoral artery occlusion. Am J Phys. 1997;273:H1255–65. https://doi.org/10.1152/ajpheart.1997.273.3.H1255.
21. Gray C, Packham IM, Wurmser F, Eastley NC, Hellewell PG, Ingham PW, et al. Ischemia is not required for arteriogenesis in zebrafish embryos. Arterioscler Thromb Vasc Biol. 2007;27:2135–41. https://doi.org/10.1161/ATVBAHA.107.143990.
22. Cai W, Vosschulte R, Afsah-Hedjri A, Koltai S, Kocsis E, Scholz D, et al. Altered balance between extracellular proteolysis and antiproteolysis is associated with adaptive coronary arteriogenesis. J Mol Cell Cardiol. 2000;32:997–1011.
23. Cheng XW, Kuzuya M, Nakamura K, Maeda K, Tsuzuki M, Kim W, et al. Mechanisms underlying the impairment of ischemia-induced neovascularization in matrix metalloproteinase 2-deficient mice. Circ Res. 2007;100:904–13. https://doi.org/10.1161/01.RES.0000260801.12916.b5.
24. Scholz D, Schaper W. Preconditioning of arteriogenesis. Cardiovasc Res. 2005;65:513–23. https://doi.org/10.1016/j.cardiores.2004.10.032.
25. Perera D, Kanaganayagam GS, Saha M, Rashid R, Marber MS, Redwood SR. Coronary collaterals remain recruitable after percutaneous intervention. Circulation. 2007;115:2015–21. https://doi.org/10.1161/CIRCULATIONAHA.106.665257.
26. Zimarino M, Ausiello A, Contegiacomo G, Riccardi I, Renda G, Di Iorio C, et al. Rapid decline of collateral circulation increases susceptibility to myocardial ischemia: the trade-off of successful percutaneous recanalization of chronic total occlusions. J Am Coll Cardiol. 2006;48:59–65. https://doi.org/10.1016/j.jacc.2005.12.079.
27. Werner GS, Emig U, Mutschke O, Schwarz G, Bahrmann P, Figulla HR. Regression of collateral function after recanalization of chronic total coronary occlusions: a serial assessment by intracoronary pressure and Doppler recordings. Circulation. 2003;108:2877–82. https://doi.org/10.1161/01.CIR.0000100724.44398.01.
28. Heil M, Ziegelhoeffer T, Wagner S, Fernandez B, Helisch A, Martin S, et al. Collateral artery growth (arteriogenesis) after experimental arterial occlusion is impaired in mice lacking CC-chemokine receptor-2. Circ Res. 2004;94:671–7. https://doi.org/10.1161/01.RES.0000122041.73808.B5.
29. Hoefer IE, van Royen N, Rectenwald JE, Deindl E, Hua J, Jost M, et al. Arteriogenesis proceeds via ICAM-1/Mac-1- mediated mechanisms. Circ Res. 2004;94:1179–85. https://doi.org/10.1161/01.RES.0000126922.18222.F0.
30. Grundmann S, Hoefer I, Ulusans S, van Royen N, Schirmer SH, Ozaki CK, et al. Anti-tumor necrosis factor-{alpha} therapies attenuate adaptive arteriogenesis in the rabbit. Am J Phys. 2005;289:H1497–505. https://doi.org/10.1152/ajpheart.00959.2004.
31. van Royen N, Voskuil M, Hoefer I, Jost M, de Graaf S, Hedwig F, et al. CD44 regulates arteriogenesis in mice and is differentially expressed in patients with poor and good collateralization. Circulation. 2004;109:1647–52. https://doi.org/10.1161/01.CIR.0000124066.35200.18.
32. Stabile E, Kinnaird T, la Sala A, Hanson SK, Watkins C, Campia U, et al. CD8+ T lymphocytes regulate the arteriogenic response to ischemia by infiltrating the site of collateral vessel development and recruiting CD4+ mononuclear cells through the expression of interleukin-16. Circulation. 2006;113:118–24. https://doi.org/10.1161/CIRCULATIONAHA.105.576702.

33. Carr AN, Howard BW, Yang HT, Eby-Wilkens E, Loos P, Varbanov A, et al. Efficacy of systemic administration of SDF-1 in a model of vascular insufficiency: support for an endothelium-dependent mechanism. Cardiovasc Res. 2006;69:925–35. https://doi.org/10.1016/j.cardiores.2005.12.005.
34. Pugh CW, Ratcliffe PJ. Regulation of angiogenesis by hypoxia: role of the HIF system. Nat Med. 2003;9:677–84. https://doi.org/10.1038/nm0603-677.
35. Bhargava M, Joseph A, Knesel J, Halaban R, Li Y, Pang S, et al. Scatter factor and hepatocyte growth factor: activities, properties, and mechanism. Cell Growth Differ. 1992;3:11–20.
36. Ferrara N, Gerber HP, LeCouter J. The biology of VEGF and its receptors. Nat Med. 2003;9:669–76. https://doi.org/10.1038/nm0603-669.
37. Pearlman JD, Hibberd MG, Chuang ML, Harada K, Lopez JJ, Gladstone SR, et al. Magnetic resonance mapping demonstrates benefits of VEGF induced myocardial angiogenesis. NatMed. 1995;1:1085–9.
38. Schwarz ER, Speakman MT, Patterson M, Hale SS, Isner JM, Kedes LH, et al. Evaluation of the effects of intramyocardial injection of DNA expressing vascular endothelial growth factor (VEGF) in a myocardial infarction model in the rat-angiogenesis and angioma formation. J Am Coll Cardiol. 2000;35:1323–30.
39. Kranz A, Rau C, Kochs M, Waltenberger J. Elevation of vascular endothelial growth factor A serum levels following acute myocardial infarction. Evidence for its origin and functional significance. J Mol Cell Cardiol. 2000;32:65–72. https://doi.org/10.1006/jmcc.1999.1062.
40. Greenberg JI, Shields DJ, Barillas SG, Acevedo LM, Murphy E, Huang J, et al. A role for VEGF as a negative regulator of pericyte function and vessel maturation. Nature. 2008;456:809–13. https://doi.org/10.1038/nature07424.
41. Silvestre JS, Tamarat R, Ebrahimian TG, Le-Roux A, Clergue M, Emmanuel F, et al. Vascular endothelial growth factor-B promotes in vivo angiogenesis. Circ Res. 2003;93:114–23. https://doi.org/10.1161/01.RES.0000081594.21764.44.
42. Li X, Tjwa M, Van Hove I, Enholm B, Neven E, Paavonen K, et al. Reevaluation of the role of VEGF-B suggests a restricted role in the revascularization of the ischemic myocardium. Arterioscler Thromb Vasc Biol. 2008;28:1614–20. https://doi.org/10.1161/ATVBAHA.107.158725.
43. Bry M, Kivela R, Holopainen T, Anisimov A, Tammela T, Soronen J, et al. Vascular endothelial growth factor-B acts as a coronary growth factor in transgenic rats without inducing angiogenesis, vascular leak, or inflammation. Circulation. 2010;122:1725–33. https://doi.org/10.1161/CIRCULATIONAHA.110.957332.
44. Zhang F, Tang Z, Hou X, Lennartsson J, Li Y, Koch AW, et al. VEGF-B is dispensable for blood vessel growth but critical for their survival, and VEGF-B targeting inhibits pathological angiogenesis. Proc Natl Acad Sci U S A. 2009;106:6152–7. https://doi.org/10.1073/pnas.0813061106.
45. Witzenbichler B, Asahara T, Murohara T, Silver M, Spyridopoulos I, Magner M, et al. Vascular endothelial growth factor-C (VEGF-C/ VEGF-2) promotes angiogenesis in the setting of tissue ischemia. Am J Pathol. 1998;153:381–94. https://doi.org/10.1016/S0002-9440(10)65582-4.
46. Onimaru M, Yonemitsu Y, Fujii T, Tanii M, Nakano T, Nakagawa K, et al. VEGF-C regulates lymphangiogenesis and capillary stability by regulation of PDGF-B. Am J Physiol Heart Circ Physiol. 2009;297:H1685–96. https://doi.org/10.1152/ajpheart.00015.2009.
47. Rissanen TT, Markkanen JE, Gruchala M, Heikura T, Puranen A, Kettunen MI, et al. VEGF-D is the strongest angiogenic and lymphangiogenic effector among VEGFs delivered into skeletal muscle via adenoviruses, Circ. Res. 2003;92:1098–106. https://doi.org/10.1161/01.RES.0000073584.46059.E3.
48. Autiero M, Waltenberger J, Communi D, Kranz A, Moons L, Lambrechts D, et al. Role of PlGF in the intra- and intermolecular cross talk between the VEGF receptors Flt1 and Flk1. Nat Med. 2003;9:936–43. https://doi.org/10.1038/nm884.
49. Carmeliet P. Fibroblast growth factor1 stimulates branching and survival of myocardial arteries: a goal for therapeutic angiogenesis? Circ Res. 2000;87:176–8.
50. Safi J Jr, DiPaula AF Jr, Riccioni T, Kajstura J, Ambrosio G, Becker LC, et al. Adenovirus mediated acidic fibroblast growth factor gene transfer induces angiogenesis in the nonischemic rabbit heart. Microvasc Res. 1999;58:238–49. https://doi.org/10.1006/mvre.1999.2165.

51. Banai S, Jaklitsch MT, Casscells W, Shou M, Shrivastav S, Correa R, et al. Effects of acidic fibroblast growth factor on normal and ischemic myocardium. Circ Res. 1991;69:76–85.
52. Watanabe E, Smith DM, Sun J, Smart D, Delcarpio JB, Roberts TB, et al. Effect of basic fibroblast growth factor on angiogenesis in the infracted porcine heart. Basic Res Cardiol. 1998;93:30–7.
53. Scheinowitz M, Kotlyar AA, Zimand S, Leibovitz I, Varda-Bloom N, Ohad D, et al. Effect of basic fibroblast growth factor on left ventricular geometry in rats subjected to coronary occlusion and reperfusion. Isr Med Assoc J. 2002;4:109–13.
54. Horrigan MC, MacIsaac AI, Nicolini FA, Vince DG, Lee P, Ellis SG, et al. Reduction in myocardial infarct size by basic fibroblast growth factor after temporary coronary occlusion in a canine model. Circulation. 1996;94:1927–33.
55. Lu H, Xu X, Zhang M, Cao R, Bråkenhielm E, Li C, et al. Combinatorial protein therapy of angiogenic and arteriogenic factors remarkably improves collaterogenesis and cardiac function in pigs. Proc Natl Acad Sci U S A. 2007;104:12140–5. https://doi.org/10.1073/pnas.0704966104.
56. Cao R, Brakenhielm E, Pawliuk R, Wariaro D, Post MJ, Wahlberg E, et al. Angiogenic synergism, vascular stability and improvement of hind-limb ischemia by a combination of PDGF-BB and FGF-2. Nat Med. 2003;9:604–13. https://doi.org/10.1038/nm848.
57. Fukuyama N, Tanaka E, Tabata Y, Fujikura H, Hagihara M, Sakamoto H, et al. Intravenous injection of phagocytes transfected ex vivo with FGF4 DNA/biodegradable gelatin complex promotes angiogenesis in a rat myocardial ischemia/ reperfusion injury model. Basic Res Cardiol. 2007;102:209–16. https://doi.org/10.1007/s00395-006-0629-9.
58. Giordano FJ, Ping P, McKirnan MD, Nozaki S, DeMaria AN, Dillmann WH, et al. Intracoronary gene transfer of fibroblast growth factor- 5 increases blood flow and contractile function in an ischemic region of the heart. Nat Med. 1996;2:534–9.
59. Frontini MJ, Nong Z, Gros R, Drangova M, O'Neil C, Rahman MN, et al. Fibroblast growth factor 9 delivery during angiogenesis produces durable, vasoresponsive microvessels wrapped by smooth muscle cells. Nat Biotechnol. 2011;29:421–7. https://doi.org/10.1038/nbt.1845.
60. Chen XH, Minatoguchi S, Kosai K, Yuge K, Takahashi T, Arai M, et al. In vivo hepatocyte growth factor gene transfer reduces myocardial ischemia–reperfusion injury through its multiple actions. J Card Fail. 2007;13:874–83. https://doi.org/10.1016/j.cardfail.2007.07.004.
61. Saeed M, Martin A, Ursell P, Do L, Bucknor M, Higgins CB, et al. MR assessment of myocardial perfusion, viability, and function after intramyocardial transfer of vM202, a new plasmid human hepatocyte growth factor in ischemic swine myocardium. Radiology. 2008;249:107–18. https://doi.org/10.1148/radiol.2483071579.
62. Pannitteri G, Petrucci E, Testa U. Coordinate release of angiogenic growth factors after acute myocardial infarction: evidence of a two wave production. J Cardiovasc Med. 2006;7:872–9. https://doi.org/10.2459/01.JCM.0000253831.61974.b9.
63. Yasuda S, Goto Y, Baba T, Satoh T, Sumida H, Miyazaki S, et al. Enhanced secretion of cardiac hepatocyte growth factor from an infarct regionis associated with less severe ventricular enlargement and improved cardiac function. J Am Coll Cardiol. 2000;36:115–21.
64. Heil M, Ziegelhoeffer T, Pipp F, Kostin S, Martin S, Clauss M, et al. Blood monocyte concentration is critical for enhancement of collateral artery growth. Am J Physiol Heart Circ Physiol. 2002;283:H2411–9. https://doi.org/10.1152/ajpheart.01098.2001.
65. Arras M, ItoWD SD, Winkler B, Schaper J, Schaper W. Monocyte activation in angiogenesis and collateral growth in the rabbit hindlimb. J Clin Invest. 1998;101:40–50. https://doi.org/10.1172/JCI119877.
66. Ribatti D. The paracrine role of Tie-2-expressing monocytes in tumor angiogenesis. Stem Cells Dev. 2009;18:703–6. https://doi.org/10.1089/scd.2008.0385.
67. Fernandez-Pujol B, Lucibello FC, Gehling UM, Lindemann K, Weidner N, Zuzarte ML, et al. Endothelial-like cells derived from human CD14 positive monocytes. Differentiation. 2000;65:287–300.

68. Arderiu G, Espinosa S, Peña E, Crespo J, Aledo R, Bogdanov VY, et al. Tissue factor variants induce monocyte transformation and transdifferentiation into endothelial cell-like cells. J Thromb Haemost. 2017;8:1689–703. https://doi.org/10.1111/jth.13751.
69. Arderiu G, Espinosa S, Pena E, Aledo R, Badimon L. Monocyte-secreted Wnt5a interacts with FZD5 in microvascular endothelial cells and induces angiogenesis through tissue factor signaling. J Mol Cell Biol. 2014;6:380–93. https://doi.org/10.1093/jmcb/mju036.
70. Yan D, Wang X, Li D, Liu W, Li M, Qu Z, et al. Macrophages overexpressing VEGF target to infarcted myocardium and improve neovascularization and cardiac function. Int J Cardiol. 2011;164:334–8. https://doi.org/10.1016/j.ijcard.2011.07.026.
71. Takeda Y, Costa S, Delamarre E, Roncal C, Leite de Oliveira R, Squadrito ML, et al. Macrophage skewing by Phd2 haplodeficiency prevents ischaemia by inducing arteriogenesis. Nature. 2011;479:122–6. https://doi.org/10.1038/nature10507.
72. Melero-Martin JM, De Obaldia ME, Allen P, Dudley AC, Klagsbrun M, Bischoff J. Host myeloid cells are necessary for creating bioengineered human vascular networks in vivo. Tissue Eng Part A. 2010;16:2457–66. https://doi.org/10.1089/ten.TEA.2010.0024.
73. Capoccia BJ, Gregory AD, Link DC. Recruitment of the inflammatory subset of monocytes to sites of ischemia induces angiogenesis in a monocyte chemoattractant protein-1-dependent fashion. J Leukoc Biol. 2008;84:760–8. https://doi.org/10.1189/jlb.1107756.
74. Gregory AD, Capoccia BJ, Woloszynek JR, Link DC. Systemic levels of G-CSF and interleukin-6 determine the angiogenic potential of bone marrow resident monocytes. J Leukoc Biol. 2010;88:123–31. https://doi.org/10.1189/jlb.0709499.
75. van Weel V, de Vries M, Voshol PJ, Verloop RE, Eilers PH, van Hinsbergh VW, et al. Hypercholesterolemia reduces collateral artery growth more dominantly than hyperglycemia or insulin resistance in mice. Arterioscler Thromb Vasc Biol. 2006;26:1383–90. https://doi.org/10.1161/01.ATV.0000219234.78165.85.
76. Schächinger V, Erbs S, Elsässer A, Haberbosch W, Hambrecht R, Hölschermann H, et al. Intracoronary bone marrow-derived progenitor cells in acute myocardial infarction. N Engl J Med. 2006;355:1210–21. https://doi.org/10.1056/NEJMoa060186.
77. Traverse JH, Henry TD, Ellis SG, Pepine CJ, Willerson JT, Zhao DX, et al. Effect of intracoronary delivery of autologous bone marrow mononuclear cells 2 to 3 weeks following acute myocardial infarction on left ventricular function: the LateTIME randomized trial. JAMA. 2011;306:2110–9. https://doi.org/10.1001/jama.2011.1670.
78. Lunde K, Solheim S, Aakhus S, Arnesen H, Abdelnoor M, Egeland T, et al. Intracoronary injection of mononuclear bone marrow cells in acute myocardial infarction. N Engl J Med. 2006;355:1199–209. https://doi.org/10.1056/NEJMoa055706.
79. Kawamoto A, Iwasaki H, Kusano K, Murayama T, Oyamada A, Silver M, et al. CD34-positive cells exhibit increased potency and safety for therapeutic neovascularization after myocardial infarction compared with total mononuclear cells. Circulation. 2006;114:2163–9. https://doi.org/10.1161/CIRCULATIONAHA.106.644518.
80. Iwaguro H, Yamaguchi J, Kalka C, Murasawa S, Masuda H, Hayashi S, et al. Endothelial progenitor cell vascular endothelial growth factor gene transfer for vascular regeneration. Circulation. 2002;105(6):732–8.
81. Schächinger V, Assmus B, Britten MB, Honold J, Lehmann R, Teupe C, et al. Transplantation of progenitor cells and regeneration enhancement in acute myocardial infarction: final one-year results of the TOPCARE-AMI trial. J Am Coll Cardiol. 2004;44(8):1690–9. https://doi.org/10.1016/j.jacc.2004.08.014.
82. Meyer GP, Wollert KC, Lotz J, Steffens J, Lippolt P, Fichtner S, et al. Intracoronary bone marrow cell transfer after myocardial infarction: eighteen months' follow-up data from the randomized, controlled BOOST (BOne marrOw transfer to enhance ST-elevation infarct regeneration) trial. Circulation. 2006;113:1287–94. https://doi.org/10.1161/CIRCULATIONAHA.105.575118.
83. Quyyumi AA, Vasquez A, Kereiakes DJ, Klapholz M, Schaer GL, Abdel-Latif A, et al. PreSERVE-AMI: a randomized, double-blind, placebo-controlled clinical trial of intracoro-

nary administration of autologous CD34+ cells in patients with left ventricular dysfunction post STEMI. Circ Res. 2017;120(2):324–31. https://doi.org/10.1161/CIRCRESAHA.115.308165.
84. Beitnes JO, Gjesdal O, Lunde K, Solheim S, Edvardsen T, Arnesen H, et al. Left ventricular systolic and diastolic function improve after acute myocardial infarction treated with acute percutaneous coronary intervention, but are not influenced by intracoronary injection of autologous mononuclear bone marrow cells: a 3 year serial echocardiographic sub-study of the randomized-controlled ASTAMI study. Eur J Echocardiogr. 2011;12:98–106. https://doi.org/10.1093/ejechocard/jeq116.
85. Tendera M, Wojakowski W, Ruzyłło W, Chojnowska L, Kepka C, Tracz W, et al. Intracoronary infusion of bone marrow-derived selected CD34+CXCR4+ cells and non-selected mononuclear cells in patients with acute STEMI and reduced left ventricular ejection fraction: results of randomized, multicentre Myocardial Regeneration by Intracoronary Infusion of Selected Population of Stem Cells in Acute Myocardial Infarction (REGENT) Trial. Eur Heart J. 2009;30:1313–21. https://doi.org/10.1093/eurheartj/ehp073.
86. Steinhoff G, Nesteruk J, Wolfien M, Kundt G, PERFECT Trial Investigators Group, Börgermann J, et al. Cardiac function improvement and bone marrow response -: outcome analysis of the randomized PERFECT phase III clinical trial of intramyocardial CD133+ application after myocardial infarction. EBioMedicine. 2017;22:208–24. https://doi.org/10.1016/j.ebiom.2017.07.022.
87. Jiang M, He B, Zhang Q, Ge H, Zang MH, Han ZH, et al. Randomized controlled trials on the therapeutic effects of adult progenitor cells for myocardial infarction: meta-analysis. Expert Opin Biol Ther. 2010;10(5):667–80. https://doi.org/10.1517/14712591003716437.
88. Jeevanantham V, Butler M, Saad A, Abdel-Latif A, Zuba-Surma EK, Dawn B. Adult bone marrow cell therapy improves survival and induces long-term improvement in cardiac parameters: a systematic review and meta-analysis. Circulation. 2012;126(5):551–68. https://doi.org/10.1161/CIRCULATIONAHA.111.086074.
89. Foubert P, Matrone G, Souttou B, Leré-Déan C, Barateau V, Plouët J, et al. Coadministration of endothelial and smooth muscle progenitor cells enhances the efficiency of proangiogenic cell-based therapy. Circ Res. 2008;103:751–60. https://doi.org/10.1161/CIRCRESAHA.108.175083.
90. Vilahur G, Oñate B, Cubedo J, Béjar MT, Arderiu G, Peña E, et al. Allogenic adipose-derived stem cell therapy overcomes ischemia-induced microvessel rarefaction in the myocardium: systems biology study. Stem Cell Res Ther. 2017;1:52. https://doi.org/10.1186/s13287-017-0509-2.

Index

M. Dorobantu, L. Badimon (eds.), *Microcirculation*,
https://doi.org/10.1007/978-3-030-28199-1